Scientific
Foundations
of Nursing

D1147849

Third Edition

Scientific Foundations of Nursing

Madelyn T. Nordmark, R.N., M.S. (N.E.)

Staff Assistant, Research, Los Angeles County Medical Center School of Nursing; formerly Research Assistant Professor, School of Nursing, University of Washington

Anne W. Rohweder, R.N., M.N.

Coordinator, Health Occupations Department, Olympic College, Bremerton, Washington; formerly Research Assistant Professor, School of Nursing, University of Washington

J. B. Lippincott Company   PHILADELPHIA New York Toronto

Third Edition

Copyright © 1975, 1967, by J. B. Lippincott Company
All rights reserved

Science Principles Applied to Nursing
First Edition, by Madelyn Titus Nordmark and Anne W. Rohweder
Copyright © 1959, by J. B. Lippincott Company

This book is fully protected by copyright and, with the
exception of brief excerpts for review, no part of it may
be reproduced in any form by print, photoprint, microfilm
or any other means without written permission from the
publisher.

Distributed in Great Britain by Blackwell Scientific Publications,
London, Oxford, Edinburgh

ISBN 0–397–54166–X

Printed in the United States of America

5 7 9 8 6 4

Library of Congress Cataloging in Publication Data

Nordmark, Madelyn Titus.
    Scientific foundations of nursing.

    First ed. published in 1959 under title: Science
principles applied to nursing.
    Bibliography: p. 13
    Includes index.
    1. Nurses and nursing.   I. Rohweder, Anne W., joint
author.   II. Title.   DNLM: 1. Education, Nursing.
WY18 N832s
RT69.N6   1975   610.73   75-1374
ISBN 0–397–54166–X

Preface

Two decades ago, the Commonwealth Fund supported a 5-year project at the University of Washington School of Nursing. The purpose of the project was to find better ways of relating basic sciences and clinical nursing. The first edition of this book, entitled *Science Principles Applied to Nursing*, reported some of the findings of that study and was intended as a guide for teachers of nursing.

In the second edition, retitled *Scientific Foundations of Nursing*, the science and nursing sections from the first edition were expanded, and the format was changed to facilitate use by students who were finding the book helpful in their nursing programs. A chapter was added for students and practitioners of nursing, suggesting ways the material might be useful to them.

The format of this, the third, edition remains basically the same. However, all sections have been updated from current science references, research data and medical and nursing texts. Science and nursing contents have been increased; new science material has been incorporated; and more supportive data has been added.

Part I, Orientation, presents a brief description of the methods used in the original study at the University of Washington and those used in the preparation of the second and third editions of this text. Also included in Part I is the section "Suggestions for Nursing Students and Practitioners," an aid to them in the use of this text.

Part II, The Biologic and Physical Sciences and Related Nursing Care, contains science content from the fields of anatomy, physiology, pathology, microbiology, physics and chemistry and from related nursing care. Each "Anatomy and Physiology" section has been rewritten to incorporate recent scientific findings and more supportive data, in more detail. For example, Chapter 3 (Nutrition) contains the most recent Recommended Daily Allowances (RDAs) of nutrients, and Chapter 5 (Electrolyte Balance) now includes the normal intra- and extracellular concentrations of specific electrolytes. All "Pathology" sections in Part II have been expanded, especially in detailing symptoms and signs. More pathophysiology is included, and associations between pathophysiology and symptoms and signs are more explicit.

"Nursing Care" sections in Part II have been rewritten to reflect new nursing applications and reorganized to be more inclusive. Each section now opens with a nursing care statement, similar in intent to the general statement which opens each chapter, summarizing the foci of nursing care covered in that chapter. Each "Nursing Care" section is itself composed of 3 subdivisions: Collection, Evaluation and Communication of Data; Promotion of Health and Prevention of Disease/Injury; Care of Patients with Specific Problems. Symptoms and signs included in the chapter's "Pathology" section are summarized at the beginning of the first part, and important areas for health teaching can be found at the beginning of the second. In the third part, nursing care of patients with disease conditions is identified.

Part III, Psychosocial Principles and Nursing Applications, has also been expanded to include new and more complete scientific information and to develop current nursing practice concerns, in particular: crisis intervention; death and dying; and the process of aging.

Crisis intervention theory has been given special play in Chapter 6 (Growth and Development, Learning and Adaptive Problem-Solving), and in Chapter 8 (Disturbances of Equilibrium). The concepts of death and dying have been particularly expanded in Chapter 9 (Sociocultural Influences on Behavior). The problem of dealing with aging has been given recognition throughout Part III, to give this phase of life attention equal to that given the life phase of birth through adolescence.

The introductions to Parts II and III explain the presentation of material in each part, set forth the limitations of the content included and identify the changes and additions made since the original study. They should be used as guides to the study of each part.

Part IV, A Guide to Use for Nursing Educators, as the title suggests, offers ideas of ways the science and nursing contents of the text may be useful to nursing educators. In effect, it is a corollary to the "Suggestions for Nursing Students and Practitioners" of Part I.

It is our sincere hope that students and instructors, alike, will continue to find this book a practical and helpful resource in the learning and teaching of nursing care based on scientific foundations.

Madelyn T. Nordmark
Anne W. Rohweder
March 1975

Acknowledgments

I am deeply indebted to Mrs. Carla Bouchard, Registered Dietitian (formerly with the Dietary Department of the Los Angeles County—University of Southern California Medical Center), for her expert assistance in the revision of the chapter on nutrition.

Special thanks go to Mrs. Hana Zemplenyi, Staff Assistant in Tutorial Services in the Los Angeles Medical Center School of Nursing (formerly Instructor in Basic Sciences for Paramedical Staff, University of Prague), who evaluated several sections of the revised science content and offered helpful suggestions for additions and changes. I also wish to acknowledge the help of Mrs. Lavina Sheetz, R.N., Director of In-Service Education in the Nursing Department of the Los Angeles County—University of Southern California Medical Center, who reviewed sections of the revised nursing content and offered suggestions relative to the format used in this edition.

I greatly appreciate the encouragement given me by faculty members in the Los Angeles County Medical Center School of Nursing during the revision process and am most grateful to Mary O. Martinetti, R.N., Director, for her continued interest and administrative support.

Lastly, I thank my husband and daughter, who were patient and understanding and helpful in so many different ways during the year of revision efforts.

—MTN.

Without the long-suffering patience of the faculty and students of the Olympic College nursing program, revision of Part III would never have been completed. There are too many of them to list by name, but they deserve public recognition for their support and willingness to work without my full participation during the critical phases of revision.

—AWR.

Contents

PART I

Orientation

Introduction

The nurse is constantly called upon to make independent decisions in the solution of such problems as those concerning patient care, safety for herself and others and interpersonal relationships. Increasingly, she is expected not only to make wise decisions for herself but to guide auxiliary personnel who perform nursing care functions. In the process of executing nursing activities, the nurse cannot always find a policy, a "rule of thumb" or a person in authority to assist her when a problem arises. Even if comprehensive sets of rules were available, the habitual use of such rules would be potentially dangerous, in that they could very likely lead to unthinking and harmful actions because of failure to understand the reasons behind the rule. As demands for nursing services increase, the professional nurse will become more and more the diagnostician of nursing care problems, expected to devise creative nursing interventions; less and less will she function primarily as a follower of medical orders and an overseer of routine procedures. It would seem vital, then, that the professional nurse be equipped to solve problems in a wise and resourceful manner.

Successful use of problem-solving methods (which, hopefully, the nurse will employ in making her decisions) implies that the problem solver has in her possession or at her disposal the facts and understanding necessary for the analysis and solution of problems. This implication leads to two significant questions: What knowledge must a professional nurse possess? How can this knowledge and its use in solving nursing problems be learned most effectively?

Recognition of the significance of these questions led the original planners of the five-year curriculum study in basic nursing education at the University of Washington School of Nursing* to select as one area for investigation the relationship

---

* Ole Sand, *Curriculum Study in Basic Nursing Education* (New York: Putnam, 1955).

between the general and the professional education of nursing students. The Commonwealth Fund first supported this separate study within the framework of the total curriculum study, and the objective of the project became finding better ways to relate basic sciences and clinical nursing.

The basic sciences were considered to include the social and the natural sciences. The former were defined as psychology, sociology and anthropology. The natural sciences were defined as the biological sciences of anatomy, physiology (including biochemistry) and microbiology, as well as the physical sciences of chemistry and physics.

Methods of Identification Used in Original Study

During the first three years of the Commonwealth Study, primary emphasis was placed on the development of methods for (1) teaching students how to apply basic science knowledge in solving nursing problems, and (2) evaluating students' abilities to do so. When the Commonwealth Fund extended its financial support an additional two years, the emphasis of the investigation shifted to identifying the basic science content that is applicable to nursing. Fundamental differences between the natural and the social sciences and their applications to nursing influenced the methods of approach to this identification. The methods used in the original study will be described briefly.

THE NATURAL SCIENCES

Early in the Commonwealth Study it was suggested that the science content generally taught to nursing students in the various science courses (anatomy and physiology, physics, chemistry and microbiology) be examined in terms of applications to nursing. Although this was feasible, the opposite approach was also thought to be advantageous, i.e., the examination of nursing itself to determine related science content.

It was the latter approach that led to experimentation with the analysis of common nursing activities, such as, for example, measurement of blood pressure and catheterization. Nursing procedures were examined in terms of facts from the natural sciences, with the assumption that these facts, when applied, would result in procedures safely and effectively performed. Although these analyses proved useful for day-to-day teaching, this method was discontinued. The specific procedures represented a limited part of total nursing care, and the analyses showed—not surprisingly—much repetition of some of the science content. For example, the fact that cleanliness inhibits the growth of microorganisms was repeated in each analysis.

At this point it was decided that a much broader view of nursing care should be considered in developing a methodology. It seemed that if the nursing care designed to meet the expected needs of patients with specific physiological problems were analyzed, the resulting science content would be more comprehensive and, perhaps, less repetitive. This method necessitated the development of nursing care plans for hypothetical patients with problems involving the different structures and functions of the body. Many faculty members contributed to the development of these care plans which proved again to be highly valuable for teaching. However, when some of the nursing care was analyzed for the related science content, the amount of science identified was so extensive that working with all the material in its interrelated and unorganized state was utterly impractical. It became obvious that some method for organization of the science content was needed.

A review of the science already identified revealed that most of it came from anatomy and physiology. Moreover, it was notable that the statements concerned with physiology tended to fall into some broad categories—categories that involved such processes as blood circulation and respiration. These two observations resulted in the use of the concept of nursing care aimed at maintaining physiological homeostasis as a basis for the determination of the content from anatomy and physiology that is important in nursing.

Ten factors involved in the maintenance of a constant internal environment were identified. These included such requirements as oxygen, blood pressure, nutrition and electrolyte balance. Seven additional factors were then identified as being necessary for effective and independent functioning of the human organism (though not essential to homeostasis). These factors included locomotion, sensory processes and certain protective mechanisms.

After each of these factors had been identified and incorporated in a general statement (that provided some indication of the import of each particular factor on the total functioning of the human organism), each factor was studied in terms of its embodiment of major facts from anatomy and physiology and the application of these facts in nursing. This process required two associated activities. Nursing care related to each of the factors had to be identified and then analyzed for related science content. Practically simultaneously, anatomy and physiology content related to the specific factor under consideration had to be reviewed, selecting facts that seemed to be applicable to patient care. Elements of pathology were also occasionally included with the anatomy and physiology.

As the material was developed, no attempt was made to associate any specific science statements with any statements of specific nursing care. Instead, the material was prepared in units: statements of nursing care related to each factor of human functioning were made, and these were followed by selected facts from anatomy and physiology. Because the human body is a whole, functioning unit, the placement of the facts about structure and function into separate sections proved a difficult and perhaps impossible task. Repetition was purposely avoided through the use of many cross-references. An attempt was made to keep the specificity levels of the science statements somewhat similar all the way through, but variations occurred, as it seemed more important to state the science content so that it could have meaning to a nurse and really serve as a guide to action.

When each of the sections of nursing care and related science had been completed, the nursing care was reviewed and criticized by both a medical specialist and a committee of clinical nursing instructors. The science statements were reviewed and criticized by a physiologist. Changes were made as recommended.

After the identification of the anatomy and physiology content had been completed, the nursing care was analyzed for the purpose of identifying any science aspects from the fields of physics and chemistry. Some of the chemistry identified, though not directly applicable in nursing, was thought to contribute to the intelligent application of some of the physiology content and was thus included. Clinical nursing instructors and professors of chemistry and physics criticized the physics and chemistry statements, and changes were made as recommended. These statements were then added to the science sections.

Nursing care concerned with the protection of patients from microbial injury provided the basis for the identification of important facts and principles from the field of microbiology. Again, nursing care was identified along with applicable science content. Clinical nursing instructors and a pathologist reviewed and criticized the nursing section, and a medical microbiologist criticized the science statements. Changes were made as recommended.

The total material was then given to a jury for evaluation. Jury members were asked to review and criticize all nursing and science sections and to evaluate the relatedness of the nursing and science in each. Their responses were used to reorganize, delete and correct the material.

THE SOCIAL SCIENCES

Since the social sciences are concerned with human behavior without respect to specific physiological illness, treatment or nursing procedures, it did not seem expedient in the original study to analyze nursing care plans or procedures to determine social science principles. Such plans and procedures are usually oriented toward physical care, toward maintaining physiological homeostasis or toward the mechanics of carrying out a procedure. Any psychosocial aspects of care that might be appended to such plans or procedures would have had to be stated in broad, relatively meaningless terms, such as "provide reassurance" or "avoid embarrassment."

The possibility of analyzing social science texts, outlines or other reference material was also ruled out as a possible methodology. It would have been difficult to arrive at defensible criteria for the selection and/or omission of concepts and principles. It also would have been extremely difficult to develop a framework from which to review the diverse theories and approaches expounded in contemporary social science literature. One finds a wide variety of theoretical approaches to man's individual and collective behavior, and not all theories are compatible. This lack of agreement was especially crucial to the original Commonwealth Study, when choices had to be made regarding terminology. The problem of terminology is discussed later in this text, with particular reference to some of the concepts and principles included in Part III.

Finally, an analysis of actual patient-nurse situations seemed the most profitable initial approach to the study of relationships between social sciences and nursing. Such analysis could provide information about the kinds of psychosocial problems that patients actually encounter in the course of illness and hospitalization, irrespective of the presenting complaint, physiological illness or the resulting care and treatment. Material collected in this way also might help to circumvent one of the major complaints about the use of social science concepts in teaching nursing students—the difficulty in arriving at specific principles to guide the nurse's behavior.

With these considerations in mind, an adaptation of Flanagan's "Critical Incident Technique"* was chosen as the primary means of collecting source material for the

---

* John C. Flanagan, "The Critical Incident Technique," *Psychological Bulletin*, Vol. 51, No. 4: 327–358.

original Commonwealth Study. This method provided for the collection of descriptions of patient and nurse behavior in operationally defined critical situations. Critical incidents were defined as nurse-patient interactions in which patients were either helped (a positive situation) or harmed (a negative situation) by some action of a nursing team member. The benefit or harm to the patient was described in terms of the patient's observable reaction to the situation.

Descriptions of nurse-patient situations were collected from nurses who were involved in giving patient care or in supervising patient care on medical, surgical and obstetrical* services of four large general hospitals. The nurses were asked to describe incidents in which they had recently been involved or which they had recently observed. These incidents then were analyzed in terms of the social science principles that seemed to be inherent in the situation. The collection and analysis of situations represented an attempt to arrive at some of the factors that influence the human being's psychosocial equilibrium while he is in a situation requiring nursing care.

A group of faculty members from the University of Washington School of Nursing, representing all clinical areas, assisted in the process of screening and analyzing patient-nurse incidents. Throughout the entire period of the original study, this faculty committee functioned in an informal advisory capacity and as a work group to assist in analysis of patient-nurse situations and formulation of statements of principle. After preliminary statements of principle had been made, they were critically reviewed by two members of the University of Washington Department of Psychology.

The final draft of the material was submitted to a group of six additional social scientists for review. This group included one psychologist, two sociologists and three anthropologists. With the exception of the anthropologists, all of the reviewers had had some experience in the health science fields. They were asked to consider the principles and hypotheses from the standpoint of: (1) the truth of the statements, (2) the relevance of substatements to major statements and (3) the relevance of the nursing section to the science sections. The responses of the reviewers were used to reorganize, delete and correct the material for publication.

Suggestions for Nursing Students and Practitioners
SUMMARY OF THE NURSE'S ROLE

The professional nurse's two major areas of action may be roughly defined as: (1) direct patient care, and (2) interaction with other health workers on behalf of the patient. Although the skills and abilities required for successful performance in both areas may overlap or be interdependent, it is still fruitful to examine them separately. A person seeks assistance in solving his health problems when some dysfunction has constituted disequilibrium or a threat to the integrity of the very intricately balanced, interlocking systems which normally keep him functioning as a healthy individual within his particular environment. When the nurse participates in a patient's problem-solving, certain assistance skills are expected of her.

---

* Since one of the hospitals did not have an obstetrical unit, material in this area was supplemented by a study using similar methods for the same purpose: Patricia Rose, "The Identification of Psychiatric Principles Inherent in the Nursing Care of a Selected Group of Maternity Patients" (unpublished masters thesis, University of Washington, 1958).

Provision for Normal Needs

When a person is hospitalized, he surrenders to the hospital the responsibility for organizing his environmental forces in such a way as to preserve normal function in areas not directly affected by his illness. Hopefully, he will not have to suffer total discontinuity in life style while temporary dysfunctions are being corrected or while he is learning adaptations necessitated by permanent functional changes.

For example, the agency the patient has entered accepts responsibility for maintaining a comfortable environmental temperature; providing for normal nutritional and fluid balance needs; providing facilities to maintain cleanliness, safety and comfort; and promoting normal social interaction. Although responsibility is delegated to the institution as a whole, and departments are created to provide some of the necessary services (e.g., housekeeping and dietary departments), the nurses in direct contact with the patient 24 hours a day, are those who observe, supervise and manipulate this environment to the best interests of the individual patient. The nurse observes and regulates the physical environment of the room, transfers from doctor to dietary department the order for a "regular diet" and supervises the distribution and patient intake of food and fluid; she supervises or participates in cleanliness and comfort procedures; she regulates social interaction, facilitates continuity of the patient's religious practices and so forth. Except in unusual circumstances, it is not necessary for the doctor to "order" nursing care of the variety described above. Such activities constitute the bulk of nursing services routinely offered to patients, and the unwritten assumption is that they are nursing responsibilities.

Provision for Therapeutic Needs

Above and beyond continuity of normal practices, the patient has special needs occasioned by his illness. In this area, his doctor is immediately responsible for diagnosis and therapeutic procedures. But again, it is the responsibility of the nursing service to see that therapeutic procedures are effectively integrated into the total care plan. This may mean that the nurse, under doctor's orders, manipulates special temperature-regulating and humidifying equipment because of the patient's problems; or the nurse may, under doctor's orders, carry out special nutritional and fluid-balance procedures, such as gavage feeding or intravenous therapy. The nurse may have to carry out or supervise adaptations of normal cleanliness and comfort procedures to adjust for immobility; or she may have to engage in special interpersonal techniques if psychological disequilibrium is severe.

Regardless of the patient's particular health problem, the nurse must be concerned with the totality of care—the integration of care to meet both normal and therapeutic needs. It is assumed that the nurse has the intelligence and preparation to function without specifically written orders from a doctor on how to bathe a patient with painful arthritis, how to prevent skin breakdown of a comatose patient, or what psychological techniques to employ when the doctor is difficult to work with.

Interaction with Others:
Planning and Coordination

In each of these examples, the nurse could take direct action or she could serve as a leader in nursing care programming. With the increasing demand for nursing services of both in- and out-patient natures, the nurse is more likely to serve as supervisor, teacher and coordinator of a corps of auxiliary nursing personnel. In addition, coordination of the activities of nursing personnel with personnel from other departments in the hospital is required. In the future there will also be an enormous increase in the cooperative contacts between nurses and community health agencies.

In all of these health personnel interactions, the nurse assumes "wellness" on the part of co-workers, and her attention is primarily directed toward maintaining the optimal functioning of a social environment set up specifically with patient care as its goal. Skills involved in this aspect of nursing are associated with such areas as communication, teaching and learning, leader and team interactions, counselling, guidance and motivation, group problem-solving and change agent functions.

No matter what the specific nursing intervention required, the nurse cannot function as a consistently effective member of the health team unless her decisions for action are based on sound scientific knowledge of human physiological and psycho-social function. No matter how creative a problem solver the nurse might be, her solutions will be only as good as the mental data she has at her command to apply to practical situations.

PRACTICAL USES OF THE SCIENCE AND NURSING SECTIONS

The material in this book is not meant to be used as a substitute "short course" for full-scale study of basic sciences. The professional nurse needs to study the sciences in depth and scope *before* attempting to organize and systematically use selected science concepts. Without such study, material as organized and presented here may be only vague and half-understood, therefore not maximally usable in immediate, acute and practical situations. For example, a conceptual statement such as "perception of a situation is unique to each individual in the situation" summarizes literally volumes of supporting evidence and detailed subconcepts or principles. The nurse does not need to have at her mental fingertips all of the supporting evidence from scientific studies nor all the detailed substatements that construct or illuminate the concept, but her full comprehension of the summarizing statement and its implications for nursing is limited without the initial encounter with such data that is obtained in collegiate basic science courses.

If this book is not a capsule course in basic sciences, how can the nursing student and the practicing nurse use the material to best advantage?

Organization of Knowledge

Perhaps the most useful function of Parts II and III is that they serve as guides to the organization of knowledge in basic science and nursing courses. In the previous example of "perception," reference was made to using the bulk of material studied in order to fully understand a given concept. Since not all of the student's reading and experimentation is necessarily pertinent to nursing action, the individual student must find a way to summarize related material, to cull out the pragmatically important from supporting or incidental data. Rote memorization of all the facts one encounters is sheer intellectual waste.

Unless the student is already provided with a study guide for the organization of learning, this book may be helpful for that purpose. For example, the student, while studying the circulatory system, can use the sections in Part II relating to circulating blood and oxygen supply as guides to selecting areas for concentrated study and as summarizing statements of detailed course learning. In addition, the student may find that particular instructors and textbooks place insufficient emphasis on given units of study that she, the student, knows will be important to her as a nurse. In such a case, the information from this book can be used to guide independent study in those neglected areas.

Transfer of Theory to Practice

Basic science courses are seldom taught concurrent with nursing courses that require the application of the particular science being studied. At best, correlation of science and nursing courses is imperfect. Unless a science instructor is teaching a course for nurses only, he makes no special effort to point out nursing applications of science data. Nursing instructors, on the other hand, often base their teaching on an assumption that the student will *recall* science concepts and principles when presented with nursing situations in which they are applicable. Every student is well aware that recall of pertinent science data is not nearly so automatic and instantaneous as might be desired!

The method of organization of basic science and nursing applications in Parts II and III can be helpful to students in the transfer of knowledge in both basic science and nursing courses. A review of nursing applications can provide examples that will make the science behind them more meaningful and therefore more easily learned. Continuing with the example of the circulatory system, if the student reviews nursing actions concerning blood pressure, she is more likely to be motivated toward developing an understanding of physiology related to the pressure of circulating blood. Later, when she is assigned to patients with circulatory problems, she can review both the science and the nursing applications as a basis for progression of learning in nursing theory and practice.

Review and Relearning

In a sense, review of past learning is not separate from the two previous examples of possible uses for this book. Review and relearning do deserve a special note, however, for the graduate who has been away from nursing for some time and for the nurse who has been working in one specialized area of practice and is transferring to another. Nurses who find themselves in these situations may use the science and related nursing care sections either as straight review material or as a guide to determining particular areas in which they need more extensive study. It may be, for example, that a nurse who has been away from bedside practice for some years discovers while reviewing that there are some serious gaps in her previous learning, or that subsequent developments in science and in nursing practice indicate a need for special references or for particular learning experiences. If educational opportunities are not readily available, the nurse can set up a self-directed learning program with this text.

Evaluation of Nursing Care

The authors would particularly like to see students and graduates use the science and nursing care sections for evaluation of individual nursing care plans. This does not mean that the nurse should sit down with the book every time she writes a care plan! It does mean that once the reader is familiar with format and content of this text, her thinking about patient needs can be directed in an organized manner. It does mean that she can look at care plans with a full awareness of what is meant by totality of care, and that her plans can be checked to see if full consideration has been given to all aspects of that care. For example, if a plan includes teaching a patient some aspect of self-care, the nurse can review the material on learning to be sure her plans are well formulated and consistent with the dynamics of human learning. Also, if she is responsible for the supervision and teaching of auxiliary personnel in the use of body mechanics, she can review both the sections on learning and on body mechanics in order to evaluate her own knowledge and supervisory and teaching behavior. In addition, it means that the student or graduate has a ready reference for checking out the validity of ideas and care plans when in doubt about their scientific soundness.

One of the most common uses of material in the first edition was as a reference for students in the writing of care plan analyses. These analyses required the student to state scientific principles that justified or led to the nursing intervention planned for the patient. Although the graduate doesn't have time for such lengthy written plans, she *must* have the science in mind and be able to verbalize it when necessary to guide the work of auxiliary personnel.

Development of a Way of Thinking

Hopefully, nurses of the present and the future, with their increased store of background knowledge, will not be poor human counterparts of data-processing computers. With all of their awe-inspiring and labor-saving characteristics, computers still are capable of only one thing—a reliable, accurate and predictable response when the right buttons are pushed. They are not capable of original thinking—of devising unique applications of old and new scientific data to changing and increasingly complex nursing care problems.

No human being can hope to compete with a machine when it comes to storing information any more than this book can contain all of the scientific information a nurse will need for planning and implementing patient care. But it is hoped that the material the book does contain, together with the format in which it is presented, will foster habits of analytical thinking. Nurses, whether students or graduates, can help develop the nursing care of the future if they learn to approach every patient care problem with such questions as these:

1. What does the patient require to maintain optimal function?
2. What do we know about human structure and function that will help determine what the patient needs and how we can help him?
3. What scientific reasons do we have for continuing a particular nursing practice?
4. Is there a better way, scientifically based, for solving this patient's problem?

In short, nurses can use computers to their own ends rather than become a human part of a computer system. Nurses of the future must be able to outgrow this or any text as they develop their own thinking habits through the solutions of patient care problems.

The Biologic and Physical Sciences and Related Nursing Care

Introduction

Part II is divided into 20 chapters.* Each chapter contains science sections and a nursing care section. Chapters 1 through 10 are concerned with essentials of physiologic homeostasis; Chapter 11, with locomotion; Chapters 12 through 15, with protective structures and functions; Chapters 16 through 18, with sensory processes, intellectual processes and speech; Chapter 19, with reproductive functions; and Chapter 20, with infection and infectious diseases. All of the chapters have been written in outline form, because this seems to provide the simplest presentation of extensive content. Although the main focus is on the nursing care of adults, some specific information about infants, children and the elderly is included, along with implications for the care of persons in these age groups.

In all chapters except the last, each science section is preceded by a general statement (in bold type) that pertains to the particular structures, functions and/or requirements of the human organism which are under consideration. The science sections consist of statements of scientific facts, principles and generalizations from anatomy and physiology, physics, chemistry and pathology. The physics and chemistry relate

---

* Unless otherwise noted, all chapter references in Part II are made only to the chapters in Part II and not to those in Part III, though the numbers may agree.

to the preceding anatomy and physiology only, and statements are sometimes repeated in different chapters. (These two sections would be greatly expanded were nursing care related to prescribed diagnostic procedures and therapeutic measures included.) The science sections are followed by "Nursing Care" sections that contain statements of nursing care related to the science content.

In the original study pathology was not considered a basic "natural science," but elements of pathology were included in the anatomy and physiology sections, and lists of symptoms and signs associated with physiologic dysfunctions were included in the nursing sections. In the second edition and in the present one, pathology content has been compiled in separate science sections.

The statements of nursing care are both general and specific. In most instances general nursing objectives are followed by examples of specific nursing actions to achieve those objectives. We recognize that nursing care must be planned and implemented in compliance with the prescribed medical regimen. Occasionally, attention is called to the fact that a particular nursing measure should be taken *within* medical orders only or that a particular nursing measure should (or may) be taken *until* medical orders are available. In some cases attention is called to the importance of following medical orders *exactly*. This is not to imply that medical orders are not to be followed exactly at other times, but it does imply that in these specific situations it is of utmost importance that everyone, including the patient, understand that the orders are to be followed *exactly*.

Many symptoms and signs have been listed in each chapter. The nurse's understanding of those associated with specific physiological dysfunctions provides for recognition of actual or potential problems that have particular implications for the physician and for nursing care. The more purposeful and comprehensive patient assessments the nurse is able to make, the more assistance she can give to patients and to physicians. In many instances the systematic patient evaluations made by the nurse are of *critical* importance. The patient and the physician both depend upon the independent, prompt and correct actions of the nurse when there are threats to vital life processes or to the future well-being of the patient.

The science portion of Chapter 20 is devoted almost entirely to microbiology. In addition to general statements about microorganisms as infectious agents and about the control, sources and transmission of disease-producing microorganisms, there is specific information about particular pathogens. The list is not exhaustive but is believed to be fairly representative. A few of the helminths are also considered briefly, for although adult worms are not microscopic in size, their eggs and some of their other forms are.

It is important that persons using this material understand that the science and related nursing care have been purposively developed in units. These units have been found to be useful in the analysis and synthesis of extensive science and nursing content. They are interrelated, and many cross-references have been made to reduce repetition. The nursing care in each chapter relates almost exclusively to the science content in that chapter.

The reader should not approach Part II with the notion that it contains all the science that is important for a nurse to understand and be able to apply to patient care. What the reader can expect to find are many of the concepts, principles, facts and hypotheses from the biologic and physical sciences that have relevancy for nursing. Similarly, the nursing care statements represent only some applications of this science content.

Many references have been used in the preparation of this edition. The major ones include:

Anderson, Linnea, *et al.*: *Nutrition in Nursing.* J. B. Lippincott Company, Philadelphia, 1972.

Beland, Irene L.: *Clinical Nursing: Pathophysiological and Psychosocial Approaches,* ed. 2. The Macmillan Company, New York, 1970.

Benenson, Abram S.: *Control of Communicable Diseases in Man,* ed. 11. The American Public Health Association, Washington, D.C., 1970.

Brunner, Lillian, *et al.*: *Textbook of Medical-Surgical Nursing,* ed. 2. J. B. Lippincott Company, Philadelphia, 1970.

Frobisher, Martin, *et al.*: *Microbiology in Health and Disease,* ed. 12. W. B. Saunders Company, Philadelphia, 1969.

Guyton, Arthur: *Basic Human Physiology: Normal Function and Mechanisms of Disease.* W. B. Saunders Company, Philadelphia, 1971.

Maxwell, Morton H., and Kleeman, Charles R., eds.: *Clinical Disorders of Fluid and Electrolyte Metabolism,* ed. 2. McGraw-Hill Book Company, New York, 1972.

Watson, Jeannette E.: *Medical-Surgical Nursing and Related Physiology.* W. B. Saunders Company, Philadelphia, 1972.

Williams, Sue Rodwell: *Essentials of Nutrition and Diet Therapy.* C. V. Mosby, Saint Louis, 1974.

Chapter 1

Volume and Pressure of Circulating Blood

The blood is a means of transport for substances to and from the cells; the volume and pressure of circulating blood must be maintained within certain limits to provide for the changing demands of tissues.

Anatomy and Physiology

THE CARDIOVASCULAR SYSTEM

1. The cardiovascular system is composed of the heart and blood vessels.
    A. The heart pumps blood into the major arteries.
    B. The arteries transport blood, under pressure, to the tissues.
    C. The arterioles (the last and smallest branches of the arterial system) act as control valves, releasing blood into the capillaries.
    D. The capillaries provide for the exchange of fluid, nutrients and catabolites between the blood and interstices and, in the lungs, for the exchange of gases between the alveoli and the blood.
    E. The venules (the last and smallest branches of the venous system) collect blood from the capillaries and join into larger veins.
    F. The veins carry blood from the tissues back to the heart.
2. The right side of the heart receives deoxygenated blood from the systemic circulation and pumps it into the pulmonary circulation. The left side of the heart receives oxygenated blood from the pulmonary system and pumps it into the systemic circulation.

3. The major artery coming from the left ventricle is the aorta, which passes down through the thorax and the abdominal cavity before bifurcating.
4. The heart muscle receives blood primarily through the coronary blood vessels, which comprise a complex and anastomotic system having an extraordinarily rich capillary network. The right and left coronary arteries branch directly from the ascending aorta.
5. The heart, enclosed in the pericardial sac, lies immediately behind the lower half of the sternum.
6. The walls of the arteries are thick and contain a large amount of elastic tissue.
   A. As arteries become smaller the amount of elastic tissue decreases while the amount of smooth muscle increases.
   B. In the aging process there are degenerative changes in the arteries, including the loss of elastic tissue.
7. Arteries lying over bone or firm tissue that are usually palpable include:
   A. The internal maxillary artery, in front of and slightly below the ear.
   B. The superficial temporal artery, in the temple region.
   C. The subclavian artery, behind the inner end of the clavicle against the first rib.
   D. The external carotid artery, in the neck.
   E. The facial artery, about an inch forward of the angle of the jaw.
   F. The brachial artery, on the inner aspect of the upper arm, about halfway between the shoulder and the elbow.
   G. The radial artery, which passes down the radial side of the front of the forearm.
   H. The femoral artery, in the mid-groin.
   I. The popliteal artery, behind the knee.
   J. The dorsalis pedis artery, below the ankle on the dorsum of the foot.
8. The walls of the veins are very thin, but they are muscular, allowing for dilatation and constriction.
   A. There are both deep and superficial veins in the extremities.
   B. Because veins are very distensible, they can store large or small quantities of blood, depending upon the needs of the body. Veins are approximately 8 times more distensible than their corresponding arteries, and their volume is 3 times greater.
   C. Many of the veins in the lower extremities have valves to prevent backflow of blood.
   D. The return of blood to the heart through the veins is brought about by the external pressures of contracting skeletal muscles (sometimes called the "venous pump"), the action of the valves and the constriction of the veins. The decrease in intrathoracic pressure during inspiration also encourages venous return.
   E. Blood is drained from the brain through large venous sinuses, which also drain blood from the scalp, the face and the mastoid region.
9. There are billions of capillaries, distributed among all functioning body cells.
   A. The most important means by which substances are transferred between capillaries and interstices or alveoli is diffusion.
   B. Excess fluid in the interstices interferes with the exchange of nutrients, gases and metabolites.

    C.   Normally, the arterioles and the precapillary sphincters regulate blood flow through the capillaries so that not all are open at one time.

    D.   The number of open, functioning capillaries increases when tissues are active.

10. A number of body organs have relatively large blood supplies and/or storage places for blood. These include the kidneys, the liver, the lungs, skeletal muscles, the skin, the spleen and the pregnant and postpartum uterus.

11. Blood is a viscous fluid composed of cells and plasma.

    A.   The hematocrit of blood is the percentage of blood that consists of cells. This is normally about 40 percent.

    B.   More than 99 percent of the cells are red blood cells.

    C.   The greater the percentage of cells, the more viscous the blood.

BLOOD VOLUME

1. The cardiovascular system is a closed system, and blood is not usually found outside of the system except as it is found in the uterus related to reproductive functions.

    A.   Approximately 60 to 240 ml. of venous blood, mixed with mucus and endometrial tissue, is lost during a normal menstrual period. (Normally menstrual blood does not clot.)

    B.   The life of a fetus depends upon the mother's blood circulating through the placenta.

    C.   Labor may be accompanied by a loss of blood-tinged mucus from the cervix.

    D.   A loss of more than 500 ml. of blood during delivery is above normal.

    E.   Following delivery there is a flow of uterine discharge from the vagina which may last from 1 week to 6 weeks. The flow is similar to a heavy menstrual flow, with the discharge changing from bloody to serous to mucous.

    F.   Following delivery, involution of the uterus occurs.

        [1]   The small blood vessels in the uterus are arranged between smooth muscle fibers in such a way that uterine muscle contractions can partially occlude these vessels.

        [2]   A well-contracted postpartum uterus prevents excessive blood loss. Mechanical stimulation (fundus massage) and suckling of the infant stimulate uterine contractions.

        [3]   Pressure exerted upward against the uterus by a full urinary bladder can interfere with proper uterine contraction.

        [4]   The fundus of the uterus should be firm and well below the umbilicus immediately after delivery. Starting at about the level of the umbilicus the first postpartum day, the fundus normally returns into the pelvis at a rate of approximately one-half inch a day. Failure of the uterus to contract and involute properly may result in bleeding and may indicate intrauterine bleeding.

2. Blood volume varies with body weight and surface area. It is estimated at about 3 liters per square meter of body surface.

    A.   In infants and children the blood volume is somewhat less per kilogram of body weight and per square meter of body surface than in adults.

    B.   The average-size adult has 5 to 6 L. of blood.

     C. The rapid loss of more than 30 percent of total blood volume often causes death.
3. Blood volume may be affected by variations in fluid balance. It increases when there is an increase in the volume of extracellular fluid and decreases when there is a decrease in extracellular fluid. (See Chapter 4 on "Fluid Balance.")

HEMOSTASIS AND BLOOD COAGULATION

1. Whenever a blood vessel is severed or ruptured, several mechanisms protect the body from significant blood loss:
   A. The wall of the blood vessel contracts immediately.
   B. A platelet plug forms at the injury site. (This mechanical barrier is of particular importance in the prevention of bleeding from very small blood vessels that are continuously being injured during common, everyday activities.)
   C. A blood clot is formed.
   D. Fibrous tissue grows into the clot to close the hole permanently.
2. Blood clotting takes place in three steps:
   A. A chemical substance, prothrombin activator, forms in response to trauma to a blood vessel or to the blood itself.
      [1] When tissues are injured, clotting is initiated by a substance from tissue extract called thromboplastin. Thromboplastin interacts with several clotting factors in the plasma to become prothrombin activator.
      [2] When the blood itself is traumatized, injured platelets release a blood clotting factor, Platelet Factor 3, that interacts with several clotting factors in the plasma to become prothrombin activator. (Blood may become traumatized by the roughened endothelial surface of a blood vessel.)
   B. The prothrombin activator, in the presence of calcium ions, catalyzes the conversion of prothrombin into thrombin.
   C. Thrombin acts as an enzyme to convert fibrinogen (a plasma protein) into fibrin threads, which form the network of the clot.
3. Prothrombin is formed continually by the liver and is utilized continually for blood clotting.
4. Vitamin K, a fat-soluble vitamin produced by the action of microorganisms on certain kinds of food in the intestinal tract, is needed for production of prothrombin.
5. The average platelet (or thrombocyte) count is approximately 250,000 per cubic millimeter of blood.
6. The blood clot is composed of a network of fibrin threads that entrap blood cells, platelets and plasma. The threads adhere to injured blood vessel surfaces. Within a few minutes after the clot is formed, it retracts and pulls the edges of the injured blood vessel together. If the clot becomes dislodged, the clotting process must be reinitiated.
7. Blood clots contain plasminogen, which can be converted to plasmin within 24 hours. Plasmin acts as a digestive enzyme to bring about the dissolution of the primary clot.
8. Blood, after it is shed, normally clots within 3 to 5 minutes (clotting time).
9. Bleeding from punctured skin capillaries normally ceases within 2 minutes (bleeding time).

10. Prothrombin time measures the activity of prothrombin in the blood. Using the Quick Test, the normal prothrombin time is 14–18 seconds. If the time is prolonged beyond 30 seconds there is a tendency to bleed.
11. Intravascular clotting is normally prevented by:
    A. A normal rate of blood flow through the blood vessels. (Stasis of blood can result in intravascular clotting.)
    B. A smooth endothelial surface.
    C. The specialized structure of the endothelium that prevents the activation of prothrombin.
    D. Heparin. (Heparin is a powerful anticoagulant produced primarily by mast cells located in connective tissue surrounding capillaries.)

BLOOD TYPES

1. The blood of different persons has antigenic and immune properties, so that the antibodies in the plasma of one person's blood react with antigens in the cells of another's. The antigens and antibodies are almost never precisely the same in any 2 persons.
2. Two groups of antigens are most likely to cause blood transfusion reactions involving agglutination and/or hemolysis of red blood cells.
   A. The O–A–B system of antigens.
      [1] Type A blood agglutinates the cells of both Type B and Type AB blood.
      [2] Type B blood agglutinates the cells of both Type A and Type AB blood.
      [3] Type AB blood does not agglutinate the cells of any other type of blood, because there is no antibody in the serum.
      [4] Type O blood is not agglutinated by any other type of blood, because there is no antigen in the blood cells.
   B. The Rh system.
      [1] When Rh factor (in red blood cells or in breakdown products of red blood cells) is injected into a person's blood that does not contain Rh factor (the Rh negative person), he becomes sensitized to the Rh factor and develops anti-Rh agglutinins.
      [2] The immune response to Rh factor varies with individuals.
      [3] Repeated exposure to Rh factor causes an increase in the development of antibodies.
      [4] If a fetus is Rh positive (this characteristic may be inherited from the father) and the mother is Rh negative, the mother develops anti-Rh agglutinins which diffuse into the bloodstream of the fetus and cause agglutination of the red blood cells. Clumps of blood cells occlude small blood vessels and hemolysis occurs.

HEART FUNCTION

1. A special excitatory and conduction system composed of specialized cardiac muscle fibers coordinates the sequences of rhythmic heart action. This system generates and transmits electrical impulses that cause contraction of the atrial and ventricular segments of the myocardium.
   A. The rate and rhythm of the contractions of the heart are dependent upon the

speed and regularity with which electrical impulses are generated by the sino-atrial node and upon the functional integrity of the conduction system.

B. The conduction system includes:

[1] The sino-atrial node, which normally acts as the pacemaker of the heart.

[2] The atrioventricular bundle, which transmits (with a very important slight delay) impulses between the atria and the ventricles.

[3] The left and right bundles of Purkinje's fibers, which transmit impulses to all parts of the ventricles.

C. The atria contract before the ventricles, pumping blood into the ventricles prior to the strong ventricular contractions.

D. There are some pacemaker cells in the atrioventricular bundle and some in other parts of the ventricles that can generate and transmit impulses, causing ventricular contractions. (When the ventricles contract on their own, the rate is only about 28 beats per minute.)

E. The sino-atrial node function can be taken over by the atrioventricular node or other hyperirritable cells in the conduction system, and this can cause cardiac arrhythmias.

[1] Stimulants such as coffee or tobacco can, if used excessively, cause hyperirritability within the conduction system.

[2] The intake of cold fluids may cause cardiac arrhythmias in a particularly irritable conduction system.

2. The adult human heart normally pumps blood at a rhythmic rate of 70 to 80 beats per minute. In general, the heart beat rate bears an inverse relationship with the size of the individual.

A. The average rate for the new born is 130–140 contractions per minute.

B. Fetal heart tones can usually be heard by the fifth month of pregnancy and average between 120–160 beats per minute.

3. The heart rate may be accelerated or depressed by the autonomic nervous system.

A. The cardiac accelerator center is located in the medulla oblongata and operates through the sympathetic division of the autonomic nervous system.

B. The cardiac inhibitor center is also located in the medulla oblongata; the vagus nerves, which are part of the parasympathetic nervous system, carry inhibitory impulses to the conduction system and heart musculature.

4. Epinephrine causes an increased heart rate.

5. In general, the rate of cardiac contraction bears a direct relationship to the metabolic rate (e.g., there is an increased heart rate with physical activity, with hyperthyroidism and with fever). (Under normal conditions the heart rate returns to normal within a few minutes after physical activity or emotional reaction. The time required for return to normal increases as aging progresses.)

6. The cardiac cycle is the period from the end of one heart contraction to the end of the next contraction. It consists of a period of relaxation called diastole and a period of contraction called systole.

7. Two heart sounds can be heard during the cardiac cycle.

A. The first sound ("lub") is relatively long and soft and has a low pitch. Factors that cause this sound include closure of the atrioventricular valves, the rush of blood from the ventricle into the aorta and the contraction of the ventricular muscles.

B. The second sound ("dup") is shorter and sharper. This sound results from vibrations in the blood and arterial walls when the aortic and pulmonary valves close.

8. Normally blood flows continually from the great veins into the atria. About 70 percent of the blood flows directly into the ventricles, but an additional 30 percent is forced into the ventricles by atrial contractions.

9. Valves prevent backflow of blood during the cardiac cycle.
    A. The atrioventricular valves (the tricuspid and the mitral) prevent backflow of blood from the ventricles into the atria during systole.
    B. The semilunar valves (the pulmonary and the aortic) prevent backflow from these arteries into the ventricles during diastole.

10. Cardiac output is the quantity of blood pumped by the left ventricle into the aorta every minute.
    A. Although the normal adult heart, under resting conditions, will permit a maximum pumping of up to 15 L. per minute, it normally pumps only about 5 L. per minute.
        [1] The difference between what the heart normally pumps and what it is able to pump is sometimes referred to as cardiac reserve power. It is determined by the extent to which the muscle fibers can lengthen and effectively pump the blood.
        [2] Cardiac reserve power decreases with aging.
    B. Cardiac output varies directly with the amount of body surface. (There is a gradual increase in cardiac output with normal growth and development up to age 10; there is a gradual decrease in adulthood and with aging.)
    C. Normally, cardiac output is regulated by all the peripheral blood flow regulations; that is, cardiac output is controlled by the tissues themselves, in proportion to their needs.
    D. Within physiologic limits, the heart pumps all the blood that comes to it without letting blood dam up in the veins.
        [1] Cardiac output is increased when there is a general increase in the body's metabolic rate.
        [2] Cardiac output is increased when tissues demand increased blood flow.

11. The amount of blood that enters the ventricular chambers to be pumped into the pulmonary and systemic circulations is determined by:
    A. The amount of venous return.
        [1] The amount of blood returned to the heart varies with the amount of blood flow required by the tissues. Increased tissue demands result in increased blood flow, and venous return is increased. Decreased tissue demands result in decreased blood flow, and venous return is reduced.
        [2] When the heart rate in the adult exceeds 150 contractions per minute the ventricles do not fill properly between contractions, so the venous return is reduced.
        [3] Venous return from the pulmonary circulation varies with the rate of blood flow through the pulmonary circuit and with the volume and pressure of blood in the left ventricle.
        [4] Venous return from the systemic circulation varies directly with the gravitational force, the arterial blood pressure and the contractions of

voluntary muscles; it varies inversely with the intrathoracic and intra-abdominal pressures.
  B. The strength of atrial contractions.
  C. The patency of the atrioventricular valves.
12. The amount of blood pumped by the ventricles into the pulmonary and systemic circulations is determined by:
  A. The stroke-volume of the ventricular contractions.
  B. The integrity of the atrioventricular valves.
  C. The patency of the semilunar valves.
13. The work of the heart depends chiefly upon the amount of blood ejected per minute against the mean pressure in the systemic and pulmonary circulations.
  A. The force of cardiac muscle contractions varies directly with the degree to which the ventricular chambers are filled with blood.
    [1] Increased venous return increases the work of the heart.
    [2] An increase in the circulating blood volume increases venous return—increasing the workload of the heart.
  B. The greater the blood pressure in the periphery and/or in the lungs, the greater the force required by ventricular contractions to maintain an adequate blood flow. (A rise in the intraabdominal pressure against the great blood vessels increases the systemic blood pressure, and the work load of the heart is increased.)
  C. The work load of the heart is increased when blood must be pumped against the force of gravity.
  D. The work load of the heart is increased when body weight is excessive. (More than usual muscular exertion is required for physical activities, and the blood volume may be greater.)
14. Physical exercise helps to keep a heart healthy: the coronary circulation is increased, and the myocardial fibers strongly contract to increase cardiac output.
15. Heart muscle adapts to continued increase in work load by hypertrophy. A greatly hypertrophied heart becomes ineffective, as muscle fibers can no longer contract forcefully and the coronary circulation within the enlarged heart becomes inadequate.

BLOOD PRESSURE AND BLOOD FLOW

1. Arterial blood pressure can be defined as the amount of pressure exerted by the blood against the walls of the arterial blood vessels.
2. Arterial blood pressure varies with:
  A. The stroke-volume of the ventricular contractions.
    [1] The greater the force, the higher the pressure.
    [2] The greater the volume, the higher the pressure.
  B. The caliber of the arterioles. (The smaller the caliber, the higher the pressure.)
  C. The elasticity of the blood vessel walls. (The more rigid the walls, the higher the pressure.)
  D. The viscosity of the blood.
    [1] The greater the viscosity, the higher the pressure.
    [2] Blood, normally, is about 5 times more viscous than water.

3. The arterial blood pressure is influenced by the extracellular fluid volume (including blood volume) that is regulated, in part, by the kidneys.
4. Arterial blood pressure can be measured by equalizing the external pressure applied against an artery with the pressure within the artery.
   A. Systolic pressure is the pressure at the time of ventricular systole.
      [1] The systolic measurement affords information about the cardiac output and reflects changes in the arterial vessels.
      [2] Taken in the brachial artery, the average range (at rest) for an infant is 55–80 mm. of Hg, and the average range for an adult is 90–145 mm. of Hg.
   B. Diastolic blood pressure is the pressure at the time of ventricular diastole.
      [1] The diastolic measurement affords information about the basic pressure in the circulatory system.
      [2] Taken in the brachial artery, the average range (at rest) for an infant is 40–50 mm. of Hg, and the average range for an adult is 60–90 mm. of Hg.
   C. Arterial blood pressure can be determined in any extremity where a blood pressure cuff can be applied closely above a point where a pulse can be felt.
   D. Blood pressure measurements may vary between right and left extremities.
   E. Visible strong pulsations of the carotid arteries may indicate a high systolic pressure.
5. The pulse is the resultant throb in an artery caused by the rise and fall of the arterial pressure as the left ventricle contracts.
   A. The pulse can be felt wherever a superficial artery can be held against firm tissue.
   B. The strength of a pulse varies with the amount of systolic discharge and the elasticity of the arterial wall.
6. The pulse pressure is the difference between the systolic and the diastolic pressures.
   A. The pulse pressure varies directly with the amount of blood ejected by the systolic discharges.
   B. The average range of pulse pressure is 30–50 mm. of Hg.
7. Strenuous physical exercise (or contemplation of it) has the greatest of all physiological effects in raising the blood pressure.
8. There is an immediate slight rise in blood pressure when the position is changed from supine to sitting or standing. This is due to the sudden decrease of blood supply to the brain that results from the change in gravitational force.
9. Blood pressure is greatly affected by the emotional state of an individual, through the association between emotions and the autonomic nervous system.
10. Central venous pressure is the pressure of blood in the right atrium of the heart. The normal pressure is approximately 2 mm. of Hg. Under abnormal conditions it can rise as high as 20–30 mm. of Hg.
    A. Central venous pressure is increased when heart action is weak and blood returned to the heart cannot be pumped adequately.
    B. Central venous pressure is increased when there is a rapid inflow of blood from the systemic veins.
11. Venous pressure everywhere in the body is directly affected by the central venous pressure. (When the central venous pressure increases by as little as 10 mm. of Hg, the neck veins begin to protrude.)

12. Because of hydrostatic pressure, the pressure in the veins of the feet (of an adult) is approximately 90 mm. of Hg when the person is standing absolutely still.
    A. Increased venous pressure within the leg veins causes increased pressure within the capillaries and fluid leaks from the capillaries into the interstitial spaces. Up to 20 percent of blood volume can be lost within 15 minutes when a person stands absolutely still.
    B. The pressure in the veins of the feet of an adult who is walking is usually less than 25 mm. of Hg. Venous return is achieved by the massaging action of leg muscles and the presence of valves.
13. When the circulatory rate is slowed beyond certain limits:
    A. The veins may become engorged with blood containing reduced hemoglobin.
    B. The walls of the veins may become weakened, with resultant varicosities.
    C. The valves in the veins may become incompetent.
    D. Edema may result.
14. There are mechanisms for regulating blood flow to tissues in accordance with their needs.
    A. Acute needs for increased blood supply in the tissues are usually answered by the sympathetic nervous system that effects vasodilatation and the opening of a larger number of capillaries.
       [1] In general, lack of oxygen in the tissues causes an increase in blood flow.
       [2] Increased blood flow in skeletal muscles is initiated at the onset of exercise and may increase up to 20 times with strenuous exercise.
       [3] Coronary blood flow is increased with sympathetic stimulation. It may be increased 4 to 5 times during strenuous exercise.
       [4] An increase of electrolytes or end products of protein metabolism in the circulating blood causes an increase in blood flow in the kidneys.
       [5] An increase in carbon dioxide in tissue fluids in the brain causes local vasodilatation.
       [6] Blood flow in the skin is controlled almost entirely by the brain, through the temperature-regulating center.
          a. The skin has 2 different kinds of blood vessels: the usual vessels concerned with nutrition and special vascular structures designed for heat regulation. Many of the latter are found on the volar surfaces of the hands and feet and in the lips, nose and ears. When these special vessels are constricted, blood flow may be decreased to almost none at all; when dilated, the flow may be increased up to 7 times.
          b. When the skin is exposed to cold the reduced blood flow may affect nutrition of the cells. Under very hot conditions cardiac output may be markedly reduced because there is so much blood in the skin.
       [7] Blood flow in the gastrointestinal tract is dependent upon local regulatory mechanisms. It is increased by glandular activity and smooth muscle activity. Sympathetic stimulation causes intense vasoconstriction (e.g., when increased blood flow is needed in skeletal muscles).
    B. Long-term needs for increased blood supply to tissues are met by increased vascularity.
       [1] The increase in the number and size of blood vessels probably occurs in response to oxygen need. The process requires days, weeks or months.

[2] The degree of response to need for increased vascularity is greater in young tissues than in old.

[3] Hyperoxia causes decreased vascularity. (If a newborn is exposed to high concentrations of oxygen over a period of time there may be a sudden and excessive increase in vascularity in the retina when the infant is exposed to normal atmospheric conditions.)

15. High metabolic rates in the brain and liver require an extremely large blood flow.
    A. The body's control systems are geared especially to maintain constant cerebral blood flow (except when there is hypoxia or hypercapnia). These controls require constant excitability of nerve cells.
    B. The total hepatic blood flow per minute in the adult is almost one-third of the total cardiac output. Large quantities of blood can be stored in the liver, because of its structure.

16. Urine secretion by the kidney requires a large blood flow.

17. In pregnancy there is a markedly increased blood flow to the uterus.

18. Tissue (cellular) functioning is impaired if the volume and pressure of circulating blood are not maintained within certain limits. When vital organs are involved there is threat to life.
    A. Impaired brain function may involve the vital centers; may result in disturbances in sensory and motor functions; and may cause behavior changes, loss of cognition and loss of consciousness.
    B. Impaired coronary circulation results in impaired heart action.
    C. Impaired pulmonary function may result in an inadequate supply of oxygen and inadequate elimination of carbon dioxide.
    D. Impaired kidney function results in oliguria or anuria, affecting fluid and electrolyte balance, the acid-base balance and the elimination of toxic catabolites from the body.
    E. Impaired liver function results in problems with the metabolism of carbohydrates, protein and fats, fluid and electrolyte balance, blood clotting and detoxification processes.

19. Inadequate circulation to muscle tissue results in severe pain in the affected muscles.

20. Inadequate circulation to peripheral nerves causes tingling and burning sensations and, eventually, loss of sensation.

21. Under normal conditions the blood flow in specific tissues is increased when:
    A. There is increased tissue functioning.
    B. There is injury to the tissue. (Following a localized injury to the body there is a brief local vasoconstriction, followed by an active hyperemia; this in turn is followed by a decrease in blood flow within the affected part.)
    C. Heat is applied to the tissue.

22. Most elderly people have some impairment of circulatory function. The degree of impairment varies with individuals and may involve any or all of the body organs.

SPECIAL CIRCULATORY CONTROLS

1. Almost all the blood vessels of the body (except capillaries) are supplied with sympathetic nerve fibers.

A. The sympathetic nerves carry both vasoconstrictor and vasodilator fibers, but the most important are the vasoconstrictor fibers.

[1] There is an extensive distribution of vasoconstrictor fibers in the kidneys, the gastrointestinal tract, the spleen and the skin.

[2] The sympathetic nerves to skeletal muscles carry sympathetic vasodilator fibers, as well as vasoconstrictor fibers, and the motor cortex excites the vasodilator system.

2. The vasomotor center is located in the lower pons and upper medulla oblongata. It is responsible for continual stimulation of vasoconstrictor fibers that maintain the blood vessels in a partial state of contraction (vasomotor tone). When vasomotor tone is not properly maintained, the vessels dilate, peripheral resistance is decreased and the arterial blood pressure falls.

3. Ischemia of the vasomotor center, due to impaired circulation to the brain, results in a powerful sympathetic vasoconstriction which causes an elevation of the systemic arterial blood pressure. This is called the C.N.S. ischemic response.

4. The vasomotor center may act as a unit (when there is physical or emotional stress) to stimulate generalized vasoconstriction, stimulate the heart and stimulate the production of epinephrine and norepinephrine, which stimulate circulation even more.

5. The body's alarm pattern, which occurs in preparation for "fight or flight" and with strenuous exercise, results from stimulation of the hypothalamus.

A. Blood flow through the skeletal muscles is increased.

B. There is extensive vasoconstriction throughout the body, increasing the systemic arterial blood pressure.

C. There is a great increase in heart activity—both rate and strength of contractions.

D. The stimulation of the central nervous system (C.N.S.) results in increased attentiveness and a feeling of excitement.

Physics

1. Gravity is the force of attraction between two objects (e.g., the earth and an object on or near the earth).

2. The law of gravitation states that any two objects in the universe are attracted to each other with a force that is proportional to the product of their masses and inversely proportional to the square of the distance between them.

3. Weight is the attraction of the body by the earth.

4. Energy is the capacity for performing work—the moving of a mass of matter through space. The amount of energy required to move mass is dependent upon the resistance offered by opposing forces (e.g., weight of object, gravity, friction, atmospheric pressure).

5. Pressure is the force exerted on a unit area.

6. Liquids at rest exert pressure. The pressure exerted by a column of liquid in a container is equal to the height of the liquid times its weight per unit volume.

7. Fluids flow from an area of higher pressure to one of lower pressure, and the rate of volume flow is directly related to the pressure gradient.

8. Viscosity (fluid friction) is the internal resistance of fluid in motion, which retards flow.
9. Gases are relatively insoluble in liquids, unless the temperature is decreased and/or the pressure is increased.

Chemistry

1. Immiscible liquids are those that will not dissolve in one another (e.g., oil and water).
2. Hemoglobin is a conjugated protein made up of heme, the red pigment, and globin, a protein. Heme contains iron.
   A. Oxyhemoglobin is scarlet in color. Reduced hemoglobin is a darkish purple color.
   B. When hemoglobin undergoes chemical breakdown, different colored pigments are formed, depending upon the extent of oxidation and reduction processes (e.g., red, green, brown, yellow).
   C. When hemoglobin undergoes chemical digestion, the heme portion forms a black pigment.

Pathology

SYMPTOMS AND SIGNS

Symptoms and signs of problems that involve or may involve the volume and pressure of circulating blood include:

1. Bleeding.
   A. Observable bleeding (except that associated with normal female reproductive functions), which includes bleeding:
      [1] From skin or mucous membrane (e.g., due to a surgical wound or a traumatic injury). Careful observations must be made under the person, under clothing, around dressings or casts and so forth.
      [2] Into the skin or mucous membrane (e.g., petechiae, ecchymosis, hematomas, purpura).
      [3] From any body opening (e.g., epistaxis, hematemesis, hemoptysis, or from the auditory canal, the anus, the vagina, the urinary meatus).
         a. Bleeding from the gastrointestinal tract may be observed as gross blood or as digested blood (coffee-ground vomitus or melena).
         b. Vaginal bleeding (including blood clots) is abnormal during pregnancy and the postpartum period.
         c. Excessive bleeding during delivery is abnormal.
      [4] In any body fluids that are eliminated normally or drained artifically.
   B. Internal bleeding (which may lead to hemorrhagic shock). Symptoms and signs may include:
      [1] Abnormally low blood pressure or a progressive drop in blood pressure.
      [2] Weak, rapid pulse.
      [3] Pale, cold, moist skin with cyanosis possibly appearing around the lips and in nail beds.

      [4] Rapid and deep respirations (air hunger).

      [5] Subnormal temperature.

      [6] Oliguria or anuria.

      [7] Thirst.

      [8] Behavioral changes such as apprehensiveness, excessive irritability, restlessness, confusion, apathy. (Apprehensiveness may be indicated by a tense, anxious facial expression, general muscular tension, excessive or very limited verbal communication, inability to concentrate, gastric discomfort and dryness of the oral mucosa. It should be noted that under different circumstances anxiety or apprehensiveness may also be indicated by elevation in blood pressure, an increase in pulse and respiration rates, frequency of urination, diarrhea and muscular tremors.)

      [9] Dizziness, visual blurring, tinnitus.

    [10] Loss of consciousness.

  C. Nonobservable bleeding within specific body parts. This includes:

      [1] Hemarthrosis (painful, tender, swollen and hot joints).

      [2] Intramuscular bleeding (painful, tender, swollen and hot muscles).

      [3] Intrapleural bleeding (dyspnea and painful respiration, splinting of chest wall, changes in heart action).

      [4] Bleeding into the respiratory tract (dyspnea, choking, wet "gurgling" cough, cyanosis, frequent swallowing, apnea).

      [5] Intraperitoneal or retroperitoneal bleeding (abdominal discomfort, distention, rigidity of abdominal musculature).

      [6] Bleeding into the gastrointestinal tract (frequent and possibly difficult swallowing, abdominal discomfort and distention in involved area).

      [7] Bleeding into uterus—postpartum (a soft, boggy uterus which can be palpated high in abdominal cavity).

      [8] Bleeding into cranial cavity (behavioral changes; loss of consciousness; neuromuscular disturbances; marked changes in vasomotor mechanisms, heart action, breathing, body temperature; blurring of vision; tinnitus).

2. Abnormally high or low arterial blood pressure.

3. Abnormal pulse rate, rhythm or character and/or an apical-radial pulse differential.

4. Discomfort.

  A. Substernal pain, which may be a dull ache, a feeling of pressure or may be acute, severe and continuous pain.

  B. Pain in either shoulder, radiating down the arms.

  C. Pounding heart, palpitations, feelings of breathlessness.

  D. Claudication, numbing, tingling in extremities, cramping of leg muscles—particularly at night, following day's activities.

  E. Feeling of heaviness in lower extremities, especially at end of day or after standing for period of time.

  F. Feeling of cramping and pressure in lower abdomen and back at onset of menstruation.

  G. General abdominal discomfort, possibly similar to indigestion.

  H. Severe and/or frequent headaches.

5. Unusual fatigue.

6. Dyspnea, orthopnea, persistent cough that may be moist, abnormal breathing patterns.
7. Changes in skin temperature (cold or hot).
8. Changes in skin color (e.g., red, pale, mottled, cyanotic).
9. Hypothermia or hyperthermia.
10. Behavioral changes (e.g., apathy, excessive irritability, apprehension, confusion, disorientation, loss of memory).
11. Loss of consciousness, possibly convulsions.
12. Swelling of feet or ankles.
13. Large, tortuous, engorged veins (e.g., in neck or lower extremities).

HEMORRHAGE

1. Hemorrhage is the escape of blood from the vascular system.
    A. It may be internal or external.
    B. It may be from arteries, veins and/or capillaries.
    C. It may be classified according to structure.
        [1] Petechiae are small, punctated hemorrhages.
        [2] An ecchymosis is larger and more diffuse (e.g., a bruise).
        [3] Purpura is a condition in which petechiae and ecchymoses are so extensive they become confluent.
    D. It may be due to a break in continuity of a blood vessel or to the oozing of blood through damaged capillary walls.
2. Conditions that affect blood vessels and may cause hemorrhage include:
    A. Trauma.
        [1] The continuity of blood vessels may be destroyed directly by outside force or indirectly by bone splinters.
        [2] A blow to the skull can result in hemorrhage within the cranial cavity. This can result in inadequate circulation to the brain tissue, and/or the bleeding can result in increasing intracranial pressure. The symptoms produced depend upon the amount of bleeding, the location of the bleeding and how rapidly blood accumulates.
    B. Chemical erosion (e.g., gastric ulcer).
    C. An inflammatory process involving tissue necrosis.
    D. An aneurysm (a sac-like dilatation caused by a structural weakness in walls of a blood vessel) may rupture with undue strain or stress. Aneurysms are apt to occur in the aorta, in the carotid artery and in cerebral vessels.
    E. Arteriosclerosis can weaken the walls of arteries and cause rupture.
    F. Hypoxia causes capillary hemorrhages (may be observed in newborns).
    G. Capillary fragility can result from Vitamin C deficiency.
    H. Dilated veins (or varicosities) may rupture. Rupture of esophogeal varices can result in serious bleeding.
3. Conditions that affect blood constituents and may cause hemorrhage include:
    A. Hemophilia, a hereditary, sex-linked disease in which there is prolonged clotting time.
    B. Thrombocytopenic purpura, a condition in which there is spontaneous hemorrhaging into the skin and mucous membranes. The bleeding time is

prolonged due to an inadequate number of platelets (usually below 50,000 per cubic millimeter of blood).
   C. Purpura, which may occur as an allergic response or as a response to septicemia or certain chemical substances.
   D. Inadequate prothrombin production due to interference with the manufacture of Vitamin K in the intestinal tract and/or absorption of Vitamin K by the intestinal tract and/or the production of prothrombin in the liver. Diarrhea, lack of bile and liver disease are all conditions that can interfere with these processes.
 4. Chronic blood loss occurs when there is chronic menorrhagia, ulcerative colitis and peptic ulcer.
 5. The body can generally compensate for chronic blood loss (such as may occur with the 3 conditions mentioned above), but the sudden loss of more than 30 percent of blood volume is often fatal.
 6. The site of bleeding is significant because of the possible effects of the pressure exerted by the accumulating blood (e.g., within the cranial cavity, within the thoracic cavity, within the pericardial sac).
 7. The degree to which vasoconstriction is possible may be limited by arteriolosclerosis.
 8. The time required for the healing process (scar formation, resorption of blood from the tissues, etc.) varies with the extent and location of the hemorrhage, the blood supply to the part and any interference with the normal healing processes. Trauma, infection and chemicals such as digestive juices may interfere with the fibrous consolidation of a thrombus.

CIRCULATORY SHOCK
 1. Circulatory shock is a condition in which cardiac output is reduced to the extent that tissues are damaged for lack of adequate blood flow. It may be caused by loss of blood volume, diffuse systemic vasodilatation and/or inadequate cardiac function.
   A. Symptoms and signs of circulatory shock include:
      [1] Abnormally low arterial blood pressure or a progressive drop in blood pressure.
      [2] Rapid, thready pulse—which may be irregular—or no pulse.
      [3] Pale, cold, moist skin with cyanosis possibly appearing around lips and in nail beds.
      [4] Rapid, shallow breathing.
      [5] Subnormal body temperature.
      [6] Behavioral changes such as apprehensiveness, confusion, apathy.
      [7] Dizziness, visual blurring, tinnitus.
      [8] Loss of consciousness, possibly convulsions.
   B. When cardiac output is suddenly reduced, the cerebrum is most sensitive to inadequate blood flow.
   C. In hemorrhagic shock, the loss of blood volume causes a decrease in the mean systemic blood pressure; there is a decrease in venous return and, consequently, a decrease in cardiac output.

[1] Approximately 10 percent of the blood can be lost without a significant effect on the arterial blood pressure or cardiac output; but after that there is a decrease in the cardiac output first and then in the blood pressure.

[2] The fall in arterial blood pressure stimulates the sympathetic vasoconstrictor system throughout the body to increase peripheral resistance and increase venous return.

[3] Heart activity increases greatly in an attempt to increase cardiac output.

[4] Adequate arterial pressure is maintained in the coronary and cerebral blood vessels (by circulatory reflexes) until the systolic arterial blood pressure falls below 70 mm. of Hg.

[5] A loss of 15–20 percent of the blood volume causes mild shock; a loss of 20–35 percent, moderate shock; a loss of over 45 percent, severe shock.

D. The loss of plasma from the blood also causes a hypovolemic shock, similar to hemorrhagic shock. This can occur when:

[1] There are severe burns and plasma is lost through denuded body surfaces.

[2] There is intestinal obstruction and plasma is lost through leaking capillaries into the intestinal walls and lumen.

E. Neurogenic shock is usually caused by a loss of vasomotor tone. There is an increase in vascular capacity and venous pooling. Venous return is greatly reduced. This type of shock can occur with brain damage and may be associated with the administration of deep general anesthetics or spinal anesthesia.

F. Anaphylactic shock is caused by a severe antigen-antibody reaction, in which damaged cells release highly toxic substances that cause sudden and diffuse vasodilatation. Venous return is greatly reduced. With this type of shock there are symptoms and signs associated with allergic response:

[1] Localized edema in area in which contact with allergen was made.

[2] Generalized edema.

[3] Itching, sneezing, prickling feelings in throat.

[4] Choking, wheezing, dyspnea, cyanosis.

G. Toxic or septic shock (also hypovolemic) occurs when there is excessive loss of blood and plasma into the tissues, due to extensive damage to capillary endothelium by a severe infection (e.g., peritonitis or septicemia).

H. Cardiac shock occurs when cardiac output falls suddenly due to interference with heart function. This may occur when there is coronary thrombosis or myocardial infarction. Symptoms and signs of myocardial infarction include:

[1] Symptoms and signs of circulatory shock.

[2] Severe substernal pain which may radiate to shoulder(s) and down arm(s).

[3] Behavior indicating fear, extreme anxiety.

[4] Dyspnea.

[5] Great weakness.

2. Circulatory shock may be classified as:

A. Compensatory, in which case automatic compensatory mechanisms are able to bring about recovery.

[1] Within minutes circulatory reflexes may be able to effect enough vasoconstriction to maintain minimally adequate circulation.

[2] Within hours, or possibly days, fluid is absorbed into the blood from the intestinal tract and interstitial spaces to compensate for loss of blood volume.

B. Progressive, in which case the structures concerned with maintaining blood circulation themselves begin to deteriorate due to inadequate blood flow.
[1] There is depression of cardiac function.
[2] The vasomotor center is depressed.
[3] Stasis of blood results in thrombosis in tiny blood vessels.
[4] There is increased capillary permeability with loss of blood volume.

C. Irreversible, in which case there is deterioration of the cardiovascular system and of the nervous system, which cannot be stopped. Death inevitably results.

3. The low arterial blood pressure that accompanies shock results in inadequate glomerular filtration pressure in the kidneys, which reduces urinary output. Further, the high metabolic rate of the kidney demands a high rate of blood flow, and when blood flow is reduced below a certain level, tubular necrosis can occur fairly quickly.

HEART FAILURE

1. Heart failure can result from any condition that reduces the ability of the heart to pump blood.

A. Cardiac arrhythmias decrease the pumping effectiveness of the heart. These are caused by abnormal functioning of the excitatory and conduction system. Abnormalities may result from actual injury to these specialized muscle fibers, from inadequate circulation or from changes in irritability which may be caused by certain chemical substances.
[1] Bradycardia is a very slow heart beat which may not provide adequate circulation. It may lead to cardiac standstill.
[2] Paroxysmal atrial tachycardia is a rapid regular heart beat that starts and stops abruptly. A very rapid rate (over 150 beats per minute in adult) does not allow for adequate filling of the ventricles before contractions.
[3] Atrial fibrillation results in a totally irregular heart beat, both in force and rhythm. The sino-atrial node has lost control, and many impulses of differing strengths originate in the atria. The ventricles respond to as many of these rapid irregular impulses as they can and as strongly as they can. Cardiac output is reduced. There is usually a pulse deficit.
[4] Ventricular tachycardia involves rapid ventricular contractions and predisposes to ventricular fibrillation. The faster the rate the more serious the problem in terms of reduced cardiac output and reduced coronary circulation.
[5] Ventricular fibrillation involves rapid, irregular and ineffective ventricular contractions. The ventricles cease to pump blood.
[6] Heart block may be partial or complete. It may be caused by problems in the atrioventricular bundle. Complete heart block may be temporary or permanent. In permanent complete heart block, the ventricles take over control and contract approximately 28 times per minute. This rate does not provide for adequate cardiac output.

B. Cardiac arrest may result from:
    [1] Anoxia (e.g., due to airway obstruction).
    [2] Depression of the nervous system by drugs or by hypercapnia.
    [3] Hypotension.
    [4] Coronary occlusion or myocardial infarct.
    [5] Neurogenic reflexes associated with heart action (e.g., stimulation of the vagus nerves).
C. Disorders or disease conditions affecting the myocardium reduce the pumping effectiveness of the heart. Myocardial weakness may result from trauma, inadequate circulation, an inflammation or an increase of potassium ions in the extracellular fluid.
D. Compression of the heart limits its capacity to receive and pump blood. Cardiac tamponade may occur when there is pericarditis with production of exudate or when there is bleeding into the pericardial sac.
E. When cardiac muscle fibers have been stretched or have hypertrophied to their limit, cardiac reserve is lost and any demands on the heart to increase output can precipitate heart failure.
    [1] Hypertrophy of the left ventricle occurs when there is increased peripheral resistance or when there is leaking or stenosis of the aortic valve or leaking of the mitral valve.
    [2] Hypertrophy of the left atrium occurs when there is mitral stenosis or weakness of left ventricle contractions.
    [3] Hypertrophy of the right ventricle occurs when there is leaking or stenosis of the pulmonary valve or when there is increased resistance in the pulmonary system (which may be due to pulmonary disease).
    [4] Hypertrophy of the right atrium occurs when there is stenosis of the tricuspid valve (rare) or weakness of right ventricle contractions.

CONGESTION

1. Hyperemia (or congestion) is a condition in which there is an excess of blood in the blood vessels because of the dilatation and engorgement of the vessels. It may be active (due to increased blood flow) or passive (due to decreased blood flow).
2. Local passive congestion may be caused by:
    A. Thrombosis (intravascular clotting).
    B. External pressure against a vein or veins (e.g., due to tumor growth, pregnancy, scar tissue formation).
    C. Back pressure, due to varicose veins.
3. General passive congestion can result from reduced blood flow through the heart chambers or through the lungs.
    A. Congestive heart failure may be related to low cardiac output or increased venous pressure. Causes of congestive heart failure include:
        [1] Hypertension.
        [2] Atherosclerosis of the coronary arteries, decreasing the blood supply to the myocardium.
        [3] Mechanical disorders of the valves due to congenital anomalies, valvular stenosis, valvular insufficiency.

a. A frequent cause of valvular stenosis or insufficiency is rheumatic fever.

b. Aortic valve insufficiency may result from syphilis infection.

[4] Increased resistance in pulmonary system due to pulmonary disease.

B. With left-sided heart failure, blood is not pumped out of the left ventricle adequately, resulting in increased pulmonary systemic pressure with pulmonary congestion. Pulmonary edema can occur.

[1] Pulmonary vascular congestion causes dyspnea, orthopnea and persistent cough.

[2] Pulmonary edema may occur rapidly. Dyspnea becomes more severe, and the cough becomes increasingly moist and productive of bloody and foamy sputum. Ventilation becomes increasingly limited.

C. With right-sided heart failure, blood is not pumped out of the right ventricle adequately, and this results in systemic congestion.

[1] Venous pressure rises in the great veins and their tributaries.

[2] The liver becomes filled with blood.

[3] There is leakage from the capillaries, resulting in dependent edema and ascites.

D. Left-sided heart failure usually leads to failure of the right side, as the right ventricle has to work harder and harder to push blood into the congested pulmonary system.

E. Fluid and salt retention are associated with chronic heart failure.

[1] Glomerular filtration is reduced because of the reduced cardiac output and reduced arterial blood pressure.

[2] There is an increase in the production of aldosterone with a resultant increase in absorption of sodium and water.

[3] Both of these effects result in an increase in the volume of extracellular fluid.

F. Circulatory overload that may occur when there is a rapid increase in blood volume can cause pulmonary congestion and pulmonary edema.

[1] Pulmonary congestion and edema may occur when parenteral fluids are administered too rapidly. This tends to happen more quickly with older people and when there is heart damage.

[2] When a person with considerable dependent edema is up and about for a period of time and then rests in a recumbent position, reabsorption of excess interstitial fluid into the blood can result in a circulatory overload.

G. A compensated heart is one in which hypertrophy of cardiac fibers has increased the contracting power of the fibers so that the heart is able to attain some degree of normal function.

[1] The amount of blood supply to a hypertrophied heart does not increase proportionately.

[2] Repeated episodes of overexertion lead to progressive congestive heart failure.

[3] The degree of compensation varies among individuals.

THROMBOSIS AND EMBOLISM

1. Thrombosis is the formation of blood clots within the vascular spaces. It may be due to:

A. Injury to the endothelium (e.g., trauma, chemicals, toxins, bacterial infections, atherosclerosis).

B. Decrease in rate of blood flow (most common in deep veins of legs and pelvis; favored by generalized passive congestion; more common in aged or debilitated).

C. Changes in blood constituents (e.g., increase in number of platelets or erythrocytes).

    [1] There is an increase in the number of platelets in the circulating blood following surgery.

    [2] Polycythemia vera is a condition in which there is a great increase in the number of erythrocytes (e.g., 8,000,000 per cubic millimeter of blood).

2. Thrombophlebitis is a condition in which venous thrombosis is associated with inflammation of the veins. It occurs most frequently in the lower extremities. The agent is usually bacterial, and the thrombus is usually firmly attached. Venous sinuses of the brain may become the site of thrombophlebitis as a consequence of mastoiditis, infections of the face or deep, infected scalp wounds.

3. Phlebothrombosis is a thrombus in a vein. It occurs most frequently in the veins of the lower extremities. The thrombus may show no effects or may cause hyperemia, edema and pain. It is often fairly loosely attached so it can become dislodged rather easily.

4. The effects of thrombosis depend upon such factors as:

A. Whether or not the thrombus completely occludes a blood vessel.

B. Location, size and type of blood vessel involved.

C. The extent of collateral circulation that already exists or develops.

D. Whether or not the thrombus breaks loose.

E. Whether or not the thrombus becomes infected.

5. The possible results of thrombosis include:

A. No observable effects.

B. Local passive congestion, edema.

C. Mechanical interference with heart function.

D. Blood infection.

E. Ischemia or infarction of tissues affected by occlusion.

F. Sudden death due to occlusion of a major artery (e.g., coronary, cerebral, pulmonary).

6. Embolism is a process wherein there is an impaction somewhere in the cardiovascular system of material brought there by the circulation. The material is called an embolus; it may be a solid, an immiscible liquid or bubbles of air.

A. Solid emboli may be composed of such substances as coagulated blood or agglutinated blood cells, tissue cells or parasites.

B. Liquid emboli may be injected intravenously by accident, or they may be introduced into the blood stream during major surgery or with extensive traumatic injuries. An example is a fat embolus.

C. Air emboli may be introduced into the blood stream accidentally during intravenous therapy, during surgery or with traumatic injury involving the neck and the chest.

D. The effects of emboli depend upon the site of the impaction and upon the size of the embolus compared to the caliber of the blood vessel.

ISCHEMIA

1. Ischemia is a condition in which the blood supply to a part is decreased. The decrease may be absolute (such as a sudden complete occlusion of a blood vessel) or relative (such as occurs with hypotension or failure to meet increased demands of tissues). Causes of ischemia, other than thromboembolism, include:
   A. Hypotension (e.g., with shock following surgery).
   B. Tissue demand for sudden increase in circulation (e.g., with strenuous physical activity).
   C. Mechanical occlusion:
      [1] Destruction of capillaries (e.g., with burns, freezing).
      [2] Restrictive devices (e.g., tourniquet or cast).
      [3] Tumor masses.
      [4] Volvulus (redundant loop of intestine); intussusception (telescoping of intestines); strangulated hernia (loop of intestine protrudes through an opening and blood supply to the involved part is cut off).
      [5] External pressure against blood vessels (e.g., pressure of body weight over bony prominences, especially when there is little adipose padding).
   D. Disease conditions of the arteries:
      [1] Raynaud's disease is a condition in which there is arterial spasm, usually in the fingers and hands. Spasms seem to be increased by cold or emotional stress. Circulation is reduced.
      [2] Thromboangiitis obliterans (Buerger's disease) is a condition in which there is inflammation of the lining of the arterial wall, often accompanied by thrombus formation. It occurs most frequently in the lower extremities. Circulation may become greatly reduced.
      [3] Atherosclerosis is both a degenerative process and an inflammatory reaction involving the arteries. There is a thickening of the intima, the cells of which are loaded with fat. Cholesterol crystals appear, the artery reacts with connective tissue formation and a plaque is formed. The lumen of the vessel is not only narrowed but roughened (which may lead to clot formation) and weakened (which may lead to aneurysm formation and/or hemorrhage).
         a. The arteries with predominantly elastic media (the aorta and its major branches, the coronary arteries and the larger arteries of the brain) tend to be involved most frequently. The condition is often associated with diabetes mellitus and hypertensive disease and tends to occur increasingly during the aging process.
         b. A high-fat diet, especially one containing large amounts of cholesterol and saturated fats, appears to increase chances of developing atherosclerosis.
      [4] Arteriosclerosis is an inclusive term which means, literally, the hardening of the arteries. It includes atherosclerosis, medial sclerosis (which involves the calcification of the medial layer of arterial walls) and hyperplastic arteriosclerosis (which involves the thickening of the medial layer of arterioles and smaller arteries and results in marked narrowing of the lumens). Hyperplastic arteriosclerosis occurs most frequently in the kidneys and ocular fundi.

E. Injury of peripheral nerves or a nerve plexus (e.g., injury of the brachial plexus can result in ischemia of the arm and hand).

F. Poor venous return from a body part can result in a decrease in circulation.

2. Possible consequences of ischemia include:

A. Atrophy of the part (e.g., skeletal muscles, brain).

B. Decreased functioning of tissues and organs affected.

C. Poor wound healing.

D. Infarction. This is a condition in which the blood supply to a part is decreased below the limits the tissue can tolerate (e.g., may result from further reduction of the blood supply or a sudden demand for increased circulation). The tissues become hypoxic; the blood vessels become atonic and congested with blood; the tissues die because of anoxia and chemical injury. Examples include:

[1] Decubitus ulcers (over bony prominences).

[2] Chronic skin ulcers (lower leg).

[3] Gangrene (e.g., of extremities, intestines).

[4] Cerebral hemorrhages.

[5] Myocardial infarct (which may lead to cardiac arrest or heart rupture).

3. The healing of an infarct involves the removal of dead tissue, the fighting of any infection that may be present, the regeneration of cells that have not been damaged too severely and the replacement by fibrous tissue of those that have been irreversibly damaged.

A. The time required for healing varies with such factors as the blood supply to the part, the nutritional status of the individual, the presence of infection, and rest for the part involved.

B. The infarct area is weak until regeneration of cells is well underway.

C. Fibrous tissue cannot function as anything but fibrous tissue; therefore, when it replaces damaged nervous tissue, muscle tissue, etc., normal functioning may be limited.

4. Ischemic pain in the heart muscle that usually occurs intermittently (but may occur continuously) is called angina pectoris.

A. Ischemia of cardiac muscle occurs whenever the work load of the heart becomes too great in relation to available coronary blood flow.

B. An angina attack may result from strenuous physical activity, emotional stress, exposure to cold or overeating.

C. Vasoconstriction resulting from the excessive use of nicotine may restrict coronary blood flow.

5. Coronary disease is sometimes associated with overweight.

HYPERTENSION

1. Hypertension is a condition in which there is sustained elevation of the systemic arterial blood pressure. In the adult elevation is usually judged to be above 140/90.

A. Hypertension may occur secondarily in a number of conditions, including certain kidney disorders, hyperthyroidism and adrenal cortical tumors.

B. An increased systolic pressure is frequently caused by rigidity of the aorta (which may develop during the aging process).

C. If the blood pressure is elevated and there is no known cause, the condition is known as essential hypertension.

[1] There is a sustained abnormal constriction of arterioles and small arteries throughout the body.

[2] The tendency to develop essential hypertension seems to be inherited.

[3] Retention of salt and water by the kidney appears to be basic cause of essential hypertension.

[4] Sometimes essential hypertension appears to be associated with excessive and/or prolonged emotional stress.

2. Headaches (sometimes severe) may occur when there is hypertension.

3. Hypertension increases the workload of the heart because of the increased peripheral resistance. The heart may become hypertrophied and eventually fail.

4. Prolonged and/or severe hypertension predisposes to kidney damage and hemorrhages in the retina and in the brain.

Nursing Care

Nursing care should be directed toward assisting the patient to attain, retain or regain the best possible circulatory function.

COLLECTION, EVALUATION AND COMMUNICATION OF DATA

1. Patients should be interviewed, observed and examined to identify symptoms and signs of actual or potential circulatory problems.

A. Circulatory problems may be indicated by:

[1] Bleeding (internal, external).

[2] Abnormalities in blood pressure and/or pulse.

[3] Abnormalities in respiratory functioning, particularly dyspnea and persistent cough.

[4] Abnormalities in color, temperature and condition of the skin.

[5] Abnormalities in body temperature.

[6] Weakness, unusual fatigue.

[7] Loss of consciousness, abnormal pupil dilatation.

[8] Abnormalities in cognitive and/or emotional behavior.

[9] Physical discomforts including pain, feeling of pressure, numbness.

[10] Edema (generalized or dependent).

[11] Symptoms and signs of impaired renal function.

[12] Abnormalities of superficial veins.

B. Systematic patient evaluation is of especial importance when the patient:

[1] Has lost or is losing a significant amount of blood.

[2] Has a diagnosed disease condition that affects:
a. The heart.
b. The blood vessels.
c. Blood coagulation.
d. The brain.
e. The kidneys.

[3] Has sustained traumatic injury (e.g., with surgery, an accident, a newborn after a prolonged and difficult labor) which involves or may involve:
a. The heart.
b. The blood vessels (especially major vessels).

     c. An organ that has a relatively large blood supply.

     d. The brain.

     e. Fractures and bone dislocations.

[4] Has sustained an injury in which there is a rapid loss of plasma (e.g., extensive burns).

[5] Has a diagnosed disease condition in which hemorrhage is a common complication (e.g., liver disease, peptic or duodenal ulcer, leukemia).

[6] Has symptoms and signs that indicate an actual or potential impairment of circulatory function (e.g., phlebothrombosis).

[7] Has a history of hypersensitivity.

[8] Has been or is receiving medication which affects:

     a. Heart action (e.g., cardiotonics, cardiac stimulants, cardiac depressants).

     b. Vasomotor mechanisms (e.g., vasodilators, vasoconstrictors, ganglionic blocking agents, sympatholytic drugs).

     c. Blood-clotting mechanisms (e.g., anticoagulants, hemostatics).

     d. The brain (e.g., C.N.S. stimulants or depressants).

[9] Is receiving therapy that may cause allergic response (e.g., transfusion, sera, desensitizing drugs).

[10] Is receiving a transfusion.

[11] Is receiving intravenous fluids (of particular importance when patient is at extremes of age and/or has limited cardiac reserve).

[12] Has a constrictive, or potentially constrictive, device applied to a body part (e.g., tourniquet, drying cast, pressure bandage, traction).

[13] Is confined to bed and/or is dependent upon others for changes of position and exercise.

[14] Is experiencing severe emotional stress.

[15] Has a proportionately large amount of blood in the peripheral circulation (e.g., with very hot bath, in hot and humid climate or when standing still for prolonged period).

[16] Is in utero.

[17] Is pregnant, in labor, delivering or within 3 weeks postpartum.

[18] Is at extremes of age: infant, especially premature newborn, and elderly.

C. Whenever a patient has symptoms and signs that indicate an actual or potential problem involving the volume and pressure of circulating blood, the blood pressure and/or pulse should be evaluated frequently.

[1] The frequency of blood pressure and pulse measurements depends upon the condition of the patient and the particular problem that is either existent or potential.

[2] The pulse should be taken over whichever artery is most convenient and easiest to palpate. Pulsations of the carotid arteries can often be observed without palpation.

[3] When the pulse is irregular or weak or when an accurate count is absolutely essential, a stethoscope should be used to listen to the apical heartbeat. Discrepancies between the apical and radial rates are significant.

[4] When a blood pressure measurement cannot be made over the brachial

artery, the ausculatory and/or palpatory methods may be used with other arteries (e.g., the radial, popliteal or dorsalis pedis).

D. Fetal heart tones should be evaluated during pregnancy, labor and delivery. This is of critical importance when the mother has problems involving the volume and pressure of circulating blood, oxygen lack or fluid and electrolyte imbalance.

E. Data collected should be evaluated not only on the basis of a single deviation from normal (e.g., a low blood pressure reading) but should also be evaluated on the basis of combinations of symptoms and signs that are commonly associated with specific circulatory problems (e.g., symptoms and signs associated with internal bleeding).

F. A patient's observable blood loss should be evaluated in relation to such factors as:

[1] The general physical condition (e.g., appearance, vital signs).

[2] Any diagnosed disorder (e.g., any bleeding in a hemophiliac patient is potentially serious).

[3] The type and rate of bleeding (e.g., from arteries or veins of different sizes or from capillaries).

[4] The estimated amount of blood loss, especially as related to the size of the patient.
   a. Whenever possible, estimation of the amount of bleeding should be made and reported.
   b. Bandages, sanitary pads, etc. may be saved for inspection.
   c. Total or partial specimens of urine, vomitus, black stools should be saved for inspection.

G. A patient's blood pressure and pulse should be evaluated in relation to such factors as:

[1] Usual blood pressure and pulse.

[2] Age.

[3] Weight-height comparison.

[4] Posture or position and/or any abrupt change in position.

[5] Physical activity.

[6] Emotional state.

[7] Any diagnosed disorder.

[8] Medications the patient is taking or has taken recently.

[9] Presence of head injury.

2. How, when and what data are communicated to the physician and/or other nursing personnel depend upon:

A. Any immediate threat to the patient's life processes (e.g., symptoms and signs of circulatory shock).

B. Any potential threat to the patient's life and well-being (e.g., symptoms and signs of phlebothrombosis).

C. Any particular implications for the physician in relation to:

[1] The patient's progress or lack of progress toward recovery (e.g., patient's circulatory response to increased physical activity).

[2] Making a diagnosis (e.g., new objective or subjective data).

[3] The patient's physical and emotional responses to specific diagnostic procedures or therapeutic measures.

D. Any particular implications for nursing care (e.g., control of physical activity).

PROMOTION OF HEALTH AND PREVENTION
OF DISEASE/INJURY

1. Health teaching to promote optimal circulatory function should be concerned with:
   A. The importance of:
      [1] A balanced, nutritious diet throughout the life cycle, with avoidance of excessive calories, saturated fats and salt.
      [2] A balanced program of exercise throughout the life cycle, with avoidance of strenuous physical exertion without proper training.
      [3] Adequate rest and sleep.
      [4] Relaxation and avoidance of excessive and/or prolonged emotional stress.
      [5] Learning to cope with unavoidable stress.
      [6] Changing position and moving about intermittently when sitting for long periods, elevating legs when possible.
      [7] Avoiding prolonged standing, crossing legs at thigh and wearing of restrictive clothing (e.g., round garters).
      [8] Avoiding excessive use of stimulants such as coffee and tea.
      [9] Not using tobacco.
   B. The importance of:
      [1] Periodic health evaluations (especially important when there is familial history of cardiovascular disease).
      [2] Prompt medical consultation when:
         a. There are early symptoms and signs of circulatory problems (e.g., dyspnea, unusual fatigue, substernal discomfort, edema).
         b. Children have tonsillitis and/or pharyngitis.
         c. There is a possibility of a syphilitic infection.
      [3] Proper obstetrical care.
   C. Accident prevention.
2. Circulation of blood to a part may be increased, within physiological limits, by:
   A. Positioning.
      [1] If increased arterial flow is desired, the part should be level with or lower than the heart.
      [2] If increased venous return is desired, the part should be level with or elevated above the heart.
   B. Active or passive exercise.
   C. Massage.
   D. Limiting loss of body heat.
   E. Local application of heat.
3. External pressure against peripheral blood vessels should be prevented by:
   A. Positioning patients in good body alignment.
   B. Providing adequate support to body parts.
   C. Avoiding pressure against the popliteal spaces when patient is in dorsal recumbent or sitting position.

4. Prolonged pressure against body parts should be prevented by:
    A. Frequent position changes (within medical orders).
    B. Use of special mattresses when possible.
5. When a patient is confined to bedrest or chair rest, it is particularly important that tissues over bony prominences be protected from any unusual or prolonged pressure by:
    A. Frequent position changes.
    B. Proper use of special devices such as foam rubber pads.
6. Restraints, blood pressure cuffs and/or tourniquets should be used with caution. They should be applied properly. They should be removed and/or released as soon as possible. Adequate circulation in the extremity must be assured.
7. If a tourniquet is applied for any length of time, it should be loose enough to allow some venous return and to provide enough circulation of blood to prevent tissue damage. It should be in full view, and any personnel caring for the patient should be made aware of its application.
8. Whenever a patient has a potentially constrictive device such as a cast (especially a drying cast), traction, a bandage or a restraint applied to an extremity, the extremity should be observed for symptoms and signs of inadequate circulation. Observations should be made for:
    A. Abnormal changes in color and/or temperature of the skin.
    B. Presence of edema.
    C. Presence of a distal pulse.
    D. Physical discomforts such as pain, tingling or numbness.
9. When a patient has a newly applied, wet cast, the involved body part should be supported and handled so as to prevent any changes in the shape of the cast which might interfere with circulation.
10. Caution should be used with the application of cold. Cold applications should be discontinued if the patient complains of pain in the area and/or if the area becomes blanched and remains so for several minutes after application has been removed.
11. The environmental temperature, clothing and bed coverings should be controlled to prevent overheating (causing peripheral vasodilatation) or chilling (causing peripheral vasoconstriction). This is of particular importance when the patient has actual or potential circulatory problems (e.g., a recently postoperative patient, a patient with known cardiovascular problems, the newborn).
12. Patients should be protected from the possibility of thrombus formation in the lower extremities by:
    A. Encouraging and assisting with periodic and effective leg exercises.
    B. Encouraging and assisting with periodic ambulation (within medical orders).
    C. Proper application of elastic stockings or ace bandages when prescribed.
    D. Preventing constriction of blood vessels by such things as garters, improperly applied ace bandages or crossing of legs at thigh.
    E. Preventing chilling of the lower extremities.
    F. Encouraging and/or providing for increased venous return by periodically elevating the legs above the level of the heart (within medical orders).
    G. Preventing traumatic or chemical injury to peripheral blood vessels (e.g., gentle handling of extremities, caution with intravenous procedures, accident

prevention). If a patient who has received or is receiving intravenous therapy has symptoms and signs of inflammatory response around the injection site, this should be reported promptly.

13. If a patient who might be prone to developing phlebothrombosis in the lower extremities should complain of localized discomfort in the calf of the leg (likely to be increased by plantar flexion of foot), the possibility of thrombus formation and resultant emboli should be considered.
    A. The patient should remain quietly in a dorsal recumbent position with the involved limb at rest.
    B. The leg should not be massaged.
    C. The physician should be notified promptly.

14. All patients should be protected from accidental injuries which may result in traumatic injury to blood vessels or loss of plasma (e.g., burns).

15. If a patient sustains severe physical injury or emotional shock, possible hypotension (with resultant decrease in circulation to the brain) should be prevented by placing the patient in the horizontal position or in a position in which the head is lower than the heart. Having the head lower than the heart may be contraindicated if there is head injury or respiratory distress.

16. When a patient has sustained injury to blood vessels and bleeding has been controlled, dislodgement of clots or disruption of sutures should be prevented by:
    A. Protecting the wound from mechanical injury.
    B. Handling the affected part gently.
    C. Controlling movement of the affected part (within medical orders).
    D. Preventing strain on the affected part by providing adequate support, applying bandages properly.
    E. Preventing sudden elevation of the systemic arterial blood pressure by encouraging and providing for physical and emotional rest. (This is most important when the injury is extensive and involves arteries.)

17. Patients should be protected from postural hypotension by:
    A. Allowing only gradual postural changes (lying to sitting to standing), observing total patient response to each change and controlling any further change in accordance with the response.
    B. Preventing pooling of blood in leg veins by the proper application of elastic stockings, ace bandages, abdominal binders or special belts before the patient stands. (This is of particular importance when the patient is ambulating after extended bedrest, is postoperative, is receiving hypotensive drugs, has had a lumbar sympathectomy, has impaired circulatory function and/or is elderly.)

18. Circulatory shock in the postoperative patient may be prevented by:
    A. Controlling pain (without depression of circulatory function).
    B. Avoiding traumatic injury.
    C. Preventing exposure to chilling with consequent vasoconstriction.
    D. Preventing generalized vasodilatation due to overheating.
    E. Detecting signs and symptoms of circulatory problems quickly and taking prompt action.

19. Immiscible liquids such as waxes or oils should never be injected into the blood stream.

20. Air should never be allowed to enter the blood stream.
21. When a patient is receiving an intravenous infusion or transfusion the amount and rate of fluid administered must be carefully regulated in accordance with:
    A. Any medical orders.
    B. Size of the patient.
    C. Patient's circulatory status (e.g., blood pressure, presence of cardiac disease, cardiac reserve).
    D. The rate of flow required to provide continuous flow of fluid through the needle.
22. Patients receiving fluids intravenously should be observed closely for signs and symptoms of circulatory overload. This is particularly important when the patient already has a normal blood volume or has impaired heart action or reduced cardiac reserve.
23. All blood used for transfusions must be positively identified before administration.
24. Patients receiving whole blood or red cells should be attended closely for the first several minutes after procedure is begun and, unless there are medical orders to the contrary, the rate of flow should be slow (e.g., 20–30 gtt. per minute). If the patient shows no indications of a transfusion reaction, the flow can then be increased to the recommended rate.
    A. If a patient receiving blood develops symptoms and signs of a hemolytic reaction (chills, fever, headache, backache, abdominal distress, drop in blood pressure), the transfusion should be stopped immediately and the physician notified.
    B. If a patient receiving blood develops symptoms and signs of hypersensitivity (e.g., urticaria, itching, wheezing), the physician may be notified, but the transfusion need not be stopped unless the symptoms increase in severity.
25. A sensitivity test should be performed before the injection of any serum.
26. When sera or antigen solutions are administered:
    A. The patient should be observed closely for any allergic response.
    B. An emergency vasoconstrictor drug (e.g., epinephrine) should be readily available for prompt administration in case of anaphylactic shock.

CARE OF PATIENTS WITH SPECIFIC CIRCULATORY PROBLEMS
Problems Related to Volume of Circulating Blood

1. When a patient has active external bleeding:
   A. The site of bleeding should be located.
   B. The type and amount of bleeding should be determined. (The amount of blood loss should be estimated as closely as possible.)
   C. Bleeding should be controlled and normal clotting encouraged by:
      [1] Applying pressure directly over the bleeding site (when possible). Exceptions include bleeding in eye, from ear and over larynx.
      [2] Immobilizing the involved part and elevating it above the level of the heart (when possible).
      [3] Protecting the bleeding site from any trauma or strain.
      [4] Using pressure point control if direct pressure is not possible:
          a. On the carotid artery, to control bleeding in the head.
          b. On the temporal artery, to control bleeding in the scalp.

      c. On the facial artery, to control bleeding around mouth and nose.

      d. On the subclavian artery, to control bleeding in shoulder and arm.

      e. On the brachial artery, to control bleeding in arm.

      f. On the femoral artery, to control bleeding in leg.

    [5] Applying a tourniquet above the bleeding site on an extremity *only* if direct pressure and pressure point control are unsuccessful in controlling bleeding.

  D. Demands on the cardiovascular system should be minimized by:

    [1] Providing and encouraging physical and emotional rest.

    [2] Keeping the patient warm but preventing vasodilatation.

  E. Close observations should be made for symptoms and signs of shock when there is extensive loss of blood.

  F. The promptness of needed medical attention is indicated by the site(s) of bleeding, the type and extent of bleeding and the general condition of the patient.

2. Uncontrolled severe bleeding (observed or suspected) is a medical emergency.

3. When epistaxis occurs, the blood supply to the area may be reduced by:

  A. Placing the patient in an upright sitting position. (If a horizontal position is indicated because of the patient's condition or injury, the patient should be placed in a prone position to prevent blood from entering the esophagus or trachea.)

  B. Applying pressure against the nose and upper lip.

4. When there is bleeding or suspected bleeding in the gastrointestinal tract, food and fluids should be withheld until medical orders are available. An exception would be a small amount of rectal bleeding.

5. When there is bleeding or potential bleeding in the pelvic region (e.g., in relation to uterus, bladder or rectum):

  A. Increased pressure within the pelvic blood vessels may be prevented by:

    [1] Discouraging the patient from being on feet, especially for extended periods of time.

    [2] Encouraging good venous return from the extremities by positioning and by effective use of prescribed elastic stockings or ace bandages.

    [3] Preventing straining with defecation.

  B. Pressure against these organs may be minimized by:

    [1] Assisting the patient in the elimination of flatus.

    [2] Preventing bladder distention.

  C. Traumatic injury should be avoided by performing any treatments that involve these organs with particular gentleness.

6. Following parturition the uterus should be maintained in a contracted state by:

  A. Uterine massage.

  B. Preventing distention of the urinary bladder.

  C. Administration of oxytocic drugs as ordered.

7. When there is bleeding or potential bleeding within the cranial cavity (e.g., with head injury, brain surgery or cerebral vascular accident):

  A. The patient should be positioned so as to provide adequate circulation to the brain but not increased pressure within the blood vessels.

  B. Demands on the cardiovascular system should be minimized by providing physical and emotional rest. (Pain-relieving drugs, such as narcotics, that may depress circulatory function should be administered with great caution.)

C. The blood pressure and pulse should be monitored frequently.
   [1] Any fluctuation in these vital signs indicates potential threat to the patient and should be reported promptly.
   [2] A rise in blood pressure and decrease in pulse rate followed by a rise in pulse rate and a fall in blood pressure indicate serious threat to the patient and should be reported promptly.

D. The patient should be observed closely for other indications of increased intracranial pressure. (See Chapter 12.)

8. When a patient shows symptoms and signs of internal hemorrhage:

A. This is a medical emergency.

B. Adequate circulation to the brain should be promoted by placing the patient in a horizontal position with the legs elevated above the level of the heart. The head should be level with the chest or may be slightly elevated.

C. Demands on the cardiovascular system should be minimized by:
   [1] Providing physical and emotional rest. (Pain should be relieved as much as possible, but any drugs that depress circulatory function must be administered only with great caution.)
   [2] Providing warmth but preventing vasodilatation.
   [3] Administering oxygen (within orders) when cyanosis is present.

D. Actions should be taken to restore blood volume by such means as:
   [1] Increasing the rate of flow of any intravenous fluids (unless this is contraindicated). The need to decrease bleeding and the capacity or effectiveness of the cardiovascular system must be taken into consideration.
   [2] Preparing for administration of intravenous fluids, blood, plasma or plasma expanders.

E. Preparation should be initiated for the control of bleeding by surgical intervention.

9. When a patient shows symptoms and signs of circulatory shock:

A. This is a medical emergency.

B. Adequate circulation to the brain should be promoted by placing the patient in a horizontal position with the legs elevated above the level of the heart.

C. Actions should be taken to restore blood volume if the problem involves hypovolemia. (See 8D, above.)

D. Preparation should be made for the administration of emergency drugs to elevate the blood pressure. When a patient is in anaphylactic shock, an immediate-acting sympathomimetic drug (e.g., epinephrine) should be administered promptly as prescribed.

E. Oxygen may be administered if this is indicated by the patient's circulatory and respiratory status.

F. Pain should be relieved as much as possible, but any drugs that depress circulatory function must be administered with great caution.

G. Kidney function should be observed closely. (See Chapter 4.)

10. When a patient has a condition in which there is a blood clotting defect (e.g., hemophilia), or when there is a potential problem with blood clotting (e.g., with

biliary disease) or when a patient is receiving (or has recently received) anticoagulant therapy:

A. Systematic evaluation for indications of bleeding should be made.

B. The presence of bleeding requires prompt medical attention. Bleeding in a hemophiliac patient or in a patient on anticoagulant therapy represents a medical emergency.

C. Traumatic injury to tissues must be prevented in every possible way (e.g., accident prevention, gentle skin care and oral hygiene, careful handling of all body parts, use of oral route for medications whenever possible).

11. When a patient is receiving anticoagulant therapy, it is essential that blood clotting tests be performed frequently. Test results should be communicated to the physican promptly when changes in drug dosage may be indicated by a reduction in prothrombin activity or a prolonged clotting time.

12. When a patient has a condition in which there is known weakness of the arterial walls (e.g., with arteriosclerosis or aneurysm) and there is danger of rupture:

A. Demands upon the cardiovascular system should be minimized by:

[1] Encouraging and providing for more than usual sleep and rest.

[2] Avoiding exposure to extremes of external temperature.

[3] Encouraging minimal desirable body weight.

B. Sudden elevation of the systemic arterial blood pressure should be prevented by such means as:

[1] Avoiding strenuous physical activity.

[2] Alleviating coughing.

[3] Preventing increases in intra-abdominal pressure that occur when there is straining with defecation.

[4] Avoiding emotionally stressful situations.

[5] Encouraging and assisting with gradual postural changes (from lying to sitting to standing positions).

13. When a patient develops circulatory overload (indicated by symptoms and signs of pulmonary congestion):

A. This is a medical emergency.

B. Any additional blood volume should be avoided (i.e., the flow of intravenous fluids should be reduced to absolute minimum rate that maintains flow through the needle).

C. Venous return from the extremities may be reduced by the effective use of rotating tourniquets, when ordered.

D. Preparation may be made for an emergency phlebotomy to reduce circulating blood volume.

E. Cardiotonic and diuretic drugs should be ready for prompt administration as ordered.

Problems Involving Heart Action

1. When a patient develops an abnormally rapid, slow or irregular heart beat:

A. This is a medical emergency.

B. Cardiac load and cardiac activity should be reduced by:

[1] Providing complete rest.

[2] Providing consistent emotional support to allay fear, anxiety.
- C. Observations should be made for symptoms and signs of circulatory failure.
- D. Any drug that might be causing this response should be withheld pending prompt notification of the physician.
- E. Cold or icy fluids should be avoided.
2. A patient subject to attacks of paroxysmal atrial tachycardia should be discouraged from using stimulants such as caffeine and tobacco.
3. Abnormally rapid, slow or irregular fetal heart tones indicate fetal distress, which represents a medical emergency. Any drug the mother is receiving that might be causing changes in the fetal heart action should be withheld pending prompt notification of the physician.
4. When a person has a cardiac arrest (there is no palpable pulse):
- A. This is an extreme medical emergency, and every effort should be made to restore circulatory function within 4 minutes. Noting the exact time of arrest is very important.
- B. Closed chest massage should be started immediately. If there is also respiratory arrest, cardiopulmonary resuscitation will be required.
  [1] For cardiac resuscitation in adults:
   a. Patient must be on a flat, firm surface.
   b. The xiphoid process should be located and eliminating it from the measurement, the sternum should be divided in half. The heel of one hand should be placed on the lower half of the sternum, directly in midline. The heel of the second hand should be placed over the first and worked together as a unit.
   c. The sternum should be compressed 1½ to 2 inches at a rate of 60 compressions a minute. The process should not be stopped for any longer than 5 seconds for any reason.
   d. Compression should be coordinated with ventilation, i.e., air should be blown in when compression on sternum is relaxed. (When working alone, 2 breaths should be blown, then 15 compressions.)
  [2] For cardiac resuscitation in children, only the heel of 1 hand should be used on the lower half of the sternum, and the rate should be about 80 compressions a minute.
  [3] For cardiac resuscitation in infants:
   a. One hand should be placed under the back to support the spinal column.
   b. The middle and index fingers should be used to compress the middle of the sternum at a rate of 100 compressions a minute.
  [4] For respiratory resuscitation in adults (when the patient is not breathing):
   a. Patient must be on a flat, firm surface.
   b. The head must be hyperextended maximally to establish airway.
   c. The mouth must be cleared of secretions and any potential obstructions (e.g., dentures) in the quickest way possible.
   d. Mouth-mouth, mouth-to-nose or self-inflating bag-mask ventilation should be begun immediately. There should be 3 to 4 quick breaths initially, and then the rate should be 12 breaths per minute.

    [5] For respiratory resuscitation in children, there should be 16 ventilations a minute.

    [6] For respiratory resuscitation in infants, there should be 20 ventilations a minute.

  C. Emergency drugs, equipment and appropriate intravenous solutions to reestablish and maintain cardiac function should be ready for immediate use.

5. In general, when a patient has impaired cardiac function:

  A. The cardiac workload and cardiac activity should be reduced by such means as:

    [1] Positioning to decrease venous return from the lower extremities.

    [2] Supporting all body parts to promote relaxation of muscles.

    [3] Providing consistent emotional support to allay fear, anxiety.

    [4] Alleviating pain as promptly and completely as possible. (Effects of pain-relieving drugs on circulatory function must be watched closely.)

    [5] Preventing strenuous physical activity.

    [6] Controlling coughing.

    [7] Preventing and discouraging straining with defecation.

    [8] Providing for more than usual rest and sleep.

    [9] Avoiding emotionally stressful situations.

    [10] Avoiding chilling or overheating.

    [11] Limiting physical activity according to medical orders and the patient's response to activity.

    [12] Encouraging weight reduction, as prescribed.

    [13] Discouraging use of stimulants such as caffeine and tobacco.

    [14] Encouraging and providing (within medical orders) small and easily digestible meals, containing no irritating foods.

  B. The best possible respiratory function should be promoted. (See Chapter 2.)

6. When a patient has congestive heart failure:

  A. The cardiac workload and cardiac activity should be reduced in accordance with the patient's circulatory and respiratory status. (See 5A, above, and Chapter 2.)

  B. The patient should be positioned for best possible respiratory function. (See Chapter 2.)

  C. Cardiotonics should be administered exactly as prescribed and with all necessary precautions.

  D. Edema should be reduced. (See Chapter 4.)

  E. The patient should be evaluated systematically for symptoms and signs of circulatory failure and respiratory distress. The latter may occur because of pulmonary congestion which may progress to pulmonary edema.

  F. Intravenous fluids should be administered with caution, and the patient should be watched closely for indications of circulatory overload.

  G. It is important that the patient learn to:

    [1] Live within the limits of his cardiac reserve.

    [2] Take prescribed medications (e.g., cardiotonics and diuretics), exactly as directed.

    [3] Prevent the development of edema by sodium restriction and control of fluid intake.

[4] Be alert for early symptoms of cardiac insufficiency and follow up with prompt medical evaluation.

7. When a patient is having an attack of angina pectoris:
    A. The coronary arteries should be dilated as quickly as possible by administration of prescribed medication (e.g., nitroglycerine preparation).
    B. Cardiac work load and cardiac activity should be reduced by:
        [1] Providing complete rest.
        [2] Providing consistent emotional support to allay anxiety, fear. (Fear and anxiety may be reduced by prompt pain relief.)
        [3] Providing warmth without causing vasodilatation.

8. When a patient is known to have impaired coronary circulation and/or is subject to attacks of angina pectoris:
    A. Unusual physical exertion should be avoided.
    B. Emotionally stressful situations should be avoided.
    C. Heavy meals should be avoided, and small, easily digestable meals should be encouraged.
    D. Generalized vasoconstriction should be avoided by preventing exposure to cold and use of tobacco.

9. When a patient suffers a myocardial infarction:
    A. This is a medical emergency, and depending upon the extent and location of the infarction, it may be an extreme emergency.
    B. The patient should be observed closely for symptoms and signs of circulatory shock. Shock may be prevented or alleviated by:
        [1] Placing the patient in a horizontal position.
        [2] Restricting unnecessary physical activity.
        [3] Administering oxygen.
    C. Pain should be alleviated as much and as quickly as possible.
    D. Cold or icy fluids should be avoided.
    E. The patient should be observed closely for symptoms and signs of cardiac failure, cardiac arrhythmias, thromboembolism.
    F. It is important that during convalescence the patient learn to:
        [1] Increase exercise and activities gradually, as prescribed.
        [2] Avoid strenuous physical activity.
        [3] Avoid emotionally stressful situations and cope with unavoidable situations.
        [4] Control diet as prescribed (e.g., in relation to weight reduction, restriction of cholestrol, salt intake).

10. When a patient has rheumatic fever, damage to the heart may be limited by providing complete rest for an extended period. Recurrences should be prevented by avoiding upper respiratory infections and by obtaining prompt medical attention if they should occur.

Problems Involving Blood Flow
Through Peripheral Vessels

1. When a patient has impaired peripheral arterial circulation (e.g., due to arteriosclerosis or thromboangiitis obliterans):

A. The best possible circulation should be provided in the involved part by:
   [1] Positioning the involved part below heart level.
   [2] Assisting with postural exercises as prescribed.
   [3] Effective use of oscillating bed, as prescribed.
   [4] Providing warmth without the application of heat.
   [5] Avoiding any restrictive clothing or external pressures around or over the involved extremity.
B. Systemic demands for circulation may be reduced by maintaining a minimal desirable body weight.
C. Extra demands for blood flow in the involved extremity should be avoided (e.g., no application of external heat, protection from injury, exercise should be limited to prevent pain).
D. The use of tobacco (a vasoconstrictor) should be discouraged.
E. The extremity should be observed closely for indications of inadequate circulation (e.g., absence of pulse; skin that is cold, cyanotic, mottled or blanched; skin breakdown).

2. When a patient has impaired venous circulation in the lower extremities (e.g., due to varicose veins, pregnancy, prolonged bed rest):
   A. Venous return should be promoted by:
      [1] Active or passive leg exercises (unless there is evidence of possible thrombus formation).
      [2] Elevation of the legs.
      [3] Avoidance of standing for prolonged periods or sitting with knees bent and/or legs crossed at thigh.
      [4] Proper use of elastic stockings or ace bandages as prescribed.
      [5] Avoidance of restrictive clothing around legs or pelvic region.
   B. The involved extremity should be protected from any type of injury.
   C. The feet and legs should be observed closely for indications of inadequate circulation.

Hypertension

1. When a patient has an abnormally elevated blood pressure:
   A. Cardiac workload and cardiac action should be reduced by:
      [1] Providing for more than usual sleep and rest.
      [2] Avoiding strenuous physical activities.
      [3] Avoiding emotionally stressful situations.
      [4] Encouraging and providing for minimal body weight.
      [5] Avoiding commonly used stimulants such as caffeine and vasoconstrictor substances such as tobacco.
   B. Any intravenous fluids should be administered at a rate that will effect smallest possible rise in blood pressure.
   C. Headaches (which may indicate a rise in blood pressure and increased pressure in the intracranial vessels) should be reported promptly.
   D. Blood pressure measurements should be made frequently, and any marked increase over the usual blood pressure should be reported promptly. Any prescribed drug to reduce blood pressure should be administered promptly.

E.   The retention of sodium and water should be alleviated and/or prevented by control of fluid intake, adherance to dietary restrictions and administration of diuretic drugs as prescribed.

F.   Symptoms and signs of possible complications of hypertension should be reported promptly (e.g., those related to retinal hemorrhage, cerebrovascular accident, impaired heart action and urinary suppression).

Chapter 2

Continuous and Adequate Supply of Oxygen

All the cells of the body require a continuous and adequate supply of oxygen.

Anatomy and Physiology

THE RESPIRATORY SYSTEM

1. The respiratory system provides for the exchange of oxygen and carbon dioxide between the atmosphere and the circulating blood.
2. The air passages include the nose, mouth, pharynx, larynx, trachea, bronchi and bronchioles.
3. The nose has two air passages separated by a cartilaginous septum.
    A. There are hairs in the nose that help to filter the incoming air.
    B. Many small superficial blood vessels within the nares help to warm the incoming air, and the mucus produced by the mucous membrane lining humidifies it.
    C. The paranasal sinuses open into the nose.
4. The respiratory tract and the alimentary tract have a common passageway in the pharynx.
    A. Normally, swallowing and breathing do not occur simultaneously.
    B. During swallowing, the larynx is raised by action of pharyngeal muscles to meet the epiglottis, and the laryngeal orifice is closed by intrinsic muscle action.
    C. Normally, pressure in the oropharynx causes swallowing by eliciting the swal-

lowing reflex. The deglutition (swallowing center) is located in the medulla oblongata and lower pons.

5. The genioglossus muscle, arising from the mandible and inserting in the tongue, pulls the tongue forward. If a person is supine and the pharyngeal muscles are relaxed (e.g., when there is loss of consciousness or paralysis), the lower jaw and tongue will fall backward and close off the air passages.

6. The pharynx has lying within it masses of lymphoid tissue, called the tonsils (palatine, lingual and pharyngeal). The function of the tonsils is to protect against infection. When these tissues become hyperactive, they become enlarged.

7. The larynx is cartilaginous and muscular. It forms the upper part of the trachea and contains the vocal cords.

8. In the adult the trachea is approximately 5 inches long and 1 inch in diameter. It divides into the right and left main bronchi; the right bronchus is shorter and wider than the left, like a vertical extension of the trachea.

9. The walls of the bronchioles contain smooth muscle that is under autonomic nervous control. Parasympathetic nerves cause bronchiolar constriction; sympathetic nerves allow relaxation.

10. There is no cartilage support in the respiratory tree below the terminal bronchioles.

11. The walls of the bronchioles and the alveoli contain elastic tissue that allows distention and provides recoil. During the aging process, some elasticity is lost and there is usually an increase of fibrous tissue in the walls.

12. The alveoli provide the respiratory surface for the exchange of gases.
    A. The alveoli are tiny sacs composed of a thin elastic tissue wall containing a network of capillaries and a thin layer of epithelial cells through which molecules of gas can diffuse.
    B. There are approximately 250,000,000 alveoli in both lungs, and normally they provide about 70 square meters of area for diffusion. (This is an area of approximately 30 × 20 feet.)

13. The lining of the respiratory tract is continuous throughout, extending from the alveoli through the air passages and including the paranasal sinuses and the eustachian tubes.
    A. With the exception of the pharynx and the alveoli, the lining is ciliated mucous membrane.
       [1] Some mucus is produced in the epithelium, but most is produced in mucosal glands located in the bronchi.
          a. Normal mucus production in a 24-hour period is about 100 ml., but in disease conditions this amount can increase to as much as 1,000 ml.
          b. The mucus is 95 percent water, with a very small amount of carbohydrate and lipid. Glycoproteins are responsible for the viscosity of sputum.
       [2] Ciliary activity decreases when there is increased mucus production or when the mucus becomes thick.
       [3] Tobacco smoke slows ciliary activity.
       [4] The mucus moistens the inhaled air and prevents drying of the membrane. The greatest amount of humidification occurs in the nose.
    B. The membrane is able to absorb only extremely small amounts of aqueous solutions.

C.   Surfactant, a lipoprotein substance, that is secreted by the alveolar epithelium, prevents the collapse of alveoli by decreasing the surface tension of fluid lining the alveoli and respiratory passages. A low concentration of surfactant in the alveoli results in a tendency toward alveolar collapse (e.g., this occurs in hyaline membrane disease in the newborn).

14. Sneezing and coughing are protective reflexes for the expulsion of foreign matter from the respiratory tract.

A.   Nerve centers in the medulla oblongata trigger these reflexes.

B.   The cough reflex, because it provides for the expulsion of foreign material from the lower tract, is very important for life itself.

[1] The cough reflex may be initiated by stimulation of afferent nerve endings in the tracheal bifurcation, the laryngeal mucosa and the lung tissue or pleura by such factors as: dryness, pressure, cold, laughing or talking excessively, smoke or other irritant fumes.

[2] Approximately 2 liters of air are inhaled; the epiglottis closes and the vocal cords shut tightly; suddenly, there is forceful expiration. The epiglottis and vocal cords open widely, and the air is forced out under great pressure (possibly as great as 75 miles per hour in velocity). The forced air carries out foreign material from the trachea and bronchi.

C.   The sneeze reflex may be initiated by stimulation of sensory receptors in the nasal or nasopharyngeal mucosa. It involves depression of the uvula and clears the nasal passages of foreign matter.

PULMONARY VENTILATION

1. Air enters and leaves the respiratory tract because of the intermittent periodic production of pressure changes in the intrapulmonic cavity.

A.   The mechanical process of breathing is accomplished by movements of the chest wall and the diaphragm and, normally, is effortless.

B.   During inspiration the diaphragm descends as it contracts, and the rib cage is lifted upward and outward by:

[1] The external intercostal muscles (in quiet breathing).

[2] The sternocleidomastoid muscles, the scalenes, the thoracohumeral and the thoracoscapular muscles (in forced breathing).

C.   During expiration the diaphragm ascends as it relaxes, and the rib cage is drawn downward and inward by:

[1] The relaxation of the diaphragm and the external intercostal muscles (in quiet breathing).

[2] The contraction of the internal intercostal muscles and the abdominal muscles (in forced breathing).

D.   Relaxation of the abdominal muscles allows for greater diaphragmatic contraction, as does the absence of abdominal distention.

E.   Most individuals use both costal and diaphragmatic breathing, but some use more of one type of breathing than the other. Costal breathing is more shallow and may indicate a problem with diaphragmatic contraction.

F.   Subatmospheric pressure changes in the intrapleural space cause similar changes in the intrapulmonic pressures. These pressure changes compress and distend the lungs.

[1] During inspiration the intra-alveolar pressure becomes slightly negative (in relation to atmospheric pressure), and air flows into the respiratory passages.

    a. In quiet breathing the intra-alveolar pressure is about −3 mm. of Hg.

    b. During maximum inspiratory effort the intra-alveolar pressure may be reduced as low as −80 mm. of Hg.

[2] During expiration the intra-alveolar pressure rises slightly, and air flows out through the respiratory passages.

    a. In quiet breathing the intra-alveolar pressure is about 3 mm. of Hg.

    b. During maximum expiratory effort the intra-alveolar pressure may be increased up to 100 mm. of Hg.

G. Collapse of lung tissue is prevented by the maintenance of an intrapleural pressure that is less than atmospheric pressure.

H. The visceral and parietal pleura are serous membranes which are kept slightly moist by serous fluid. The serous fluid helps to prevent friction during the respiratory movements, and it helps to provide surface tension between the two layers of pleura.

I. The expansibility of the lungs and thorax are sometimes referred to as compliance.

[1] Lung compliance is decreased by any condition that prevents normal expansion and compression of the lungs (e.g., fibrosis, edema, blocking of alveoli).

[2] Thoracic cage compliance is reduced by deformities of the chest cage, fibrotic pleurisy and/or abnormalities of the respiratory muscles. It may be restricted by casts and dressings.

2. The internal and external intercostal muscles are innervated by spinal nerves arising from the thoracic level of the spinal cord.

3. The diaphragm is innervated primarily by the phrenic nerve, which arises from the cervical level of the spinal cord.

4. The auxiliary respiratory muscles of the chest are innervated by spinal nerves that arise at the cervical and thoracic levels of the spinal cord.

5. Normal quiet breathing requires from 5–10 percent of the total body energy expenditure; however, when there is increased airway resistance (e.g., as with obstructive pulmonary diseases), breathing may require up to 30 percent energy expenditure.

6. The maximum volume to which the lungs can be expanded includes:

A. The tidal volume. (This is the air inspired and expired with each normal breath. It averages 300–400 ml. in the adult and may be as high as 500 ml. in the young adult male.)

B. The inspiratory reserve volume. (This is the air that can be inspired over and above the tidal volume and may be up to 3,000 ml. in the young adult male.)

C. The expiratory reserve volume. (This is the air that can be expired after normal tidal expiration and is approximately 1,000 ml. in the young adult male.)

D. The residual volume. (This is the air remaining in the lungs after the most forceful expiration, averaging 1,200 ml. in the young adult male. The residual air allows for aeration of the blood between respirations.)

7. Pulmonary volumes and capacities average 20 to 25 percent less in the female than in the male.

8. Vital capacity is the total amount of air that can be exhaled after a maximal inspiration.
   A. The vital capacity of the young adult male averages 4,600 ml.; in the female the capacity averages 3,100 ml.
   B. The major factors that affect vital capacity are:
      [1] The position of the person. (Vital capacity is reduced by 200–300 ml. in the supine position.)
      [2] The strength of the respiratory muscles.
      [3] The compliance of the lungs and the thoracic cage.
   C. Effective breathing in the adult requires a vital capacity of at least 1,000 ml. If the vital capacity is reduced below 700 ml., there is respiratory failure.
   D. The normal vital capacity is equal to 70 ml. per kg. of body weight.

9. The forced expiratory volume (FEV) (in 1 second) is normally 75 percent of the vital capacity. An FEV below 75 percent indicates increased airway resistance.

10. The 1 minute respiratory volume is equal to the tidal volume multiplied by the respiratory rate. A greatly increased tidal volume can compensate for a very slow respiratory rate.

11. The respiratory center in the brain stem adjusts the rate and depth of pulmonary ventilation to meet body needs.
    A. The inspiratory and expiratory nerve centers are located in the medulla oblongata; the pneumotaxic center is in the pons. The inspiratory center initiates inspiration; the expiratory center causes expiration; and the pneumotaxic center acts as an inhibitor of inspiration.
    B. The respiratory center is greatly stimulated by an increase in either carbon dioxide or hydrogen ion concentration in the fluids of the respiratory center.
    C. Peripheral chemoreceptors (mostly in the aortic and carotid bodies) are stimulated by oxygen lack and in turn stimulate the respiratory center. (When a prolonged hypercapnia ceases to stimulate the respiratory center, it is oxygen lack that must stimulate the center.)
    D. Oxygen lack depresses all the vital centers in the brain.
    E. Exercise causes an increase in the rate and depth of respirations.
    F. The respiratory rate may increase up to 5 respirations per minute with each degree rise in body temperature.
    G. The respiratory rate and depth can be controlled to a limited extent by volition.
    H. The respiratory rate and depth are affected by emotions. (In hysteria, for example, respirations can be rapid and shallow.)

12. The average respiratory rate of a person at rest varies with age.
    A. The average rate for a newborn is 30–50 respirations per minute.
    B. The average rate for an adult is 12–16 respirations per minute.

13. The normal pattern of ventilation includes 6 to 10 deep breaths or sighs every hour, as tidal volume breathing is not enough to prevent some collapse of lung tissue.

14. Depending to some extent upon the depth of the respirations, a respiratory rate of less than 8 respirations per minute may fail to provide an adequate supply of oxygen.

15. Dead space within the respiratory tract contains air that is not involved in alveolar ventilation.
    A. Anatomic dead space is in the respiratory passages, and the volume of air involved is approximately 150 ml.
    B. Alveolar dead space is created when there are nonfunctioning alveoli.
    C. The total (or physiologic) dead space includes both anatomic and alveolar dead space. If the volume of air involved becomes more than 1/3 of the tidal volume, ventilation must be increased to maintain adequate respiratory function.
    D. Because of the dead air space in the respiratory passages, shallow breathing fails to provide adequate ventilation.
16. To maintain proper levels of oxygen and carbon dioxide in the alveoli and in the blood, there must be adequate blood flow and adequate diffusion, as well as adequate ventilation.
    A. The functional circulation in the lungs is derived from the pulmonary arteries, which arise directly from the right ventricle. The oxygenated blood returns through the pulmonary veins to the left atrium.
       [1] Any abnormal shunting interferes with the adequate oxygenation of the blood.
       [2] If hydrostatic pressure in the pulmonary vessels becomes greater than atmospheric pressure, fluid will leak from the capillaries into the alveoli.
    B. The diffusion of gases (both oxygen and carbon dioxide) through the respiratory membrane depends upon:
       [1] The thickness of the membrane.
       [2] The surface area of the membrane.
       [3] The diffusion coefficient of the gas in water. (Carbon dioxide diffuses about 20 times more rapidly than oxygen.)
       [4] The pressure difference between the 2 sides of the membrane.
          a. Normally, oxygen diffuses from the alveoli into the blood because the partial pressure of oxygen (pO_2) in the alveoli is approximately 100 mm. of Hg, while the partial pressure in venous blood is only about 40 mm. of Hg.
          b. Normally, carbon dioxide diffuses from the blood into the alveoli because the partial pressure of carbon dioxide (pCO_2) in the venous blood is about 45 mm. of Hg, while the partial pressure in the alveoli is only 40 mm. of Hg.
    C. Any conditions that alter the exchange of gases between the alveoli and the capillaries may result in an inadequate supply of oxygen to the cells (hypoxia), a decreased concentration of oxygen in the blood (hypoxemia), an increased concentration of carbon dioxide in the blood (hypercapnia) and/or a decreased concentration of carbon dioxide in the blood (hypocapnia).
    D. Adequate alveolar ventilation maintains alveolar and arterial pCO_2 at 40 mm. of Hg and arterial pO_2 at 95–100 mm. of Hg.

TRANSPORTATION OF OXYGEN TO THE TISSUES
1. Most of the oxygen carried to the body cells is in combination with hemoglobin.
    A. The amount of oxygen that can be carried by a given volume of blood is dependent upon the amount of hemoglobin contained in the red blood cells in

that volume of blood. Only very small amounts of oxygen can be dissolved in plasma under normal pressure and temperature conditions.

B. Red blood cells are produced in red bone marrow (in long bones until puberty, but only in short and flat bones in the adult).

   [1] Normal erythropoiesis requires adequate amounts of iron, Vitamin B_{12}, folic acid and pyridoxine.

   [2] As a normal red blood cell matures, it loses its nucleus and is able to contain a larger amount of hemoglobin. (Erythroblasts are immature red blood cells and contain very little hemoglobin.)

   [3] The normal, nonanemic adult produces about 200,000,000,000 new red blood cells every day. Healthy bone marrow can produce many times this number if the need exists.

C. Erythrocytes are functional for about 4 months and then are eliminated by the reticuloendothelial system, of which the spleen is a part.

D. Excessive (abnormal) breakdown of erythrocytes causes jaundice, as the breakdown of the heme portion of hemoglobin results in the accumulation of bilirubin in the body tissues and fluids.

E. The normal red blood cell count for adults is about 4,500,000 to 5,000,000 per cubic millimeter of blood. The count in a newborn is approximately the same as that in an adult. In early life, there is a slight decline in this number, but it gradually increases to the normal adult count by the age of 12 years.

F. The normal range of hemoglobin in the adult is 12–15 Gm. per 100 ml. of blood (12–15 Gm. percent). The newborn normally has between 15 and 18 Gm. percent, but this amount decreases during early life. The amount of hemoglobin then gradually increases to reach the normal adult level by the age of 12 years.

G. The average volume of red blood cells after the blood has been centrifuged is 40 percent of the total volume.

H. Under normal conditions hemoglobin is 97 percent saturated with oxygen in the lung capillaries. Increasing the concentration of oxygen in the alveoli causes a very slight increase in the amount of oxygen that can combine with the hemoglobin.

2. Reduced hemoglobin in the skin capillaries below 5 Gm. percent usually gives the skin a grayish-blue hue (cyanosis).

A. Cyanosis is more clearly evident in regions where the skin is thin and unpigmented (e.g., around the mouth, the lips, in the nail beds).

B. In the newborn there may be cyanosis in the hands and feet prior to the development of good peripheral circulation; thus cyanosis in the face and trunk is more indicative of respiratory problems in the newborn.

3. Partial pressure differences between the interstitial fluid and the arterial blood cause oxygen to diffuse into the interstitial fluid. Since oxygen is always being used by the cells, the pressure of the intracellular oxygen is always lower than that of the interstitial fluid.

UTILIZATION OF OXYGEN BY THE CELLS

1. The oxygen requirements of the cells vary directly with cellular metabolic rates.

A. Metabolic rates vary directly with the amount of thyroid hormone, the amount of cellular activity and the body temperature.

   B.   At rest the human body uses oxygen at the rate of about 200 ml./minute.
2. An individual can live only a few minutes without oxygen.
   A.   The cells of the cerebral cortex may be damaged after as little as 30 seconds
        without oxygen and are usually irreparably damaged after 4 to 5 minutes
        without oxygen.
   B.   The cells of the brain stem are generally irreparably damaged after 25–30
        minutes without oxygen.
3. Cellular metabolism varies directly with available oxygen.
   A.   Cellular functions are impaired when there is insufficient oxygen.
   B.   Striated muscle can build up some oxygen debt, but nerve tissue and cardiac
        tissue cannot.
   C.   Hypoxia causes increased capillary permeability.
4. In respiratory failure, arterial pO_2 falls below 60 mm. of Hg. An individual with
   chronic hypoxia may be able to tolerate this concentration at rest, but when there
   is an increased need for oxygen, respiratory failure occurs.
5. When an individual's supply of oxygen becomes inadequate, anxiety results—with
   all associated symptoms and signs.
6. Mitochondria, numbering from hundreds to many thousands, are present in the
   cytoplasm of all cells. The number in a cell depends upon the amount of energy the
   cell needs to perform its functions. When nutrients and oxygen come in contact
   with oxidative enzymes in the mitochondria, they combine to form carbon dioxide
   and water. The energy that is liberated is used to synthesize adenosine triphosphate (ATP), which diffuses throughout the cells and releases its stored energy
   as cell functioning requires it. ATP is used to promote:
   A.   Membrane transport (e.g., transport of glucose and electrolytes).
   B.   Synthesis of chemical compounds (e.g., proteins and cholesterol).
   C.   Mechanical work (e.g., muscle contraction, ciliary action and ameboid move-
        ment).
7. When there is oxygen lack, some cells are able to revert to anaerobic glycolysis.
   Lactic acid is an end product of this process, and it accumulates in the tissues.
8. Some poisons interfere with the utilization of oxygen by the cells.
9. Large amounts of carbon dioxide are formed in the cells and diffuse very rapidly
   into the interstitial fluid and into the capillaries. Most of the carbon dioxide is
   transported in the form of bicarbonate ion (HCO_3^-). The remainder is carried in
   loose combination with hemoglobin.

Physics

1. Atmospheric pressure is the pressure exerted by the "sea of air" above the earth
   and is approximately 14.7 lbs./sq. in. or 760 mm. of Hg at sea level.
2. Fluids (or gases) flow from an area of higher pressure to one of lower pressure. The
   rate of volume flow of fluids (or gases) is directly related to the differences in pressure (or pressure gradient).
3. The pressure exerted by gas molecules within an enclosed area (e.g., the lungs) is
   reduced if the size of that area is increased (e.g., by enlargement of the thoracic
   cavity and resultant lung expansion).

4. Pressure is the force exerted on a unit area.
5. Gravity is the force of attraction between two objects (e.g., the earth and an object on or near the earth).
6. The law of gravitation states that any 2 objects in the universe are attracted to each other with a force that is proportional to the product of their masses and inversely proportional to the square of the distance between them.
7. Gases are relatively insoluble in liquids unless the temperature is decreased or the pressure is increased.
8. The size of molecules allowed to pass through a membrane depends upon the permeability of the membrane.

Chemistry

1. The atmosphere at sea level contains approximately 20 percent oxygen and 0.04 percent carbon dioxide.
2. Hemoglobin is a conjugated protein made up of heme and globin. Heme contains iron. Hemoglobin and oxygen form a rather unstable compound, oxyhemoglobin, which is scarlet in color. Reduced hemoglobin is purple in color.
3. The oxidation of carbon and hydrogen in nutrients (e.g., glucose) is an energy-liberating chemical reaction. When oxidation is complete, carbon dioxide and water are produced.
4. Carbon monoxide and hemoglobin combine to form carboxyhemoglobin which is a more stable compound than oxyhemoglobin. Disassociation of carboxyhemoglobin in the lung capillaries can be increased by increasing the oxygen tension in the alveoli.

Pathology

SYMPTOMS AND SIGNS

Symptoms and signs of problems that involve or may involve the supply of oxygen to body cells include:

1. Abnormal respirations.
   A. Dyspnea, orthopnea.
   B. Rapid, shallow breathing.
   C. Very slow or very deep breathing. (Very slow and very deep breathing is sometimes referred to as Kussmaul breathing and is associated with metabolic acidosis.)
   D. Periodic breathing. (Hyperpnea followed by a period of apnea is sometimes referred to as Cheyne-Stokes respirations and may be associated with increased intracranial pressure.)
   E. Apnea.
   F. Noisy breathing (e.g., snoring, grunting, crowing or stridor, wheezing, gurgling sounds, rales).
   G. Unusual respiratory movements which may be associated with dyspnea (e.g., sternal and/or intercostal retraction, strong contractions of accessory muscles of respiration, limited movement on one side of chest, paradoxical movement).

2. Skin color changes (e.g., pallor, cyanosis).
   A. Color changes can generally be seen best and earliest in the nailbeds and around the mouth.
   B. In the newborn color changes can be noted best in the face and trunk.
   C. Hypoxia can exist without cyanosis.
   D. Pallor may also be noted in mucous membrane.
3. Rapid, thready pulse; palpitations.
4. Coughing, choking, sneezing, excessive yawning.
5. Hoarseness.
6. Abnormal secretions or drainage (mucus, sputum, hemoptysis).
7. Chest pain (e.g., may be sharp, dull, localized, generalized and associated with coughing or respiratory movements).
8. Apprehensiveness, restlessness.
9. Confusion, dizziness, loss of consciousness.
10. Excessive irritability, headache, anorexia.
11. Inappropriate fatigue, listlessness, lack of muscle tone.
12. Jaundice (especially in newborn).

HYPOXIA
1. Causes of hypoxia include:
   A. Hypoventilation, which may be due to:
      [1] Obstruction within the air passages (e.g., as with infections, aspiration of foreign materials, asthma or presence of secretions).
      [2] External pressure against the air passages (e.g., by tumors).
      [3] Neuromuscular disorders (e.g., as with chest injuries, poliomyelitis, brain injury, tetanus).
      [4] Loss of elasticity of lung tissue and possibly fibrosis (e.g., as occurs in aging process and with inflammatory diseases such as pneumoconiosis and tuberculosis).
      [5] Compression of lung tissue (e.g., as with pleural effusion, pneumothorax, hemothorax, tumor growth).
   B. Decrease in area of respiratory surface available for gas exchange, which may be due to:
      [1] Pulmonary diseases such as pneumonitis, atelectasis and pulmonary emphysema.
      [2] Retained secretions, exudates.
      [3] Pulmonary edema.
      [4] Bleeding within the lower respiratory tract.
      [5] Surgical removal of lung tissue.
      [6] Compression of lung tissue (e.g., as with pleural effusion, pneumothorax, hemothorax, tumor growth).
   C. Venous to arterial shunts (intrapulmonary or intracardial).
   D. Inadequate transport and delivery of oxygen to the cells, which may be due to:
      [1] Anemia.
      [2] Hemolytic disorders (e.g., sickle cell disease, erythroblastosis fetalis or malaria).
      [3] Carbon monoxide poisoning.

[4] Blood loss (acute or chronic).

[5] General circulatory deficiency (e.g., due to heart failure).

2. Inflammation of the tissues and organs involved with pulmonary ventilation can cause hypoventilation and/or a decrease in diffusion capacity of the respiratory membrane.

   A. Inflammation may be caused by:

   [1] Trauma. This may be due to:

   a. Inhalation of dust particles.

   b. Aspiration of foreign objects.

   c. Intubation.

   d. Crushing injuries.

   e. Penetrating injuries.

   [2] Physical agents such as excessive heat or cold.

   [3] Chemical agents that may be introduced into the body by means of the blood stream; into the respiratory tract by inhalation or aspiration; or into the thoracic cavity by a disease process or an accidental injury. These may include such agents as:

   a. Fumes, gases, small particles such as silicon.

   b. Allergens (which may be microorganisms).

   c. Gastric juices (e.g., in vomitus).

   d. Material from injured cells; blood.

   e. Some medications (e.g., some anesthetics, oily nose drops).

   [4] Microorganisms (i.e., viruses, rickettsia, bacteria, fungi).

   B. Inflammatory responses that can occur within the respiratory tract include:

   [1] Congestion and edema of injured tissue.

   [2] Excessive production of mucus.

   [3] Production of inflammatory exudates:

   a. Catarrhal, fibrinous, membranous, purulent, sanguineous (or hemorrhagic).

   b. The exudates formed in the respiratory tract may be eliminated through the process of resolution. This process involves phagocytosis with liquification, absorption into the lymphatic system and expulsion of material through sneezing and coughing.

   [4] Fibrosis, possibly calcification.

   [5] Destruction of cells, tissues.

   C. Inflammatory responses to injury involving the pleura include:

   [1] Congestion and edema.

   [2] Excessive production of serous fluid.

   [3] Production of inflammatory exudates (serous, fibrous, purulent, sanguineous).

   [4] Fibrosis.

   [5] Destruction of cells, tissue.

3. Many microorganisms can cause injury to the tissues and organs involved with respiratory function.

   A. The nose and mouth are common portals of entry (and exit) for pathogenic microorganisms.

   B. The body's responses to respiratory infections vary, depending upon the causative organism(s), the number of organisms, the location of the inflammation (i.e., the tissues involved), the duration of the inflammation and the resistance of the host.

C. The common cold is a communicable viral disease which may affect the paranasal sinuses, the nasal passages, the nasopharynx, the larynx, the trachea and the major bronchi. It causes congestion and edema, excessive mucus production, and the production of catarrhal and fibrous exudates. If the infection is complicated by other microorganisms (e.g., staphylococci), a purulent exudate may also be produced. If the infection is very severe the exudate may become sanguineous.

[1] Inflammation of the nasal passages, nasopharynx and paranasal sinuses may necessitate mouth-breathing, which prevents proper conditioning of the air before it goes to the lungs.

[2] Upper respiratory infections may descend downward in the respiratory tract, causing laryngitis, tracheobronchitis and pneumonitis.

[3] Severe laryngitis or tracheobronchitis can result in acute airway obstruction. Laryngospasm may occur with a severe laryngitis or in croup and can cause asphyxia. Inflammation of the vocal cords results in hoarseness and voice loss.

[4] Acute bronchitis usually begins with a dry, irritating cough that eventually becomes increasingly productive of mucoid sputum and then purulent sputum. In young children bronchitis can cause serious airway obstruction.

[5] Chronic bronchitis is a progressive disease condition in which inflammatory exudate fills and obstructs the bronchioles. It usually follows acute respiratory infections and is frequently associated with excessive smoking. There is a persistent productive cough and increasing shortness of breath. Injury to the respiratory bronchioles and alveoli may lead to bronchiectasis and pulmonary emphysema.

D. Diphtheria is a communicable disease caused by the *Corynebacterium diphtheriae*. It affects the mucous membrane of the upper respiratory tract, causing congestion, edema and the production of a membranous exudate. The swelling and the exudate obstruct the airway.

E. Pertussis is a communicable disease caused by the *Hemophilus pertussis*. Following catarrhal symptoms there is production of a fibrous exudate in the bronchi and the bronchioles. The exudate is very difficult to expel, and there are severe paroxysms of coughing with typical "whooping."

F. Pneumonia (or pneumonitis) is a condition in which the alveoli become filled with inflammatory exudate that becomes consolidated. Not only is there loss of available aerating surface, but there is inadequate ventilation in some areas of the lungs.

[1] Consolidation of involved lung tissue occurs as capillary permeability increases and serum and red blood cells collect in the alveoli. As capillary permeability increases still further, fibrinogen leaks into the alveoli and a fibrous exudate is formed.

[2] An entire lobe may be involved, or the inflammatory process may be scattered through lung tissue.

[3] The condition is generally caused by microorganisms, but it may result from chemical irritation (e.g., lipids). Any condition that allows retention of secretions in the bronchi or bronchioles predisposes to pneumonia.

[4] Pneumonia caused by bacterial agents generally has a rapid onset with persistent and painful cough, tachypnea, increasing dyspnea, possible cyanosis, rapid pulse and pain with inspiration. Sputum which may be clear at first commonly becomes sanguineous (assuming a rusty color) and tenacious.

[5] Atypical (viral) pneumonia involves a diffuse infection throughout the respiratory tract. There is a persistent dry cough that gradually becomes productive. The exudate is mucopurulent.

G. Pulmonary tuberculosis is a communicable disease caused by the *Mycobacterium tuberculosis*. The invasion of lung tissue by these bacilli results in the formation of tubercles that are nodular masses of granular tissue surrounded by a dense fibrous capsule. The tubercles may have soft, cheesy centers, or they may be dense and fibrous. They can become calcified or even ossified. The inflammatory process may result in cavity formation (because of necrosis), extensive fibrosis and, possibly, hemorrhage. The infection may predispose to pneumonia. Symptoms include fatigue, weight loss, chronic productive cough, chest pain and hemoptysis. Pulmonary ventilation is reduced, there is a loss of aerating surface, and there is considerable variation in the amount of blood flow in involved lung tissue.

H. Tetanus is a disease condition caused by the *Clostridium tetani*. The organisms produce a toxin which causes nervous tissue to become hypersensitive. The result is severe muscle spasm. If the respiratory muscles go into spasm, breathing is impaired.

I. Rabies is a viral infection that affects the brain. It can cause severe laryngeal and pharyngeal muscle spasms.

J. Poliomyelitis is a communicable viral disease that affects the central nervous system. The viruses invade the anterior horn cells, and they may invade the medulla oblongata. The latter is called bulbar poliomyelitis and may result in paralysis of the respiratory muscles and the pharyngeal muscles.

K. Encephalitis is a disease condition that may be caused by a specific virus or may be a complication of acute communicable diseases (e.g., measles). The brain is injured, and if areas involved in respiration are affected, respiratory difficulty will result.

4. Pleurisy (pleuritis) is a disorder in which the pleural membranes have responded to injury (e.g., lung infection or chest trauma) by congestion, edema and the production of fibrous exudate. This causes friction during the respiratory movements. Pain is usually severe, and breathing is impaired.

A. Pleural effusion is a condition in which the pleural membranes have responded to injury not only as they do in pleurisy but also with the production of serous or serosanguineous exudate. The exudates accumulate in the pleural cavity and interfere with respiratory movements and lung expansion.

B. In pleural empyema the pleural membranes have responded to injury (infection) with the production of a purulent exudate that accumulates in the pleural cavity and interferes with respiratory movements and lung expansion.

5. Pneumoconiosis is a condition caused by the inhalation of dust particles, frequently silicon, into the lungs. The resulting physical and chemical injury causes the formation of fibrotic nodules, usually associated with lymphatic tissue. The nodules interfere with the flow of blood and the diffusion of gases; they decrease vital capacity and predispose to pneumonia and emphysema.

6. Bronchiectasis is a condition in which there is permanent abnormal dilatation of one or several bronchi. There may be congenital weakness of the bronchial walls, but the condition is generally associated with chronic irritation of the tract due to infections or the irritation of smoke. These irritations result in the accumulation of exudates. There is persistent productive coughing, and the volume of mucopurulent sputum may be excessive. The injured bronchial walls and epithelial lining and the retained exudates all predispose to acute and chronic pulmonary infections.

7. Atelectasis is a condition in which areas of the lungs are collapsed, with no air in the alveoli. It may occur at birth if the lungs fail to expand properly. It may result from obstruction due to mucus plugs, inflammatory exudates or aspirated material followed by absorption of air from the alveoli. It can also be caused by external compression of lung tissue or by lack of surfactant in the alveoli. The condition may occur gradually or suddenly and can involve a localized area, a lobe or even an entire lung. Blood flow in the affected lung tissue is greatly restricted. The amount of respiratory embarrassment depends upon how much lung tissue is involved and how rapidly the atelectasis develops.

8. Pulmonary emphysema is a lung disease in which air flow through the terminal bronchioles is obstructed and lung tissue is destroyed. The disease is usually associated with smoking, inhalation of dusts and/or chronic lung infections. The terminal bronchioles and alveoli become greatly dilated, elastic tissue is lost, and the alveoli coalesce.
   A. These pathologic changes reduce available respiratory surface, and the air that remains in the alveoli obstructs air flow and gas exchange. Emphysema, when advanced, results in hypoxia and hypercapnia (leading to respiratory acidosis).
   B. The respiratory center may be depressed by the increased concentration of carbon dioxide in the blood and stimulated only by the hypoxia.
   C. Because normal lung elasticity cannot force air out of the alveoli, expiration requires increased muscular effort. The chest wall becomes fixed in an over-inflated inspiratory position. There is shortness of breath and increasing dyspnea.
   D. Secretions tend to increase and are retained because forceful coughing is no longer possible. The condition predisposes to acute and chronic lung infections.
   E. Pulmonary emphysema may progress rapidly, causing death, or may become chronic, with the outcome dependent upon the support of remaining pulmonary function and prevention of other pulmonary disease.

9. Allergic responses that involve the respiratory tract include:
   A. Edema of the glottis (occurs in severe hypersensitivity and infections, and when severe may cause asphyxia).
   B. Constriction of the bronchioles (e.g., as in bronchial asthma).

C.   Congestion and edema of the mucous membrane lining (occurs with hay fever, with vasomotor rhinitis and in bronchial asthma).

D.   Excessive production of mucus (occurs in vasomotor rhinitis and asthma).

E.   Production of catarrhal exudate (e.g., as in hay fever).

10. Asthma may develop as an allergic response to inhaled antigens and/or in association with bronchial infections. Asthmatic symptoms may also result from emotional disturbances. The smaller bronchioles become congested, and there is spasm of the smooth muscle. Mucus is secreted into the bronchioles. The obstructed airway causes shortness of breath, expiratory dyspnea, wheezing and cough.

A.   If the attack is severe and/or prolonged, the effort required to maintain ventilation is extremely tiring, placing considerable strain on the heart.

B.   Asthma attacks are anxiety-producing, and the anxiety tends to cause even greater respiratory difficulty.

11. Disorders with emotional components can be causes of respiratory difficulties (through effects on the autonomic nervous system). Emotional states can affect:

A.   The rate and depth of respirations.

B.   The blood supply to the various tissues (vasomotor mechanisms).

C.   The production of mucus.

D.   The diameter of the bronchioles.

12. Abnormal growths such as tumors or polyps can occur within the respiratory tract or within the chest cavity. Their location, number and size determine the extent to which they interfere with respiration.

13. If the part of the diaphragm through which the esophagus passes is not properly developed or becomes weakened, part of the stomach can protrude into the chest cavity. This interferes with lung expansion.

14. Lung expansion can be decreased by the presence of air or fluids in the chest cavity. When the intrapleural pressure is increased to atmospheric pressure the lung will collapse. If the pressure becomes great enough it can cause a mediastinal shift, affecting both circulation and respiration.

A.   Spontaneous pneumothorax may occur as a complication of pulmonary disease or following lung surgery.

B.   A sudden large pneumothorax causes severe chest pain and great respiratory distress.

C.   Hemothorax occurs when there is bleeding into the chest cavity.

D.   Pneumothorax and hemothorax frequently occur with traumatic chest injuries.

15. The accumulation of fluids within the lungs rapidly interferes with pulmonary ventilation.

A.   Gross bleeding into the lower respiratory tract may occur with trauma or may be associated with severe inflammations that cause tissue destruction.

B.   Pulmonary edema occurs when congestion within the pulmonary blood vessels becomes so great that fluid leaks through the capillary walls and permeates the air passages. This may occur as a result of such conditions as heart failure, the inhalation of irritant gases or circulatory overload. Symptoms include dyspnea, persistent coughing, frothy sputum and tracheal rales.

16. If the foramen ovale or the ductus arteriosus fails to close after birth, there will be inadequate oxygenation of blood. There is a mixing of oxygenated and deoxy-

genated blood in the ventricles (with a patent foramen ovale) and in the aorta (with a patent ductus arteriosus).

17. The functioning of the muscles of respiration may be impaired because of traumatic injuries.
    A. Penetrating wounds of the chest wall cause injury to muscle tissue and blood vessels.
    B. Crushing wounds of the chest may result in injury to muscle tissue; fractures of the ribs, the sternum, the clavicle, the thoracic vertebrae; and injury to blood vessels.
    C. Head injury, injury to the cervical spinal cord (e.g., with fractured cervical vertebrae) and traumatic injury to spinal nerves that innervate the respiratory muscles can cause respiratory problems.

18. Abnormal respirations and respiratory failure may result from injury to the respiratory center.
    A. The respiratory center may be injured by trauma, inadequate blood flow, electric shock, certain drugs and certain microorganisms.
    B. Increased intracranial pressure can cause injury to the respiratory center by interfering with normal blood flow within the brain. If the intracranial pressure becomes great enough, the medulla oblongata may be pressed downward into the foramen magnum, cutting off the blood flow in the medulla.

19. Inadequate blood supply to lung tissue (e.g., due to obstruction by emboli) interferes with pulmonary function. Pain may be severe when there are pulmonary emboli. Lung infarct may occur.

20. Anemia reduces the oxygen-carrying capacity of the blood.
    A. Anemia is a condition in which there is an abnormally low number of mature erythrocytes and/or a decreased concentration of hemoglobin in the circulating blood.
    B. Possible causes of anemia include:
       [1] Bleeding (acute or chronic).
       [2] Excessive hemolysis of red blood cells.
           a. Infections involving the blood (e.g., bacteremias, malaria) may result in excessive hemolysis.
           b. Hemolysis of red blood cells may result from immune reactions (e.g., with transfusions and in erythroblastosis fetalis). (See Chapter 1.)
           c. Trauma to red blood cells can cause hemolysis (e.g., in extensive thermal burns).
       [3] Failure of the bone marrow to produce and release an adequate number of mature erythrocytes, as occurs in hypoplastic anemia or when the bone marrow function has been depressed by chemical injury (e.g., drugs), chronic infections, radioactivity or tumor growth.
       [4] Nutritional deficiencies.
           a. In iron-deficiency anemia the amount of iron ingested or absorbed is not sufficient to meet the iron requirements for an adequate concentration of hemoglobin. The erythrocytes are hypochromic.
           b. In pernicious anemia there is a deficiency of Vitamin B_{12}, which is required for normal maturation of erythrocytes. This macrocytic type of

anemia is generally caused by inadequate absorption of this vitamin in the lower ileum, due to a deficiency in intrinsic factor in the gastric juices. Some intestinal disorders may also interfere with absorption.

c. Another macrocytic anemia may result from a deficiency in folic acid, which may occur when there is gastric cancer or poor absorption of food from the small intestine.

C. The more rapidly the anemia develops, the more severe are the symptoms. Symptoms generally include pallor, increased respiratory and pulse rates, possibly dyspnea, inappropriate fatigue and general muscular weakness. There may be impairment of mental functions. In pernicious anemia there are generally gastrointestinal symptoms (such as anorexia, indigestion, diarrhea or constipation) and progressive neurological symptoms (including tingling, burning and numbness of extremities; loss of position sense, irritability, amnesia; depression and delirium).

D. Sickle-cell disease is a hereditary hemolytic disorder occurring almost exclusively in the black race. When each parent has a defective Hemoglobin–S gene (sickle-cell trait), the child develops sickle-cell disease. The erythrocytes are sickle-shaped and rigid, and their membranes rupture easily. There is a chronic, severe anemia, and the peculiarly shaped cells cause obstruction in the microcirculation.

21. Carbon monoxide poisoning reduces the oxygen-carrying capacity of the blood because the gas combines (irreversibly) with the hemoglobin in the red blood cells.

22. When the basal metabolic rate is increased, as in fever or with thyrotoxicosis, there is an increased need for oxygen. If the respiratory and circulatory systems fail to meet the increased need, hypoxia results.

Nursing Care

Nursing care should be directed toward assisting the patient to attain, retain or regain the best possible respiratory function.*

COLLECTION, EVALUATION AND COMMUNICATION OF DATA

1. Patients should be interviewed, observed and examined for symptoms and signs of actual or potential respiratory problems.

A. Respiratory problems may be indicated by:

[1] Abnormalities in breathing, including postures assumed to overcome them.

[2] Coughing, sneezing.

[3] Abnormal discharges or blood from respiratory tract.

[4] Hoarseness.

[5] Physical discomfort, including chest pain (which may or may not be associated with respiratory movements) and numbness or tingling in extremities.

[6] Inappropriate fatigue.

---

* Although respiration includes the production, transportation and elimination of carbon dioxide, this chapter is concerned primarily with oxygen supply. Carbon dioxide is considered more extensively in Chapters 6 and 7.

[7] Loss of consciousness.

[8] Abnormalities in cognitive or emotional behavior.

[9] Jaundice, particularly in the newborn.

B. Systematic patient evaluation is of especial importance when the patient:

   [1] Has or may have acute airway obstruction.

   [2] Has a diagnosed disease condition that affects:

      a. The respiratory passages.

      b. The lungs.

      c. The pulmonary or systemic circulation.

      d. The production and/or destruction of red blood cells.

      e. The brain, especially the medulla oblongata.

      f. The thoracic cage, including respiratory muscles.

   [3] Has sustained traumatic injury (e.g., surgery, accident) which involves or may involve:

      a. The respiratory passages, the lungs, the pleura.

      b. The thoracic cage and/or respiratory muscles.

      c. The brain.

      d. Blood loss.

      e. Destruction of red blood cells (e.g., in thermal burns).

   [4] Has symptoms and signs that indicate actual or potential impairment of circulatory function.

   [5] Has a history of hypersensitivity (e.g., bronchial asthma).

   [6] Is receiving oxygen therapy.

   [7] Has a tracheostoma.

   [8] Is on a mechanical respirator.

   [9] Has chest drainage/suction.

  [10] Has severe pain, especially in chest, abdomen.

  [11] Is receiving or has been receiving drugs that are central nervous system depressants (e.g., general anesthetics, sedatives, narcotics).

  [12] Is receiving intravenous fluids (of particular importance when patient is very young or elderly and/or has limited cardiac reserve).

  [13] Is receiving a transfusion.

  [14] Is very young (especially the premature newborn) or elderly.

  [15] Is confined to bed rest, especially if dependent upon others for position changes and exercise.

C. Whenever a patient has symptoms and signs that indicate an actual or potential problem involving respiratory function, the respirations and the pulse should be evaluated frequently.

   [1] The frequency of evaluation depends upon the condition of the patient and the particular problem presented.

   [2] The respiratory rate can be counted most accurately when the patient is unaware that this is being done.

D. Data collected should be evaluated not only on the basis of a single deviation from normal (e.g., tachypnea) but should also be evaluated on the basis of combinations of symptoms and signs that are commonly associated with specific respiratory problems (e.g., symptoms and signs associated with chronic airway obstruction).

[1] A patient's respirations should be evaluated in relation to such factors as:
  a. His age.
  b. His usual respirations.
  c. His posture or position.
  d. Any physical activity.
  e. His emotional state.
  f. The environmental temperature.
  g. The presence of pain.
  h. The presence of fever.
  i. The diagnosed disease condition.
  j. Medications the patient is taking or has taken recently.

[2] A patient's cough should be evaluated in relation to such factors as:
  a. Frequency.
  b. Time of occurrence.
  c. Sound.
  d. Sputum production.

[3] A patient's sputum should be evaluated in terms of:
  a. Volume.
  b. Color.
  c. Odor.
  d. Consistency.
  e. Presence of blood or particles.

2. How, when and what data are communicated to the physician and/or other nursing personnel depend upon:
  A. Any immediate threat to the patient's life processes (e.g., indications of acute airway obstruction).
  B. Any potential threat to the patient's life and well-being (e.g., symptoms and signs of pneumonia).
  C. Any particular implications for the physician in relation to:
    [1] The patient's progress or lack of progress toward recovery (e.g., patient's respiratory response to increased physical activity).
    [2] Making a diagnosis (e.g., new objective or subjective data).
    [3] The patient's physical and emotional responses to specific diagnostic procedures or therapeutic measures.
  D. Any particular implications for nursing (e.g., in relation to positioning).

PROMOTION OF HEALTH AND PREVENTION OF DISEASE/INJURY

1. Health teaching to promote optimal respiratory function should be concerned with:
  A. The importance of:
    [1] Good posture and deep breathing exercises.
    [2] A balanced, nutritious diet with avoidance of excessive calories.
    [3] Supplemental iron in diet for female—during growth periods, from onset of menses to menopause, during pregnancy.
    [4] Adequate rest and sleep.
    [5] Chewing food adequately before swallowing, not eating too fast and avoiding laughing and talking with food in mouth.

[6] Keeping small objects out of reach of infants and small children; not giving them food they are unable to chew properly.

[7] Protecting children from suffocation in plastic bags and in airtight containers such as discarded refrigerators.

[8] Avoiding:
   a. Excessive use of alcohol.
   b. Inhalation of tobacco smoke.
   c. Inhalation of air contaminants such as sand, dust, fumes, allergens, smog.

B. Prevention of upper respiratory infections through such means as:
   [1] Humidification of dry air.
   [2] Avoidance of crowds, especially when there is epidemic of a respiratory infection.
   [3] Avoidance of chilling, fatigue.
   [4] Effective oral hygiene.

C. Prevention of spread of upper respiratory infections through such means as:
   [1] Prompt and proper treatment of upper respiratory infections.
   [2] Covering nose and mouth when sneezing or coughing.
   [3] Handwashing and proper tissue technique.
   [4] Isolation from others as much as possible during acute infection (especially from infants, young children, elderly).

D. Importance of:
   [1] Periodic health evaluations.
   [2] Routine vaccinations against diphtheria, pertussis, tetanus, poliomyelitis and against influenza when indicated.
   [3] Tuberculin skin testing.
   [4] Prompt medical consultation when there are early symptoms and signs of respiratory disorders (e.g., dyspnea, persistent coughing, sputum production).
   [5] Genetic screening for sickle-cell trait in black couples.
   [6] Rh determination for pregnant women.

E. Learning to perform pulmonary resuscitation (mouth-to-mouth breathing).

2. Adequate pulmonary ventilation should be promoted and hypostatic pulmonary congestion prevented.
   A. This is of critical importance when the patient:
      [1] Already has impaired respiratory function.
      [2] Is postoperative and has had a general anesthetic.
      [3] Is very young or elderly.
      [4] Is a heavy smoker.
      [5] Is unconscious.
      [6] Is immobilized, debilitated and/or bedridden.
      [7] Is obese.
   B. Positioning should allow the best possible lung expansion.
   C. Position changes (within medical orders) should be made frequently and on a regular schedule.
   D. A clear airway must be maintained (e.g., by encouraging and assisting with effective coughing on a regular schedule and using nasopharyngeal suctioning as necessary).

    E.   Patients should be encouraged and assisted with deep breathing exercises on a regular schedule.

    F.   Patients should be encouraged to do or should be assisted with active and/or passive exercise (within medical orders). Ambulation, when possible, is particularly important.

    G.   Physical discomfort associated with breathing should be alleviated (e.g., by splinting chest, administering analgesics).

    H.   Abdominal distention should be prevented or alleviated.

    I.   An adequate fluid intake helps to liquify respiratory secretions.

    J.   Great caution should be used in the administration of any prescribed drugs that are central nervous system depressants.

    K.   Great caution must be used when there are chest tubes and water-sealed drainage.

        [1] If air or fluid starts to enter the chest cavity, the tube must be clamped off immediately.

        [2] When a chest tube does not appear to be draining properly this should be investigated and remedied promptly.

3. Obstruction of the air passages should be avoided by:

    A.   Preventing the aspiration of food, fluids, vomitus, respiratory secretions, blood and/or foreign objects.

        [1] An unconscious person should never be given anything by mouth.

        [2] Only *very* small amounts of physiologic saline solution should be used in tracheostomy care.

        [3] Infants should not be left alone while feeding from a bottle.

        [4] When a patient has difficulty with swallowing, he should be carefully assisted with eating and drinking and observed closely for swallowing ability. Food and fluids should be withheld if swallowing is greatly diminished.

        [5] All possible safety measures should be used in gavage feedings.

        [6] Food and fluids should be withheld prior to administration of a general anesthetic.

        [7] Food and fluids should be withheld when there is violent coughing.

        [8] When there is likelihood of vomiting in an unconscious or helpless person, the patient should be positioned so as to prevent aspiration (e.g., prone, side-lying, slight Trendelenburg unless contraindicated).

        [9] Patients who are unconscious, helpless or have lost their swallowing or coughing reflex should be positioned for adequate drainage of secretions from the mouth and respiratory tract.

      [10] Patients should be encouraged and assisted to cough effectively and to eliminate respiratory secretions or exudates. This is particularly important when the patient has a condition in which there are excessive secretions or exudates, when activity is restricted or when respiratory movements are limited.

      [11] Nasopharyngeal suctioning (or suctioning of tracheostomy) should be done promptly and effectively as needed.

      [12] When there is gross bleeding into the respiratory tract (e.g., following a head injury, tonsillectomy or in advanced tuberculosis):

          a. This is a medical emergency.

       b. The patient should be positioned to promote drainage from the mouth.

[13] Dentures should be removed prior to administration of a general anesthetic or when a patient is unconscious or has lost his swallowing reflex.

[14] Nebulizers should be used properly.

[15] Small children should not be allowed to play with small objects which they may put into their mouths; children must be watched closely at all times to prevent this.

B. Preventing the tongue from falling back against the pharynx (e.g., by positioning the patient in prone position or on side or by holding the mandible up and forward).

C. Keeping the mechanical airway in the anesthetized patient in place until pharyngeal reflexes return.

D. Preventing hyperextension of the cervical spine.

4. Injury to the respiratory tract should be prevented.

  A. This is of especial importance when the patient:

    [1] Already has a respiratory disorder.

    [2] Has cardiac disease.

  B. Aspiration of food, fluids, vomitus, respiratory secretions, blood or foreign objects should be prevented.

  C. Any nursing procedures that involve the respiratory tract should be performed with great gentleness, utilizing every possible safety measure.

  D. Patients should be discouraged from smoking.

  E. Patients should be protected from respiratory infections, and these should be treated promptly.

  F. Coughing should be alleviated when it is nontherapeutic.

  G. Oily substances should not be used in procedures involving the nose or pharynx (e.g., lubrication of tubes).

5. Proper intrathoracic pressure should be maintained by using every precaution in the care of chest tubes.

6. Patients with increased intracranial pressure should be kept supine and quiet to prevent pressure conus.

7. Following thoracic surgery the positions in which the patient may lie should be specified by the physician, and orders must be followed exactly. Unless the patient has had a pneumonectomy, he can usually be turned from back to operative side.

CARE OF PATIENTS WITH SPECIFIC RESPIRATORY PROBLEMS

1. When a patient has respiratory failure:

  A. This is a medical emergency.

  B. The length of time the patient is without ventilation is of critical importance.

  C. Pulmonary resuscitation measures should be started immediately and continued as long as necessary.

    [1] See Chapter 1 in regard to cardiopulmonary resuscitation.

    [2] The patient should be placed on a mechanical respirator as soon as possible.

    [3] Respiratory stimulants should be ready for immediate administration.

[4] When available, oxygen may be administered when breathing is reestablished by resuscitative measures.
2. When a patient has an obstruction in the upper airway:
   A. Any foreign material in the mouth or throat should be removed immediately.
   B. Suction, when available, should be used to remove blood or vomitus.
   C. Positioning should promote drainage from the mouth.
   D. The patient may be placed over a chair or edge of bed (a child may be held upside down) and hit on the back to dislodge an object.
   E. When available, oxygen may be administered if the patient is gasping.
   F. Mouth-to-mouth or mouth-to-nose resuscitation may be attempted.
   G. Preparation should be made for emergency tracheotomy.
3. When a patient has aspirated foreign material into the bronchi, preparation should be made for emergency bronchoscopy.
4. When a patient has sustained a traumatic injury to the chest:
   A. Breathing should be restored as quickly as possible and oxygen administered as needed.
   B. Sucking wounds should be quickly and tightly covered with a compression bandage.
   C. The patient should be kept quiet, with chest stabilized.
   D. Any imbedded objects should not be removed.
5. When a patient has symptoms and signs of spontaneous pneumothorax or tension pneumothorax:
   A. The patient should be positioned on the affected side.
   B. Close observations should be made for indications of cardiorespiratory failure.
   C. Preparation should be made for emergency thoracentesis and/or surgery.
6. When pulmonary circulation is impaired and the patient develops symptoms and signs of pulmonary edema:
   A. Tourniquets should be ready for use (three for rotating).
   B. Cardiotonics should be ready for immediate administration.
   C. Preparation should be made for emergency phlebotomy.
7. When a patient has symptoms and signs of pulmonary embolism:
   A. This is a medical emergency.
   B. Oxygen should be administered as needed.
   C. Every attempt should be made to relieve as much anxiety as possible as quickly as possible.
8. When a baby does not begin to breathe upon delivery, the skin may be stimulated by slapping or contrast baths may be used to initiate respirations.
9. When a patient shows symptoms and signs of an acute asthma attack:
   A. Prescribed medications (bronchodilators) should be administered promptly.
   B. Any possible emotional components preceding the attack should be noted and reported/recorded appropriately.
   C. Oxygen may be administered as needed.
10. When patients have hypoxia:
   A. Tissue demands for oxygen should be reduced by providing and encouraging physical and emotional rest.

    B. Positioning should provide the best possible ventilation with greatest comfort and support for patient.

    C. The airway should be kept clear.

    D. Oxygen should be available and administered properly as needed and within medical orders. Oxygen is helpful when the patient's condition involves:

        [1] Loss of aerating surface.

        [2] Deficiency in circulation.

        [3] Decreased ventilation due to obstruction.

        [4] Neuromuscular difficulties or reduced vital capacity.

        [5] Severe anemia.

        [6] Carbon monoxide poisoning.

    E. Exercise should be regulated according to tolerance.

    F. Pain should be alleviated as much as possible.

        [1] Splinting the chest wall may be helpful.

        [2] Pain-relieving medications should be used with caution to prevent depression of the respiratory center.

    G. Abdominal distention should be prevented and/or alleviated.

    H. The diet should consist of fluids or easily digestable small meals.

    I. Anxiety should be reduced as much as possible.

11. When a patient has an irritated respiratory tract (which may be indicated by persistent coughing, sneezing, excessive respiratory secretions or hoarseness):

    A. This should be medically investigated.

    B. The patient should be encouraged to restrict smoking.

    C. Warmed, humidified air may be helpful.

    D. Coughing may be alleviated by such methods as administration of cough syrups and hot fluids, avoiding cold air, or sucking on hard candy or cough drops.

    E. Possible causes (e.g., allergens, infection, smoke) should be investigated and reported.

    F. The patient should be observed closely for symptoms and signs of respiratory distress.

12. When a patient has a disease condition in which there are retained secretions in the lungs, it is extremely important that the following be performed precisely, thoroughly and on a regular schedule (within medical orders):

    A. Postural drainage.

    B. Chest percussion, vibration.

    C. Coughing.

13. When a patient has pulmonary emphysema:

    A. Breathing exercises should be performed properly and frequently to improve ventilation and increase lower costal and diaphragmatic breathing.

    B. Physical activities or emotional stresses that cause dyspnea should be avoided.

    C. Relaxation and slow breathing should be encouraged.

    D. Great caution should be used in administration of prescribed oxygen.

        [1] A high concentration of oxygen should never be used.

        [2] The patient should be watched closely for indications of respiratory depression.

14. Patients with deficiency anemias should be helped to understand, accept and follow through with prescribed treatment. This is of critical importance for the patient with pernicious anemia.

15. When a patient is receiving drugs that depress the central nervous system, the respiratory rate should be observed closely. If the rate slows significantly (e.g., below 12 breaths per minute in an adult), the medication should be withheld pending prompt notification of the physician.

16. When carbon dioxide is administered the procedure must be carried out with great caution, and the patient must be observed closely for indications of respiratory distress.

Chapter 3

Nutrition

All the body cells require adequate amounts of essential nutrients in order to live and to function properly.

Anatomy and Physiology

NUTRITIONAL NEEDS

1. Sufficient amounts of carbohydrates, fats, proteins, vitamins and minerals are necessary in the diet to provide for:
   A. The building, maintenance and repair of body tissues.
   B. The synthesis of substances necessary for the regulation of body processes (i.e., enzymes and hormones).
   C. The synthesis of substances necessary for proper body functioning (e.g., hemoglobin and antibodies).
   D. The production of energy.

2. A person's nutritional status is determined by the adequacy of the nutrients ingested, absorbed and utilized for that individual's needs.
   A. An optimum nutritional state is when the essential nutrients are supplied and utilized to maintain optimum health.
   [1] Factors that affect daily dietary requirements, in health, include:
      a. Age. (The effect is related largely to growth pattern. There are greater requirements for almost all nutrients from birth through adolescence, in comparison to adulthood. Past middle age, smaller amounts of some nutrients are needed.)
      b. Sex. (The effect is related partly to physical build. The daily dietary requirements for males tends to be somewhat larger; a notable exception is the need for iron, which is greater in the female.)

78

      c. Quality and quantity of daily physical activity. (There is a direct relationship between increased physical activity and increased caloric need.)

      d. Pregnancy and lactation. (In pregnancy the calcium requirement is increased by 50 percent, whereas most other nutrients are increased by 20 percent.)

      e. Climate. (The environmental temperature and humidity affect nutritional needs.)

  [2] The requirements of certain nutrients may be increased during some disease processes or when there is stress or need for extensive tissue repair.

B. The nutritionally balanced diet contains food from the meat group, the milk group, the vegetable and/or fruit group and the bread and cereal group. The nonpregnant adult needs daily:

  [1] From the meat group, 2 servings.

  [2] From the milk group, 2 servings.

  [3] From the fruit and/or vegetable group, 4 servings.

  [4] From the bread and cereal group, 4 servings.

3. Carbohydrates are essential nutrients in the diet.

A. Carbohydrates have many important functions.

  [1] Carbohydrate is the most readily available source of energy, each gram yielding 4 calories.

  [2] Glucose is the only source of energy for nerve cells.

  [3] Carbohydrate is broken down before protein, thus protein is saved for functions other than energy production.

      a. Ingested carbohydrate is used for energy before ingested protein.

      b. Glycogen (storage form of carbohydrate) is used for energy before stored protein is broken down for energy.

  [4] Carbohydrate is essential for proper fat metabolism. Without adequate carbohydrate in the diet, by-products of fat metabolism accumulate in the blood.

B. Adults require approximately 75 to 100 grams of carbohydrate daily to prevent the accumulation of by-products of fat metabolism in the blood (ketosis).

C. Carbohydrates are classified as polysaccharides (complex, such as starch), disaccharides (double sugar units, such as lactose) and monosaccharides (simple sugars, such as glucose).

  [1] Starch is the most abundant source of carbohydrate in the diet.

  [2] Carbohydrates must be hydrolyzed to monosaccharides (glucose, fructose, galactose) before they can be absorbed from the gastrointestinal tract into the blood.

D. Carbohydrates are found in almost all foods except for meat, fish and poultry.*

E. In addition to being an essential nutrient, carbohydrate also plays an important role in elimination.

  [1] Cellulose (an indigestible carbohydrate), along with other carbohydrates, gives bulk to the food moving through the gastrointestinal tract.

---

* Sources of important nutrients have been included in the Anatomy and Physiology section rather than in the Chemistry section because it seemed that their inclusion here might be most useful to the reader.

[2] Lactose (milk sugar) encourages growth of bacteria in the gastrointestinal tract, which is important for proper digestion and elimination.

4. Fat is an essential nutrient in the diet.
   A. Fats (or lipids) have many important functions.
       [1] Fats are the most concentrated source of energy, yielding 9 calories per gram.
       [2] As adipose tissue, fat can be directly oxidized for energy.
       [3] Much of the fat in the body is deposited in adipose tissue.
            a. In the subcutaneous layer, the adipose tissue acts as an insulator.
            b. Found around many body organs, adipose tissue acts as a cushion and support.
       [4] Ingested fats are needed for the proper absorption of fat-soluble vitamins.
   B. Phospholipids (lecithins, cephalins, sphingomyelins) are formed mostly in the liver. They have specific functions.
       [1] They are important in maintaining the structural integrity of the cells and regulating cell permeability.
       [2] They are a component of the myelin sheath which insulates nerve tissue.
       [3] They are necessary for the formation of thromboplastin, which is essential for blood clotting.
       [4] They provide phosphate ions when these are needed for chemical reactions.
       [5] They are needed for the formation of various cell structures.
   C. Cholesterol, a derived lipid, is present in the diet and is also formed in body cells, primarily in the liver. It has specific functions.
       [1] Cholesterol is necessary for the formation of the steroid hormones (secreted by the adrenal cortex and gonads), of bile salts and of provitamin D.
       [2] Cholesterol in the skin prevents the evaporation of water from the outer body surface and increases skin resistance to both the absorption of water and chemical injury.
   D. Approximately 25 percent of a person's total calories should come from fat, with 1 to 2 percent essential fatty acid (e.g., linoleic acid). Essential fatty acids cannot be synthesized in the body so must be ingested. These are necessary for normal growth, reproduction and healthy skin.
   E. Ingested fat must be hydrolyzed to fatty acids and glycerol before it can be absorbed from the gastrointestinal tract into the blood.
       [1] Glycerol may be converted into glucose.
       [2] Fatty acids can be oxidized for energy.
   F. There are both animal and plant sources of lipids. Animal sources include milk products, meat, poultry, fish and eggs. Plant sources include vegetable oils, nuts, avocadoes and olives.
   G. Hydrocarbons are oily substances that are not true lipids. When ingested they cannot be hydrolized and absorbed from the gastrointestinal tract. Mineral oil is an example of a hydrocarbon. Its use is discouraged because it binds with fat-soluble vitamins, preventing their absorption.

5. Protein is an essential nutrient in the diet.
   A. Protein has many important functions.
       [1] Protein is essential for the building, maintenance and repair of all body tissues.

[2] Protein is necessary for the synthesis of many essential compounds, such as enzymes, nucleoproteins, antibodies, hormones, hemoglobin and plasma proteins (albumin, globulin and fibrinogen).

    a. Albumin, essential for normal colloidal osmotic pressure, is formed in the liver.

    b. Globulins are the antibodies responsible for natural and acquired immunity; they are also involved with enzymatic activities in the blood. About half are formed in the liver, and the remainder are formed in reticuloendothelial tissue.

    c. Fibrinogen, needed for the formation of blood clots, is formed in the liver.

    d. Plasma proteins may be lost from the body in the urine when there is renal disease or from body surfaces when denuded by burns.

    e. The synthesis of plasma proteins depends upon the concentration of amino acids in the blood.

[3] Protein is a source of energy, yielding 4 calories per gram.

[4] Proteins provide an important buffer system in the blood, helping to maintain a proper pH environment.

B. Proteins are composed of amino acids.

  [1] There are 21 amino acids present in the body in significant amounts.

  [2] Essential amino acids are those that the body is unable to synthesize and therefore must be supplied in the diet. Adults need 8 essential amino acids in the diet.

  [3] Complete proteins contain all the essential amino acids in proportions capable of maintaining life and promoting growth (e.g., eggs).

  [4] Partially complete proteins contain all the essential amino acids in amounts necessary to maintain life but not to support growth (e.g., wheat).

  [5] Incomplete proteins are lacking in 1 or more amino acids and so are unable to support life or growth (e.g., gelatin).

C. Daily protein requirements, in health and under normal conditions, are:*

  [1] For infants, 2 grams per kilogram of body weight.

  [2] For children, 20–36 grams.†

  [3] For adolescents, 44–54 grams.

  [4] For adults, 46–56 grams.

D. There are animal and plant sources of protein. Plant sources are partially complete and incomplete proteins. These include flour and cereal products, dry beans, peas, nuts, fruits and vegetables. Animal sources are usually complete proteins.

E. Proteins must be hydrolyzed into amino acids before they can be absorbed from the gastrointestinal tract into the blood.

F. Normally a balance is maintained among the amino acids in the blood, the plasma proteins and tissue proteins. When out of balance, tissue proteins have priority.

6. Although carbohydrates, fat and protein are all sources of energy, no one of these should be used exclusively for energy.

---

* All recommended daily allowances (RDAs) from here through page 85 were issued by the National Academy of Science Food and Nutrition Board in 1973.

† Highest amounts are for the males of the age group.

7. The caloric need of the body depends primarily upon the basal metabolic rate (B.M.R.) and physical activity.
   A. The basal metabolic rate is affected by:
      [1] Height. (The smaller the person, the higher the B.M.R. per unit. However, overall, the larger person has a higher B.M.R.)
      [2] Sex. (Women have a slightly lower B.M.R. than men.)
      [3] Age. (The metabolic rate in the newborn is about twice that of an adult. The B.M.R. decreases with age.)
      [4] Sleep. (Sleep decreases the B.M.R. by 10 percent.)
      [5] Body temperature. (There is a 7–10 percent increase in the B.M.R. with every degree Fahrenheit rise in body temperature.)
      [6] Thyroid hormone. (In hyperthyroidism the B.M.R. may be increased up to 100 times.)
      [7] The state of nutrition. (An undernourished person has a decreased B.M.R.)
      [8] Pregnancy and lactation. (The B.M.R. increases up to 25 percent during the last trimester of pregnancy and up to 60 percent during lactation.)
   B. Physical activity is an important factor that determines energy needs. Caloric needs depend upon:
      [1] The amount of work done.
      [2] The intensity of the work done.
      [3] The size of the body.
   C. Recommended daily dietary allowances to meet energy needs through the life cycle are:
      [1] For infants up to 6 months, 117 calories per kilogram of body weight.
      [2] For infants from 6 months to 1 year, 108 calories per kilogram of body weight.
      [3] For children, from 1,300 calories (age 1 year) to 2,400 calories (age 10 years).
      [4] For male adolescents, from 2,800 to 3,000 calories (increasing with age). For female adolescents, from 2,400 to 2,100 calories (decreasing with age).
      [5] For male adults, from 3,000 to 2,400 calories. For female adults, from 2,100 to 1,800 calories. Requirements decrease with age.
8. Many minerals are required for efficient cellular functioning and for the production of essential compounds. These include:
   A. Calcium.
      [1] Calcium is important in:
         a. Formation of bones and teeth.
         b. Normal neuromuscular irritability.
         c. Cell wall permeability.
         d. Activation of enzymes.
         e. Blood coagulation.
      [2] Recommended daily allowances are:
         a. For infants, 360–540 mg.
         b. For children, 800 mg.
         c. For adolescents and adults, 1,200–800 mg. (decreasing with age).
      [3] Primary sources of calcium are milk products and green, leafy vegetables.
   B. Phosphorus.

[1] Phosphorus is important in:
   a. Formation of essential body compounds, such as the phosphates, concerned with energy-producing reactions.
   b. Buffering action in the blood.
   c. Formation of bones and teeth.
[2] Recommended daily allowances are:
   a. For infants, 240–400 mg.
   b. For children, 800 mg.
   c. For adolescents and adults, 1,200–800 mg. (decreasing with age).
[3] Primary sources of phosphorus include protein-containing foods (e.g., milk, meat and eggs).

C. Iodine.
[1] Iodine in the form of thyroxine is important in the regulation of body metabolism and is needed for normal growth.
[2] Recommended daily allowances are:
   a. For infants, 35–45 micrograms.
   b. For children, 60–110 micrograms.
   c. For adolescents and adults, 150–100 micrograms (decreasing with age).
[3] Primary sources are iodized salt and seafoods.

D. Iron.
[1] Iron is important as a component of hemoglobin and myoglobin and in cellular oxidation.
[2] Recommended daily allowances are:
   a. For infants and children, 10–15 mg.
   b. For male adults, 10 mg.
   c. For female adults, 18 mg.
[3] Primary sources of iron include liver, meats, eggs, cereal products and dark vegetables.

E. Magnesium.
[1] Magnesium is important in:
   a. Neuromuscular activity.
   b. Synthesis of protein.
   c. Activation of enzymes.
   d. Formation of bones and teeth.
[2] Recommended daily allowances are:
   a. For infants, 60–70 mg.
   b. For children, 150–250 mg.
   c. For adults, 300–400 mg.
[3] Primary sources of magnesium are whole grains, nuts, meat and milk.

F. Zinc.
[1] Zinc is an important constituent of enzyme systems and insulin.
[2] Recommended daily allowances are:
   a. For infants, 3–5 mg.
   b. For children, 10 mg.
   c. For adults, 15 mg.
[3] Primary sources are liver and seafoods, but zinc can be found in most all foods.

G. Traces of other minerals are needed as constituents of enzymes or as enzyme activators and are important in interrelationships of ions. They also have various other functions in the body.

9. Definite amounts of other inorganic substances, such as sodium, potassium and chlorine (as chloride), are required for cells to live and to function properly. These chemicals are discussed in other chapters. (See especially Chapter 5.)

10. Vitamins are organic compounds that are needed in very small quantities for normal metabolic processes. They are classified as fat-soluble or water-soluble.

11. Fat-soluble vitamins are stored in the body and therefore can be toxic. They include:

A. Vitamin A.
   [1] Vitamin A is needed for:
      a. Normal growth of all body cells.
      b. Normal structure and function of epithelial cells.
      c. Formation of rhodopsin, which is necessary for vision in dim light.
   [2] Recommended daily allowances are:
      a. For infants, 1,400–2,000 IU.*
      b. For children, 2,000–3,300 IU.
      c. For adults, 4,000–5,000 IU.
   [3] Primary sources of Vitamin A are liver, dairy fats, green and yellow vegetables and fruits.

B. Vitamin D.
   [1] Vitamin D is important for absorption and regulation of calcium and phosphorus in the bones and other body tissues.
   [2] The recommended daily allowance up to age 50 is 400 IU.
   [3] Vitamin D is synthesized in the skin by the action of ultraviolet rays on chemical precursors of this vitamin. Other sources are fish oils and irradiated foods such as fortified milk.

C. Vitamin E.
   [1] Vitamin E is an antioxidant for Vitamin A and unsaturated fatty acids. It is necessary for hematopoiesis and, in premature infants, prevents anemia.
   [2] Recommended daily allowances are:
      a. For infants, 4–5 IU.
      b. For children, 7–10 IU.
      c. For adults, 12–15 IU.
   [3] This vitamin is prevalent in nearly all food man eats.

D. Vitamin K.
   [1] Vitamin K is essential for the production of prothrombin, which is necessary for blood clotting.
   [2] The vitamin is synthesized by bacterial flora of the gastrointestinal tract. It is found in green leafy vegetables, eggs and liver.

12. Water-soluble vitamins are not stored in the body to any appreciable extent, so they cannot be toxic. Excess amounts are excreted in the urine. Water-soluble vitamins include:

A. Vitamin C (ascorbic acid).

---

* IU = International Unit.

[1] This vitamin is needed for:
  a. Synthesis of collagen.
  b. Formation and maintenance of firm capillary walls.
  c. Proper wound healing.
  d. Improved absorption of folic acid and iron.
[2] Recommended daily allowances are:
  a. For infants, 35 mg.
  b. For children, 40 mg.
  c. For adults, 45 mg.
[3] Primary sources of Vitamin C are citrus fruits, tomatoes and other fruits and vegetables.
  B. The B vitamins.
[1] The B vitamins include: thiamine, riboflavin, niacin, pyridoxine (B_6), cobalamin (B_{12}), folic acid, pantothenic acid and biotin.
[2] These vitamins seem to function mainly in metabolism and blood formation.
  a. The vitamins involved in red blood cell formation are pyridoxine, cobalamin and folic acid.
  b. Thiamine, niacin and pyridoxine are important in carbohydrate metabolism.
  c. Niacin, pyridoxine, cobalamin and folic acid are important in protein metabolism.
  d. Niacin and pyridoxine are important in fat metabolism.
[3] The following chart shows the recommended daily allowances for B vitamins for infants, children and adults.

AGE GROUPS	THIA-MINE (mg.)	RIBO-FLAVIN (mg.)	NIACIN (mg.)	PYRI-DOXINE (mg.)	FOLIC ACID (μg.)[a]	COBAL-AMIN (μg.)[a]
Infants	0.3–0.5	0.4–0.6	5–8	0.3–0.4	50	0.3
Children	0.7–1.2	0.8–1.2	9–16	0.6–1.2	100–300	1.0–2.0
Adults	1.0–1.5	1.2–1.8	13–20	1.6–2.0	400	3.0

[a]μg. = microgram.

[4] The B vitamins are widely distributed throughout the major food groups.
13. In starvation, people use up their supply of carbohydrates first, then their fat, then protein. The loss of protein greatly impairs cellular function, and cellular death ensues. Vitamin stores are rapidly depleted. Mild deficiencies can occur within days. Within weeks deficiencies are usually severe.

REGULATION OF FOOD INTAKE
1. Food is needed almost continuously, but intake should be at a rate that can be accommodated by the gastrointestinal tract.
2. There are hunger/feeding and satiety centers in the hypothalamus.

A. The hunger (or feeding) center initiates a search for food, while the satiety center appears to inhibit the feeding center.
B. The feeding center is geared to the nutritional status of the individual and is particularly sensitive to a decrease in the normal concentration of blood sugar.
C. Hunger contractions, which may lead to hunger pangs, occur when a person hasn't had food in the stomach for many hours. The stomach contracts regularly and with intensity.
  [1] Hunger contractions are experienced as a tight and gnawing sensation in the stomach.
  [2] Hunger pangs cause acute pain.
  [3] Hunger is usually accompanied by a feeling of restlessness and tension. These sensations occur when there is hypoglycemia.
D. Daily eating habits play an important role in determining when a person feels hungry.
E. Distention of the gastrointestinal tract, especially the stomach, reduces the desire for food.
F. A feeling of satiety usually follows a full meal and is normally experienced when a person's nutritional status is good. The sensation of satiety may be associated with eating habits learned in childhood.
G. Higher centers in the cerebral cortex are involved in the control of appetite and in the selection of both quantity and quality of food.
  [1] Appetite may be decreased by:
    a. A person's emotional state (e.g., fear, depression).
    b. Visceral discomforts such as nausea and distention.
    c. The presence of pain anywhere in the body.
    d. Environmental stimuli such as unpleasant odors and sights.
    e. The effects of smell, taste, texture or appearance of certain foods on individuals. (Sometimes these are due to cultural influences.)
    f. The presence of physical illness.
    g. A dry, bad-tasting mouth and inability to chew food.
    h. A conscious effort to reduce eating.
    i. Loss of taste, smell.
  [2] Appetite may be increased by:
    a. Thinking about eating, especially foods that are enjoyed.
    b. A person's emotional state (e.g., excitement, feeling of tension).
    c. The pleasing smells, tastes and appearances of certain foods.
  [3] Food likes and dislikes are learned.
  [4] Eating habits are learned.
  [5] For some people, eating may be a means of tension release.
3. Short-term regulation of food intake (related to eating habits and stomach distention) ideally should be in accordance with the long-term regulation that is related to overall nutritional needs.
4. Obesity occurs when an excessive amount of fat is stored; there is a condition of overweight.
  A. Obesity occurs when the caloric intake is greater than the amount of energy expended in physical activity.
  B. Obesity that is related to overeating may be associated with:

[1] An abnormal feeding regulating mechanism.

[2] Psychogenic factors that affect the feeding center.

[3] Social factors.

THE DIGESTIVE TRACT AND ACCESSORY STRUCTURES

1. The gastrointestinal tract and accessory structures function to:
   A. Move food through the tract slowly enough to allow for adequate digestion and absorption and fast enough to provide the necessary nutrients for the cells.
   B. Digest food (involving both mechanical and chemical actions).
   C. Absorb nutrients from the alimentary canal into the blood or lymphatic system.
2. The alimentary canal has the same basic structure throughout. The walls have 4 layers: the mucosa, the inner connective tissue layer, the muscular layer and the outer connective tissue layer.
   A. The smooth muscle of the gastrointestinal tract is stimulated primarily by the myenteric nerve plexus that extends throughout the tract.
      [1] Normally, peristalsis (which is stimulated by distention within the tract) pushes food toward the rectum. Antiperistalsis may occur when there is an intestinal obstruction.
      [2] Parasympathetic stimulation increases the motility of the entire tract.
      [3] Sympathetic stimulation inhibits motility and excites the ileocecal sphincter. Strong sympathetic stimulation can block the movement of food along the entire gastrointestinal tract.
      [4] The movements of the gastrointestinal tract pass food along the tract, mix it with the digestive juices and provide for optimal absorption.
   B. Several types of glands produce the different secretions within the digestive tract.
      [1] Billions of single-cell mucous glands secrete mucus to protect the mucosa.
      [2] Goblet cells produce a thick and alkaline mucus that acts as a lubricant and protects the mucosa from chemical injury (due to hydrochloric acid and the digestive enzymes).
      [3] Epithelial cells produce serous fluids, digestive enzymes and hydrochloric acid.
      [4] Normally almost all the secretions are reabsorbed into the blood (or lymphatics) before reaching the colon. This includes secretions produced in accessory structures.
      [5] Parasympathetic stimulation increases secretions, and sympathetic stimulation decreases secretions.
   C. Blood flow in the digestive tract increases during digestion and absorption and decreases during strenuous exercise and under strong sympathetic stimulation (e.g., with alarm pattern).
3. Food is taken into the mouth, chewed as necessary and swallowed. Starch digestion begins in the mouth.
   A. The chewing of food is accomplished by the action of the jaw and the teeth; it is facilitated by saliva and the tongue.
      [1] Chewing is accomplished by the up and down movements of the mandible. The tongue moves food around in the mouth.

      a. The muscles of mastication originate on the zygomatic arch of the skull and insert in the mandible.

      b. The tongue is a muscular organ that is under voluntary control.

  [2] There are 3 types of teeth: the incisors and the canines, which are designed for biting, and the molars, which are adapted for grinding.

  [3] Teeth appear in 2 sets: first the deciduous, and later the permanent teeth.

      a. There are 20 deciduous teeth. These begin to erupt 6 to 9 months after birth and usually have erupted completely by the end of the second year.

      b. At about age 6, the 32 permanent teeth begin to erupt, and usually all the permanent teeth have erupted by age 18.

      c. The teeth are composed of dentine (the exquisitely sensitive, bony basis of the tooth); enamel (the white insensitive covering of the crown of the tooth that is composed largely of calcium phosphate salts); and pulp (the fibrous material projecting up into the dentine that contains nerves, blood vessels and lymphatics).

      d. The teeth are held in place by cementum, a bony substance, and by collagen fibers.

B. The salivary glands are stimulated to produce saliva by the presence of food in the mouth and by seeing, smelling and thinking about food.

  [1] There are three pairs of salivary glands, all of which have ducts opening into the mouth. The parotid glands lie below and in front of the ears.

  [2] The functions of saliva are:

      a. Lubrication of both food and the mouth, which facilitates chewing and swallowing.

      b. Dissolving food, which provides for taste.

      c. Cleansing the mouth.

      d. Beginning the digestion of starch.

  [3] There are salivatory nuclei in the brain stem that regulate the secretion of saliva.

      a. Parasympathetic stimulation increases secretion; sympathetic stimulation decreases secretion.

      b. The pressure of objects within the mouth and agreeable stimuli (e.g., the smell or sight of food that is enjoyed) can cause the production of large amounts of saliva.

      c. Disagreeable stimuli may inhibit the production of saliva.

  [4] The adult produces approximately 1,000 to 1,500 ml. of saliva daily. The pH is 6.0–7.0.

  [5] Saliva consists of:

      a. A serous secretion that contains ptyalin (salivary amylase), which begins the digestion of starch. (Digestion begins in the mouth and continues in the stomach.)

      b. A mucous secretion that protects and lubricates.

C. During proper mastication food is broken down into smaller pieces that can be more easily acted upon by the digestive juices.

D. The esophagus is a muscular tube that extends behind the trachea and through the diaphragm, ending at the cardiac orifice of the stomach.

[1] The upper portion of the esophagus is skeletal muscle but is not under voluntary control. The lower portion is smooth muscle under autonomic control.

[2] The mucous membrane lining of the esophagus secretes small amounts of mucus.

[3] At the lower end of the esophagus is a circular muscle called the gastro-esophogeal constrictor or cardiac sphincter. Normally it relaxes to allow food to pass into the stomach.

    a. The sphincter prevents gastric contents from being pushed up into the esophagus.

    b. Pressure of gastric contents can sometimes cause regurgitation into the esophagus. The highly acid chyme is very irritating to the esophageal lining.

E. Swallowing involves both voluntary and involuntary muscle action.

[1] The voluntary stage occurs when the tongue pushes food back to the pharynx.

[2] The pharyngeal stage is primarily a reflex action that involves striated muscle and pushes food into the esophagus.

[3] The esophageal phase, which is involuntary, primarily involves the peristaltic movement of smooth muscle. Food is moved into the stomach both by the peristaltic action and by gravity.

[4] The deglutition (swallowing) center is located in the lower pons and medulla oblongata.

4. The stomach is a musculomembranous pouch located between the esophagus and the duodeunum.

A. The stomach is able to store large quantities of food until it can be moved into the small intestine.

[1] The adult stomach can normally hold about 1 liter before pressure begins to build inside the stomach.

[2] Gastric distention inhibits stomach motility.

B. Peristaltic contractions of the stomach muscle mix food with the gastric secretions to produce a semifluid mixture called chyme.

C. Regular peristaltic waves push (or pump) very small amounts of chyme through the pylorus into the duodenum. The rate at which the stomach empties depends upon the fluidity of the chyme and upon peristaltic activity.

[1] The fluidity of the chyme is determined by the type of food eaten, how well the food has been masticated and how well it has been mixed in the stomach.

[2] Gastric emptying is inhibited by the enterogastric reflex, which is initiated by:

    a. High pressure in the duodenum.

    b. The presence of irritants in the small intestine.

    c. Abnormalities of the chyme (e.g., hyperacidity).

[3] The hormone enterogastrone, which is extracted from the duodenal and jejunal mucosa by chyme, inhibits gastric motility.

    a. Fatty food, especially fatty acids, inhibits gastric emptying the most; protein has an intermediate effect; and carbohydrate has the least effect.

b. A fatty meal may delay emptying of the stomach by as much as 3 to 6 hours.

[4] After a normal-sized mixed meal the stomach empties in approximately 4 hours.

D. Gastric glands secrete mucus, digestive enzymes and hydrochloric acid.

[1] Approximately 2,000 ml. of gastric juices are secreted each day, and the pH is 1.0–3.5.

[2] The gastric glands are continuously active; but nervous, mechanical and chemical factors can modify their activity. Secretion is stimulated by:
   a. The parasympathetic nervous system (through the vagus nerves).
   b. The hormone gastrin, which is secreted by gastric mucosa in response to food in the stomach. Both bulk and secretagogues (such as caffeine, low concentrations of alcohol and polypeptides) in various food substances stimulate secretion of gastrin.
   c. The presence of food in the mouth and the sight, smell and thought of food.

[3] The major digestive enzyme in the gastric juice is pepsin, a proteolytic enzyme that functions best at a pH of 2.0–3.0.

[4] Hydrocholoric acid provides the pH environment needed for the activation of pepsin.

[5] Gastric lipase is a weak enzyme that splits some fats into fatty acids and glycerol.

[6] In infants, another gastric enzyme is of importance. Renin causes the coagulation of milk protein (casein) so that it remains in the stomach longer, to be acted upon by pepsin.

[7] The secretion of a viscid and alkaline mucus is very important, as the mucus protects the stomach lining from the highly acidic content of the stomach.

5. The small intestine is a convoluted tube that extends from the pylorus to the ileocecal valve. Its main functions are the digestion and absorption of nutrients.

A. In the adult the small intestine averages 20–25 feet in length.

B. The mucosa consists of a layer of simple columnar epithelium supported by a thin layer of connective tissue.

[1] Villi, formed from the mucosa, contain capillaries and a lacteal.

[2] Mucosal folds and the villi provide an extensive surface for absorption of nutrients.

C. Glands in the small intestine secrete mucus and succus entericus.

[1] There are many mucus-secreting glands in the duodenum. Mucus is especially important in this area because it protects the duodenal lining from the highly acidic chyme.

[2] The small intestine of the adult secretes approximately 3,000 ml. of succus entericus each day. The pH is 7.8–8.0.

[3] The succus entericus is almost pure extracellular fluid that supplies a watery solution for absorption of nutrients.

[4] Intestinal enzymes are found largely within mucosal cells and appear to act there. The enzymes include:
   a. Peptidases (to break polypeptides into amino acids).

      b. Three enzymes that split disaccharides into monosaccharides.

      c. Intestinal lipase.

  [5] Secretion of succus entericus is stimulated by the distention and/or irritation of the small intestine.

D. Normally peristaltic activity moves the chyme through the small intestine at a slow rate, to provide for digestion and absorption.

  [1] It requires from 3 to 10 hours for chyme to be moved through the length of the small intestine.

  [2] Peristaltic activity increases in rate and intensity following a meal (gastroenteric reflex) and when the intestinal tract is irritated or distended.

E. The ileocecal valve (sphincter) allows contents of the ileum to enter the cecum but normally prevents backflow of fecal material from the colon into the ileum.

  [1] In the adult only about 450 ml. of chyme empty into the cecum each day.

  [2] Retention of chyme in the ileum is important, to increase time for absorption.

  [3] Pressure and chemical irritation of the ileum relaxes the ileocecal sphincter and increases peristalsis.

  [4] Pressure and chemical irritation of the cecum stimulates the valve to constrict and inhibits peristalsis.

6. The pancreas secretes enzymes needed for the digestion of carbohydrates, fats and protein.

  A. Approximately 1,200 ml. of pancreatic secretions are emptied into the duodenum each day. The pH is 8.0–8.3.

  B. The hormone secretin, which is produced in the upper small intestine in response to the pressure of the highly acidic chyme, stimulates the pancreas to secrete large quantities of fluid containing a high concentration of sodium bicarbonate.

  C. Pancreatic secretion contains proteolytic enzymes (primarily trypsin), pancreatic amylase and pancreatic lipase.

  D. If the pancreas is damaged or the pancreatic duct becomes blocked and there is pooling of secretions within this gland, the trypsin may become activated and digest the pancreas.

7. The liver secretes bile, which is important in the digestion and absorption of lipids.

  A. Bile, a brown or greenish-brown fluid, is formed continuously in the liver and stored and concentrated in the gall bladder.

  [1] Hepatic cells produce 600–700 ml. of bile each day. The pH is 7.8.

  [2] Bile may be carried directly into the duodenum, but usually it flows into the gall bladder, which lies underneath the liver.

  [3] The gall bladder is a small sac with a smooth muscle wall lined with mucosa. Its normal volume is between 40–70 ml. The bile is concentrated in the gall bladder by the absorption of water and electrolytes.

  B. Bile contains bile salts, cholesterol, bilirubin (pigment), fatty acids and some electrolytes.

  [1] The bile salts are important for the proper digestion and absorption of fats. With no bile salts in the intestinal tract up to 40 percent of the ingested lipids are lost because they cannot be digested and absorbed properly.

       a. The bile salts emulsify fats so they can be acted upon by intestinal lipases.

       b. The salts help to make the end products of fat digestion more soluble, which facilitates absorption.

       c. Bile salts facilitate absorption of fat-soluble vitamins.

    [2] Most of the bile salts are reabsorbed and resecreted by the liver.

    [3] Sometimes cholesterol is precipitated in the gall bladder, and gall stones are formed. Precipitation may be caused by:

       a. An excessive amount of cholesterol in the bile, due to a high dietary intake.

       b. An increased rate of bile concentration.

  C. Fat in the small intestine extracts the hormone cholecystokinin from the mucosa, and this hormone causes the gall bladder to contract and empty its contents into the duodenum.

8. Although the daily secretions of gastric juices vary greatly, the average daily volume of gastrointestinal secretions (including saliva, gastric juice, hepatic bile, pancreatic juice and succus entericus) totals between 7,000 and 9,000 ml. in the adult. Normally all but about 200 ml. are reabsorbed.

9. During the aging process several changes may occur in the digestive tract and accessory structures to degrees varying with individuals.

  A. There may be decreased senses of smell and taste.

  B. Degenerative changes in the mucous membrane of the mouth may allow it to be traumatized more easily.

  C. Teeth may be lost.

  D. There is usually a decrease in the secretion of the digestive juices, bile and hydrochloric acid.

  E. There is usually decreased motility of the gastrointestinal tract, which interferes with proper digestion and absorption.

NAUSEA AND VOMITING

1. Nausea is a physical sensation in which there is gastric discomfort, revulsion toward food and the feeling of impending vomiting. There may be hypersalivation.

2. Vomiting is the forceful expulsion of gastric contents through the esophagus and mouth. The stomach, cardiac sphincter and esophagus relax, and strong contractions of the abdominal muscles cause the stomach contents to be ejected.

  A. Vomiting is usually preceded by nausea. Projectile vomiting, which is sometimes associated with brain pathology, is sudden and forceful and is not preceded by nausea.

  B. The vomiting center, located in the medulla oblongata, may be stimulated by:

    [1] Afferent impulses from the stomach (e.g., due to irritation or overdistention).

    [2] Intense sensations, especially if disagreeable (e.g., pain, bad odors/tastes).

    [3] Strong emotional reactions such as rage.

    [4] Afferent impulses from parts of the body concerned with equilibrium (e.g., from the visual cortex, cochlea or cerebellum).

    [5] Pressure on the vomiting center itself.

    [6] Some emetic drugs.

3. Gagging may occur from mechanical stimulation of the pharynx or uvula and can cause vomiting.

DIGESTION AND ABSORPTION

1. Carbohydrate digestion is begun by the action of ptyalin contained in the saliva, but most carbohydrate digestion is accomplished by the action of enzymes in the small intestines. The end products are glucose, fructose and galactose. These substances are absorbed through the intestinal epithelium into the capillaries by diffusion and active transport and thus enter the portal circulation.
2. Protein digestion is accomplished by pepsin in the stomach and proteolytic enzymes in the small intestines. The end products are amino acids. The amino acids are absorbed through the intestinal epithelium, into the capillaries (primarily through diffusion and active transport) and thus enter the portal circulation.
3. Fat digestion is accomplished through emulsification by bile salts; then the fat is hydrolyzed into glycerol and fatty acids primarily by the action of pancreatic lipase. Most of the end products are absorbed through the intestinal epithelium into the central lacteals in the villi and are then carried by lymphatic vessels to the large veins. Small amounts may be absorbed directly into the portal circulation.
4. Vitamins and minerals are absorbed through the intestinal epithelium, into the capillaries and lymphatics.
   A. Vitamins A, D, E and K are fat-soluble, so their absorption is related to the absorption of fatty acids.
   B. Polyvalent minerals, such as calcium, magnesium and iron, are poorly absorbed. Vitamin D and acidity promote the absorption of calcium and iron.
   C. Electrolytes are absorbed through the intestinal wall and into the capillaries by active transport.
5. Water diffuses into the capillaries by osmosis.

METABOLISM

1. Metabolism is the sum of all the chemical reactions that occur in the body cells. Metabolism includes anabolism and catabolism.
   A. Anabolism is that aspect of metabolism in which cellular substances are synthesized from the nutrients that are provided.
   B. Catabolism is that aspect of metabolism in which substances are broken down and energy is released.
   C. The metabolism of carbohydrates, fats and protein involves the storage and release of energy and the synthesis of body tissue substances and secretions.
      [1] The amount of energy released in a cell is controlled by the activity in the cell.
      [2] The energy released in a cell is used for many cellular functions that involve chemical, mechanical and/or osmotic processes. These functions include:
         a. Synthesis of cellular components.
         b. Muscle contractions.
         c. Membrane transport (e.g., impulse conduction in nervous tissue, active absorption in the small intestines and kidney tubules and glandular secretions).

2. Carbohydrate metabolism is concerned primarily with the maintenance of a constant blood concentration of glucose and with the storage and release of energy.
   A. A constant blood concentration of glucose is necessary to meet the body's energy requirements.
      [1] Many mechanisms are needed to maintain a constant amount of blood glucose.
      [2] The normal blood glucose level is between 70–110 mg. per 100 ml. (percent) of blood.
      [3] Only rarely does the concentration rise above 140 mg. percent, even after a meal high in carbohydrates.
   B. The liver converts fructose and most of the galactose to glucose. Some galactose is utilized in synthesis of body tissues.
   C. Glucose may be oxidized by the cells to produce energy for cellular functions, or it may be stored as glycogen and converted to glucose when needed.
      [1] All cells can store some glycogen, but the liver and skeletal muscles can store the most.
      [2] Glucagon, a hormone secreted by the pancreas in response to hypoglycemia, increases the breakdown of liver glycogen.
   D. Energy is released from glucose mainly by glycolysis and then by oxidation of the products of glycolysis (the citric acid or Krebs cycle).
      [1] About 40 percent of the energy released by the breakdown of glucose is transferred to adenosine triphosphate (ATP), which is formed from adenosine diphosphate (ADP) present in the cells. Energy can then be released from the ATP as needed for cellular functions.
      [2] The remainder of the energy is changed to heat.
      [3] The end products of glucose oxidation are water, carbon dioxide and energy.
      [4] When oxygen is not available or the supply is inadequate, the energy-releasing processes can continue anaerobically for a few minutes. Lactic acid is produced and diffuses out of the cells.
   E. When glucose is not required for energy and cells are saturated with glycogen, extra glucose is converted to fat and stored in adipose tissue.
   F. Carbohydrate metabolism is regulated by the interactions of a number of hormones. These include: adenohypophyseal hormones, glucocorticoid hormones, epinephrine and norepinephrine, thyroxine and insulin. (See Chapter 8.)
   G. Insulin increases the transport of glucose through cell membranes.
      [1] In the absence of insulin the blood glucose concentration rises very high, but glucose is not available to the cells. When the renal threshold for glucose is reached, glucose spills over into the urine.
      [2] An excess of insulin results in hypoglycemia.
   H. When the body's store of carbohydrates is below normal, some glucose can be formed from amino acids and the glycerol portion of lipids. Glucocorticoids and glucagon (the hormone secreted by the pancreas in response to hypoglycemia) increase conversion of amino acids to glucose.
   I. In the absence of adequate glucose or insulin, most of the body's energy needs are supplied by the oxidation of fatty acids.
3. Protein metabolism is concerned primarily with the synthesis of body tissue substances and secretions.

A. Proteins and amino acids are continually being interchanged in the body.
B. Amino acids cannot be stored to any extent; when they are not utilized as such the body converts them to glucose and fat. Deamination of amino acids takes place mainly in the liver. Ketone acids and ammonia are formed. Ammonia is converted to urea in the liver. The ketone acids are eventually oxidized for energy production.
C. Protein metabolism is regulated by hormones.
   [1] The growth hormone increases the rate of protein synthesis.
   [2] The glucocorticoids cause a decrease in tissue protein and an increase in amino acids in the blood; they also increase the plasma proteins.
   [3] Testosterone increases the amount of protein in the body tissues, mainly muscle protein.
   [4] Thyroxine increases the metabolic rate of all cells.
4. Fat metabolism is concerned with the synthesis of body tissue substances and secretions, energy production and fat storage.
  A. Glycerol and fatty acids are used to form many of the body tissues and compounds.
  B. Fatty acids can be oxidized for energy production.
   [1] In starvation and diabetes mellitus there is an increased rate of fat utilization for energy.
   [2] Fatty acids must be degraded into other acid forms (ketone acids) to enter the citric acid cycle in the cells.
    a. The degrading process occurs mainly in the liver.
    b. The ketone bodies include aceto-acetic acid, beta-hydroxybutyric acid and acetone.
    c. An accumulation of these ketone acids in the blood leads to metabolic acidosis. (See Chapter 6.)
  C. Fat that is not used for energy production or for synthesis of body substances is stored in adipose tissue.
  D. Fat metabolism is regulated by hormones.
   [1] Insulin lack increases the utilization of fats for energy.
   [2] Glucocorticoids increase the rate of fat utilization; a lack depresses utilization of fat.
   [3] Corticotropin and growth hormone increase the mobilization of fat for utilization.
   [4] Thyroxine causes rapid mobilization of fat for utilization.
   [5] Epinephrine and norepinephrine increase mobilization of fat for utilization.
5. The liver plays a major role in the metabolism of carbohydrates, fats and protein.

Physics

1. Energy, as possessed by an object, is the ability or capacity to do work.
2. Heat is a form of energy.
3. A nutritional calorie is the amount of heat needed to raise the temperature of 1 Kg. of water (2.2 lbs.) by 1° C.
4. Gravity is the force of attraction between two objects.
5. The rate of all chemical reactions increases as the temperature rises.

Chemistry

1. Enzymes are organic catalysts.
2. The hydrolysis of food involves its chemical breakdown into simpler substances by reaction with water.
3. Starch is a polysaccharide that can be hydrolyzed to the disaccharide, maltose.
4. Maltose, sucrose and lactose are disaccharides that can be hydrolyzed to monosaccharides.
   A. Maltose is hydrolyzed to glucose.
   B. Sucrose is hydrolyzed to glucose and fructose.
   C. Lactose is hydrolyzed to glucose and galactose.
5. Lipids are esters of fatty acids and glycerol or other alcohols. Simple lipids can be hydrolyzed to fatty acids and alcohols.
   A. The lowering of surface tension aids in the emulsification of lipids. The surface tension of water may be decreased by bile salts.
   B. Simple lipids include fats, oils and waxes.
   C. Compound lipids include phospholipids and glycolipids.
   D. Lipids are insoluble in water.
   E. Mineral oil is a hydrocarbon—not a lipid—and is not digestible.
6. Proteins are very complex molecules that always contain nitrogen; they may be hydrolyzed to polypeptides, to peptones and, finally, to amino acids.

Pathology

SYMPTOMS AND SIGNS

1. Symptoms and signs of actual or potential nutritional problems include those related to specific nutritional deficiencies, those related to disorders of the gastrointestinal tract and accessory structures and those related to improper utilization of food.
2. Calorie and protein deficiency cause weight loss, weakness, apathy, loss of muscle tone, retarded growth and development, lowered resistance to infection and poor wound healing.
3. Protein deficiency causes weight loss, retarded growth and development, edema, diarrhea, lowered resistance to infection and poor wound healing.
4. Fat deficiency causes dermatitis, poor growth and symptoms and signs of deficiencies of the fat-soluble vitamins.
5. Symptoms and signs of fat-soluble vitamin deficiencies include:
   A. Vitamin A: night blindness, symptoms and signs of eye inflammation, and changes in the epithelial tissue (skin and mucous membranes).
   B. Vitamin D: abnormal bone development, stunted growth and deformities.
   C. Vitamin E: symptoms and signs of anemia and dermatitis in newborns and premature infants.
   D. Vitamin K: bleeding tendency.
6. Symptoms and signs of water-soluble vitamin deficiencies include:
   A. Vitamin C (ascorbic acid): swollen and bleeding gums, loosening of teeth, skin hemorrhages, poor wound healing.

B. The B vitamins:
   [1] Thiamine: digestive disturbances, neuritis, cardiac failure, edema.
   [2] Riboflavin: cracking at corners of mouth, skin eruptions.
   [3] Niacin: neuritis, weakness, confusion, scaly dermatitis, sore tongue, digestive disturbances.
   [4] Pyridoxine: symptoms and signs of anemia, neuritis, hyperirritability, convulsions, dermatitis.
   [5] Cobalamin and folic acid: symptoms and signs of anemia.
7. Symptoms and signs of mineral deficiencies include:
   A. Calcium: abnormal bone and tooth development, abnormal muscle contractions.
   B. Phosphorus: abnormal bone and tooth development.
   C. Sodium and potassium: symptoms and signs of electrolyte imbalance. (See Chapter 5.)
   D. Iodine: symptoms and signs of hypothyroidism, including goiter. (See Chapter 8.)
   E. Iron: symptoms and signs of anemia. (See Chapter 2.)
8. Hypoglycemia causes headache, excessive perspiration, pallor, faintness, muscle tremors, hunger, loss of consciousness.
9. Symptoms and signs associated with problems of the gastrointestinal tract and accessory structures include:
   A. Dental caries, malocclusion, loss of teeth.
   B. Nausea, vomiting, regurgitation, eructation, halitosis, difficulty in swallowing.
   C. Abnormal stools (e.g., diarrhea; stools containing undigested foodstuffs, blood, mucus, pus, fat).
   D. Excessive flatulence, abdominal distention.
   E. Physical discomforts including epigastric distress; feeling of fullness; gnawing, burning or aching pain; abdominal tenderness; cramping pain.
   F. Jaundice.
10. Symptoms and signs associated with acute abdominal inflammation include:
    A. Generalized abdominal pain that may become localized, may be severe.
    B. Tense and tender abdominal musculature.
    C. Nausea and vomiting.
    D. Rapid pulse.
11. Symptoms and signs associated with perforation of the gastrointestinal tract include:
    A. Sudden sharp abdominal pain.
    B. Generalized abdominal pain and tenderness.
    C. Rigid abdomen.
    D. Rapid and shallow respirations.
    E. Symptoms and signs of circulatory shock.
12. Symptoms and signs associated with obstruction of the intestinal tract include:
    A. Vomiting, which may be projectile, fecal, in large amounts.
    B. Acute pain, which may be cramping.
    C. Abdominal distention.
    D. Constipation.
    E. Symptoms and signs of fluid and electrolyte imbalance. (See Chapters 4 and 5.)

13. Symptoms and signs associated with improper utilization of food are included in section entitled "Problems Related to the Utilization of Food" (see pages 103–104).

MALNUTRITION AND ITS CAUSES
1. Malnutrition is a highly complex condition in which the body's nutritional needs are not adequately met.
2. Malnutrition may result from problems related to: the intake of food, the digestion and absorption of food, the utilization of food and/or an increased need for food.

Problems Related to Food Intake
1. Dietary deficiencies are related to the quantity and the quality of food eaten and the times at which food is eaten.
    A. Starvation is a condition of overall deficiency of essential nutrients.
    B. Marasmus is a condition in which there is severe caloric and protein undernutrition in infancy. There is extreme emaciation and wasting.
    C. Kwashiorkor is a condition caused primarily by a deficiency of protein. It is manifested by apathy, a general wasting, retarded growth and development and cirrhosis of the liver.
    D. Beriberi results from lack of thiamine. (See 6B[1] under Symptoms and Signs above.)
    E. Pellagra is the condition caused by deficiency of niacin. (See 6B[3] under Symptoms and Signs above.)
    F. Scurvy is caused by lack of Vitamin C. (See 6A under Symptoms and Signs above.)
    G. Rickets is a nutritional and metabolic disease of infancy and early childhood, in which there is abnormal calcification of bones. It is usually caused by a deficiency of Vitamin D and/or calcium and phosphorus. Bones become softened and deformed. This is seen most frequently in the thoracic cage and in the lower extremities (causing bowing of legs, knock-knees and enlargement of ankles).
    H. Osteomalacia is a disease of adulthood similar to rickets in children. (See G above.) Fractures occur easily, and bone deformities may develop.
2. Undernutrition may occur when there is alcoholism or when there are psychiatric problems in which individuals do not eat properly.
3. Obesity is a condition in which there is an excessive deposit of fat.
    A. A deviation of 15–25 percent above desirable body weight is indicative of obesity.
    B. Obesity can result from either or both of two factors: increased caloric intake and decreased expenditure of energy.
    C. An obese person is not necessarily a well-nourished person.
4. Anorexia and nausea interfere with food intake.
    A. Anorexia is characterized by the lack of desire for food. It may be caused by emotional upsets, drugs, certain disease conditions (frequently those involving the gastrointestinal tract) and psychogenic disorders.
    B. With nausea there is a feeling of revulsion toward food.
5. The intake of food may be limited by difficulties in chewing and/or swallowing food.

A. Teeth may be painful because of dental caries. Teeth may be lost because of dental problems such as periodontal disease, malocclusions, caries or traumatic injuries.

   [1] Dental caries may develop because of the poor quality of tooth enamel, the presence of certain types of bacteria in the mouth and/or the particular pH of the saliva.

   [2] The development of dental caries is sometimes associated with high sugar intake.

B. Stomatitis is an inflammation of the mouth that may be caused by vitamin deficiencies (e.g., niacin), systemic diseases, local injuries due to chemicals, excessive heat or microorganisms. The microorganisms may be specific pathogens or opportunists. The irritated, swollen, painful mucosa interferes with chewing.

C. Parotitis is an inflammation of the parotid glands that may result from inactivity (e.g., when a person does not chew solid food for a prolonged period) or from infection (e.g., the virus of mumps or opportunists). There is a decreased production of saliva, swelling and discomfort. There may be a purulent exudate. All interfere with chewing and swallowing.

D. Inadequate salivation causes difficulty with both chewing and swallowing. It may be caused by disorders of the salivary glands, by suppressive action of certain drugs (e.g., parasympatholytics) or by strong sympathetic stimulation (e.g., when there is fear).

E. Cleft lip or cleft palate (or a combination) results from a failure of growth and union of the body and soft tissue structures on one or both sides of the palate and upper jaw, occurring in the embryo. It can cause problems with feeding as well as problems of aspiration.

F. Abnormal growths within the mouth, traumatic injuries involving the jaw or injury to nerves innervating the muscles of the tongue or jaw can interfere with chewing.

G. Difficulty with swallowing may result from injuries to the muscles involved in swallowing or to nerves that innervate those muscles (e.g., occurs with rabies, tetanus and sometimes with cerebrovascular accidents).

H. Chewing and swallowing solid food may be an unlearned behavior in mentally retarded children.

I. The passage of food through the esophagus into the stomach may be obstructed by:

   [1] Congenital anomalies such as atresia or stenosis.

   [2] Inflammation and ulceration of the esophagus due to chemical or traumatic injury, possibly due to swallowing very hot liquids. Children may accidentally drink strong chemicals that can cause severe esophageal damage.

   [3] Achalasia, a condition in which the lower part of the esophagus fails to relax during swallowing. It is usually due to damaged or absent myenteric plexus in the area.

   [4] Esophageal spasm, which may be due to nerve damage or emotional problems.

   [5] Abnormal growths within the esophagus or pressing against it. Esophageal

obstruction results in a feeling of fullness, regurgitation of food, dysphagia. As food dams up, the esophagus becomes dilated and may be injured by chemical reactions of retained food or by infections.

Problems Related to Digestion and Absorption

1. Hyposecretion of digestive juices and/or abnormal motility of the gastrointestinal tract may result from inflammation of the digestive tract and accessory structures, emotional disturbances, inherited abnormalities, obstructions, inadequate circulation, nutritional deficiencies and abnormal growths.
2. The inflammatory responses of the gastrointestinal tract to injury include:
    A. Active hyperemia, edema, congestion.
    B. Decreased function or loss of function (e.g., secretion, motility).
    C. Increased peristaltic activity.
    D. Production of inflammatory exudates (mucous, purulent, fibrous).
    E. Destruction of tissue (erosion, ulceration).
3. The extent to which vomiting affects nutrition depends upon the amount and frequency of vomiting. Vomiting may occur as a result of:
    A. Specific disorders of the gastrointestinal tract.
    B. Emotional disturbances.
    C. Increased intracranial pressure.
    D. Effects of drugs either on the brain or on the tract.
    E. Effects of toxic substances produced in the body or ingested.
    F. Allergic response.
    G. Effects of early pregnancy.
    H. Disturbances of equilibrium.
4. Gastritis is an inflammation of the stomach mucosa. It may be caused by injury due to eating and drinking irritating foods, by certain drugs or by microorganisms and/ or their toxins. There is usually epigastric pain, nausea and vomiting.
5. Peptic ulcer is a condition in which there is destruction of mucosa and possibly submucosa of the distal esophagus, the stomach or the duodenum.
    A. Changes in the blood supply and in the gastric secretions appear to be related to the development of peptic ulcer, and these changes seem to be related to such factors as:
       [1] Emotional stress.
       [2] Irregular or poor eating habits.
       [3] Chemical or traumatic injuries.
       [4] Some drugs.
    B. The hydrochloric acid injures the damaged mucosa, and both the acid and the damaged area cause pain.
    C. There is usually a dull, gnawing pain in the epigastric region that occurs 1 to 3 hours after meals and is relieved by food. If the pylorus becomes obstructed, there may be nausea and vomiting.
    D. The ulcer(s) may be superficial or deep. If deep, they may cause bleeding (which can be severe) and/or perforation (in which case the gastric contents are spilled into the abdominal cavity, causing abscess formation or generalized peritonitis).
6. Pancreatitis is an inflammation of the pancreas and may be acute or chronic. The

condition may be caused by an obstruction of the flow of pancreatic secretions within the ducts or by an infection or traumatic injury.

  A. Acute pancreatitis is usually characterized by severe abdominal pain, nausea and vomiting, diarrhea with stools containing undigested fat and protein foods. There may be abdominal distention and rigidity when peritonitis occurs. Pancreatic destruction may progress very rapidly, as proteolytic enzymes digest tissue.

  B. If the inflammation becomes chronic there may be fibrosis and calcification and permanent impairment of pancreatic function. Digestive disturbances persist, causing anorexia and weight loss.

  C. Insulin production may be affected when there is pancreatitis.

7. Regional enteritis is a nonspecific inflammation of the small intestine, in which there is ulceration and thickening of the walls with scar formation. This interferes with absorption and may result in perforation and in the formation of fistulas and adhesions. At the onset of the inflammatory process there is cramping abdominal pain, diarrhea, nausea and vomiting.

8. Appendicitis is an inflammation of the appendix, which may be caused by a fecalith (a small, hard mass of feces), a foreign body or an infection.

  A. The inflammatory process causes distention of the tissue and results in necrosis.

  B. Symptoms include abdominal pain (which may be generalized at first and then localized in the right lower quadrant), nausea and vomiting.

  C. If the inflammation does not subside and the appendix is not removed promptly, the appendix will rupture, spilling its contents into the abdominal cavity. This results in abscess formation or generalized peritonitis.

9. An inadequate supply of bile in the small intestine may be the result of liver disease or obstruction of the bile ducts by calculi or inflammation.

  A. If the common bile duct is blocked, jaundice results.

  B. If the gallbladder is injured (due to pressure of accumulating bile, infection or stones), there is congestion, swelling and possibly necrosis and perforation.

  C. Disorders of the bile ducts and the gall bladder cause abdominal pain which may be very severe. The pain may be associated with ingestion of fatty meals.

  D. An inadequate supply of bile causes digestive disturbances such as flatulence and nausea and vomiting. These symptoms tend to occur when fatty foods are ingested.

10. Proper digestion and absorption of nutrients are prevented by increased motility of the gastrointestinal tract that does not allow adequate time for these processes to occur.

  A. There are two major causes of increased motility:

    [1] Injury to the tract, which may be caused by chemical irritation, mechanical irritation or microorganisms.

    [2] Excessive parasympathetic stimulation, which may be associated with psychogenic factors.

  B. Diarrhea is a common result of increased motility.

    [1] Diarrhea is a condition of frequent stools that may be of varying fluid consistency.

    [2] Diarrhea may be caused by:

       a. Specific intestinal diseases.

       b. Emotional disturbances.

       c. Mechanical irritation of the tract (e.g., by highly fibrous foods).

       d. Chemical irritation of the tract by drugs or certain foods or food components.

       e. Allergic response.

       f. Changes in the normal intestinal flora.

     [3] Severe diarrhea may cause problems with fluid, electrolyte and acid-base balances, in addition to nutritional deficiencies.

C. Ulcerative colitis is an inflammatory disease of the mucosa of the colon, involving ulcerations and the production of mucous, purulent and sanguineous exudates.

     [1] Possible causative factors include emotional stresses, infections, allergic response (auto-immune reaction).

     [2] There is severe diarrhea (often bloody), colicky abdominal pain, dehydration, anorexia and malnutrition.

     [3] Perforation of ulcers can occur and result in peritonitis.

D. Specific microorganisms can invade the intestinal tract and cause diarrhea. These include:

     [1] Species of *Salmonella*, which cause a type of "food poisoning."

     [2] Species of *Shigella*, which cause bacillary dysentery.

     [3] *Vibrio comma*, which causes cholera.

     [4] *Entamoeba histolytica*, which causes amebic dysentery.

11. The amount of absorption of the end products of digestion depends not only on the rate of the motility of the tract but also on the amount of surface area available for absorption.

  A. Inflammatory processes may damage mucosa (temporarily or permanently) and reduce the amount of available surface area.

  B. Surgical removal of small intestine (especially ileum) reduces the surface available for absorption.

  C. Celiac disease in children (sprue in adults) is a condition in which the intestinal villi are damaged.

     [1] The condition is associated with an intolerance to gluten.

     [2] There are frequent, loose and foul-smelling stools which are fatty, also general weakness and weight loss.

12. Obstructions within the gastrointestinal tract may cause problems with digestion and absorption.

  A. Passage of food from the stomach into the small intestine may be obstructed by pyloric stenosis (congenital or acquired through scarring), spasms of the pyloric sphincter or lack of gastric motility.

     [1] Pyloric obstruction may occur as a complication of peptic ulcer.

     [2] Pyloric obstruction causes gastric discomfort, which may become increasingly painful as stomach contractions attempt to push contents through the pyloric sphincter. Increasing gastric distention results in loss of motility. Large quantities of gastric contents may be vomited. Vomiting may be projectile. There may be problems with fluid, electrolyte and acid-base balances, along with nutritional deficiencies.

B.   Obstruction may occur in the small or large intestine. The cause may be within the intestinal wall, within the lumen or the result of compression of the tract.

[1] Mechanical obstruction (blockage of the tract) may be caused by congenital anomalies, inflammatory processes, tumor growths, adhesions, volvulus, intussusception, strangulated hernia, a large bolus of undigested or unchewed food or a foreign body.

[2] Neurogenic obstruction results from the inhibition of peristalsis due to problems involving innervation of the tract.

a. There may be an imbalance between the parasympathetic and sympathetic stimulation, or the myenteric plexus may be injured.

b. Peristalsis is decreased when the intestinal tract becomes overdistended by accumulation of fluids and/or gases or when the tract is injured by trauma or infection.

[3] Obstruction may be due to interference with the blood supply to or blood flow in the intestinal wall. Interference with blood supply may occur when there is portal congestion or mesenteric thrombosis.

[4] Symptoms and signs of small bowel obstruction include:

a. Abdominal pain caused by smooth muscle spasms.

b. Abdominal distention caused by accumulation of fluid and gases.

c. Symptoms and signs of fluid and electrolyte imbalances and of hypovolemic shock caused by loss of fluid in vomiting and seepage of plasma from damaged capillaries into intestinal lumen.

13. Enzyme deficiency or inactivity may interfere with proper digestion and absorption (e.g., lack of lactase prevents proper digestion and absorption of lactose, the carbohydrate of milk).

Problems Related to the Utilization of Food

1. Impaired liver function interferes with normal metabolism of carbohydrates, fats and proteins; with the storage of some vitamins and minerals; and with the formation of plasma proteins.

A. The liver may be injured by inadequate circulation, malnutrition, chemical processes, trauma and microorganisms.

B. Cirrhosis of the liver is a condition in which there is degeneration of liver cells. Injury to the liver causes an increase in connective tissue and fibrosis, which interferes with the complex circulation of blood through the liver. The hepatic cells do not have an adequate blood supply, and portal venous congestion develops. Bile pigments are not properly eliminated in the bile.

[1] Cirrhosis of the liver may be caused by dietary deficiencies, chronic obstruction to bile flow and severe inflammation of the liver.

[2] Symptoms and signs include:

a. Malaise, anorexia, nausea and vomiting, flatulence and weight loss.

b. Ascites, which is related to portal hypertension.

c. Generalized edema, which is related to depressed production of plasma proteins.

d. Symptoms and signs of esophogeal varices, which are caused by portal congestion.

      e. Jaundice, which is caused by distribution of bile pigment throughout the body tissues and fluids.

      f. Neurologic symptoms, which are caused by accumulation of toxic substances in the blood (normally detoxified by the liver). Problems such as apathy and forgetfulness may progress to loss of consciousness.

  C. Viral hepatitis is an infection of the liver caused by specific viruses. The inflammatory process may cause fibrosis and atrophy, degeneration and possibly necrosis of liver cells. Early symptoms include anorexia, nausea, and vomiting and discomfort in the region of the liver.

  D. Liver abscesses may result from infections caused by infectious agents that have found their way into the liver from the blood, through the gastrointestinal tract or during traumatic injury.

2. Diabetes mellitus is a chronic disease condition which affects carbohydrate, protein and fat metabolism. It is caused by insufficient secretion of insulin or by the ineffectiveness of the insulin that is secreted.

  A. Carbohydrate metabolism is depressed in diabetes mellitus, because adequate amounts of glucose cannot be transported from the blood to the cells. The concentration of blood glucose rises; without adequate glucose, the cells are unable to function properly, if at all.

  B. Heredity and obesity are predisposing factors in the development of diabetes mellitus.

  C. Diabetes mellitus can occur secondarily to other endocrine disorders (e.g., hypersecretion of adrenal cortical hormones) or may be associated with injury to the pancreas.

  D. Early symptoms and signs include:

    [1] Weakness and fatigue, due to improper carbohydrate metabolism.

    [2] Loss of weight, due to utilization of fat and protein for energy production.

    [3] Excessive eating (polyphagia), due to improper food utilization.

    [4] Passage of large volumes of urine (polyuria), caused by kidney excretion of excess glucose in the blood.

    [5] Excessive thirst (polydipsia), due to increased urinary output.

  E. If diabetes is not controlled there are:

    [1] Symptoms and signs of fluid and electrolyte imbalances. (See Chapters 4 and 5.)

    [2] Symptoms and signs of metabolic acidosis. (See Chapter 6.)

  F. Over time there usually are degenerative changes in blood vessels.

Problems Related to Increased
Need for Nutrients

1. Fever increases the metabolic rate, which increases the need for nutrients. If the increased need is not met, nutrition may not be adequate. This problem tends to occur in chronic conditions involving prolonged fever.

2. Bodily injuries requiring tissue replacement and/or repair (e.g., burns, fractures, hemorrhage, surgery) cause increased nutritional needs. There is increased need for protein, particularly. Wound healing and/or tissue replacement may be delayed and inefficient if the increased need is not met.

3. Hyperthyroidism is a condition involving excessive secretion of thyroid hormones, which accelerates the metabolic rate of most body cells. Unless food intake keeps pace with metabolism there is weight loss, weakness and fatigue.
4. In kidney disease, when there is loss of plasma proteins in the urine (primarily the albumin which is needed for proper colloidal osmotic pressure of blood), there may be need for increased protein intake.
5. Prolonged bed rest and inactivity result in loss of protein from the body tissues, producing a negative nitrogen balance. This increases the body's need for protein.
6. If increased nutritional needs during pregnancy and lactation are not adequately met, both the mother and baby may have nutritional deficiencies.

Nursing Care

Nursing care should be directed toward assisting the patient to attain, retain or regain the best possible nutritional status.

COLLECTION, EVALUATION AND COMMUNICATION OF DATA
1. A patient's dietary intake should be evaluated for both quantity and quality.
2. Patients should be interviewed, observed and examined for symptoms and signs of actual or potential nutritional problems.
   - A. Problems may be indicated by:*
     - [1] Symptoms and signs related to specific nutritional deficiencies.
     - [2] Symptoms and signs related to disorders of the gastrointestinal tract and accessory structures.
     - [3] Symptoms and signs related to improper utilization of food.
   - B. Systematic patient evaluation is of especial importance when the patient:
     - [1] Has or has had a dietary intake that is inadequate to meet normal nutritional requirements.
     - [2] Has a condition (normal or pathologic) in which there are increased nutritional requirements.
     - [3] Has a disorder that interferes with normal chewing and swallowing of food (e.g., loss of teeth, paralysis).
     - [4] Has a diagnosed disorder or traumatic injury that affects the digestion and absorption of food.
     - [5] Has a disorder in which there is or may be improper utilization of food (e.g., liver disease).
     - [6] Has persistent vomiting and/or diarrhea.
     - [7] Is elderly.
     - [8] Is not responsible (e.g., infants and small children, mentally incompetent individuals).
   - C. Whenever a patient has symptoms and signs that indicate an actual or potential nutritional problem, the dietary intake and any loss of food from the gastro-

* See also Symptoms and Signs, under Pathology, this chapter.

intestinal tract (e.g., with vomiting) should be evaluated and reported/recorded accurately.

D. Data collected should be evaluated not only on the basis of a single deviation from normal (e.g., vomiting) but should also be evaluated on the basis of combinations of symptoms and signs that are commonly associated with specific nutritional problems (e.g., symptoms and signs associated with peptic ulcer).

E. A patient's overall nutritional needs should be evaluated in relation to:
[1] Age and normal growth patterns.
[2] Weight and body build.
[3] Amount and type of physical activity.
[4] Condition of pregnancy or lactation.
[5] Presence of fever.
[6] Any diagnosed disorder or injury.

F. A patient's eating habits should be evaluated in relation to:
[1] The quality of food eaten.
[2] The quantity of food eaten.
[3] Frequency and location of eating.
[4] Rate of eating.
[5] Adequacy of chewing.
[6] Food intolerances.

G. Vomiting should be evaluated and reported/recorded in terms of characteristics of the vomiting and the vomitus.
[1] Important characteristics of vomiting include: type (e.g., projectile); frequency; relationship to food intake; possible relationship to administration of drugs; whether or not there was nausea.
[2] Important characteristics of the vomitus include: the amount, color, odor and consistency (e.g., watery, bloody, presence of undigested food).

H. Diarrhea should be evaluated and reported/recorded in terms of:
[1] Frequency of stools.
[2] Amount of each stool.
[3] Color and odor of stool.
[4] Consistency of stool (e.g., watery, mucous, bloody, presence of undigested foods).
[5] Time of occurrence in relation to ingestion of food or administration of drugs.

3. How, when and what data are communicated to the physician and/or other nursing personnel depend upon:
A. Any potential threat to the patient's life and well-being (e.g., symptoms and signs of intestinal obstruction).
B. Any particular implications for the physician in relation to:
[1] The patient's progress or lack of progress toward recovery (e.g., the patient's tolerance of diet change).
[2] Making a diagnosis (e.g., new objective or subjective data).
[3] The patient's physical and emotional responses to specific diagnostic procedures or therapeutic measures (e.g., the prescribed diet).
C. Any particular implications for nursing (e.g., method of feeding).

**PROMOTION OF HEALTH AND PREVENTION
OF DISEASE/INJURY**

1. Health teaching to promote proper nutrition and proper gastrointestinal function should be concerned with:
   A. The nutritionally balanced diet.
   B. The importance of:
      [1] A balanced, nutritious diet throughout the life cycle, with avoidance of excessive calories or other nutrient substances that could be toxic (e.g., Vitamins A and D).
      [2] Proper nutrition during pregnancy and lactation and other growth periods.
      [3] Regular mealtimes, with enough time for eating and adequate chewing.
      [4] Relaxation and avoidance of emotional stresses before, during or following meals.
      [5] Learning to cope with unavoidable stress.
      [6] Avoiding:
         a. Foods that are particularly irritating or known to upset the individual's digestive tract.
         b. Excessive use of tobacco or alcohol.
         c. Ingestion of mineral oil.
         d. Self-medication for gastrointestinal disturbances.
   C. Prevention of infections by personal hygiene measures, especially in relation to food preparation, food service and eating.
   D. Oral hygiene and proper dental care.
   E. The importance of a balanced program of exercise throughout the life cycle.
   F. Accident prevention (especially in relation to children).
   G. The importance of:
      [1] Periodic health evaluations, especially:
         a. Frequent diabetic screenings when there is familial history of diabetes mellitus.
         b. When weight reduction is being carried out under medical supervision.
      [2] Prompt medical evaluation when there are early symptoms of:
         a. Nutritional problems (e.g., loss of weight, lack of energy).
         b. Gastrointestinal problems (e.g., abdominal pain, persistent digestive disturbances).
2. Patients should be provided (insofar as possible) with a well-balanced, nutritious diet encompassing a variety of properly prepared foods that are compatible with individual and cultural tastes.
   A. The food provided should be in accordance with dietary orders.
   B. In cases of food intolerances, the diet should be altered according to the patient's needs.
3. Patients should be encouraged to eat the food as provided and especially to eat those foods that are most nutritious.
4. Adequate chewing of food should be encouraged.
   A. Patients with dental problems should be referred appropriately.
   B. Dentures should be properly fitted and used as necessary.
5. Foods of appropriate consistency for chewing or swallowing abilities should be provided.

6. Adequate time for eating should be provided.
7. Relaxation before, during and after meals should be provided and encouraged.
8. Stress-producing situations (physical or emotional) should be avoided at mealtimes if at all possible.
9. Optimal positioning for comfort during and after eating should be provided (within medical orders).
10. Patients should be protected from communicable enteric diseases and "food poisoning." (See Chapter 20.)
11. Appetite may be improved by such means as:
    A. Providing a generally pleasant atmosphere and attractive service of food.
    B. Providing foods at temperatures and with seasonings according to individual tastes (within medical orders).
    C. Eliminating unpleasant sights, noises, odors.
    D. Alleviating physical discomforts as much as possible.
    E. Providing for and assisting with oral hygiene to assure that the mouth is clean, moist and fresh-tasting as possible. This is of particular importance when the patient:
       [1] Has been vomiting.
       [2] Has been raising sputum.
       [3] Has inflammation in the oral cavity.
       [4] Has decreased salivary secretions.
    F. Providing for physical activity (within medical orders).
12. Patients should be provided or assisted with effective oral hygiene after meals and at bedtime.
13. Nursing procedures that involve the mouth, pharynx, esophagus (e.g., oral hygiene, tube feedings, gastric aspirations) should be performed with all necessary precautions to prevent physical, chemical or traumatic injury and infections.
14. When a tube is draining fluid from any part of the gastrointestinal tract or from accessory structures:
    A. The amount and type of drainage should be reported/recorded accurately.
    B. Abnormal amounts or types of drainage should be reported promptly, and total or partial specimens saved for inspection.
    C. The function of the tube should be maintained.
    D. If a tube is ordered closed for a period of time, it should be opened for drainage if untoward symptoms occur (e.g., distention, pain, nausea and vomiting), and this should be reported.

CARE OF PATIENTS WITH SPECIFIC NUTRITIONAL AND/OR GASTROINTESTINAL PROBLEMS

1. Prescribed therapeutic diets should be followed specifically.
    A. Patients should be provided and encouraged to eat/drink those foods or substances that are prescribed and should be prevented and discouraged from eating/drinking those foods or substances that should be avoided.
    B. Modifications of the normal diet which may be prescribed include:
       [1] Changes in consistency (e.g., a liquid diet, high or low fiber diet).
       [2] Increase, decrease or maintenance in energy value (e.g., high caloric diet, reduction diet, diabetic diet).

[3] Increase or decrease in specific food components (e.g., high potassium, sodium restriction, increase in a specific vitamin).

[4] Omission of specific food(s) (e.g., allergy diet, no protein).

[5] Adjustment in ratio or balance of various food constituents (e.g., high protein, low fat, diabetic diet).

[6] Rearrangement of number and frequency of meals (e.g., hypoglycemic diet, peptic ulcer diet).

2. When there are increased nutritional requirements (e.g., pregnancy, lactation, rapid physical growth, hyperthyroidism, fever, tissue repair), the diet should include foods high in nutrients.

3. When a patient is underweight, both food intake and total caloric intake should be increased; when a patient is overweight or obese, caloric intake should be restricted. In either instance, the patient's specific dietary needs and any diagnosed disorder must be taken into consideration.

4. If a patient has difficulty in chewing or swallowing:
   A. The types and consistency of foods should be in accordance with chewing and swallowing abilities as well as the condition of the mouth (e.g., acid foods should be avoided when there are open lesions).
   B. The mouth should be moist but free of abnormal or excessive secretions.
   C. Positioning should provide optimal swallowing (as possible).
   D. The quality of the food should be increased as the quantity is decreased.
   E. Special feeding methods may be required (e.g., bottle and nipple, medicine dropper, gavage feeding). These should be performed so as to assure adequate dietary intake.

5. Nausea, vomiting or regurgitation may be prevented or limited by:
   A. Not eating or drinking too much, too fast.
   B. Avoiding foods or other substances that are known to cause digestive disturbances in the individual (e.g., fatty foods, spicy foods, highly acidic foods).
   C. Assisting patient to belch any air swallowed during feeding.
   D. Restricting the ingestion of food or fluids while nausea or vomiting persist.
   E. Limiting physical activity immediately after eating.
   F. Avoiding exaggerated Trendelenburg's position for 2 to 3 hours after meals (e.g., as in postural drainage).
   G. Avoiding motions conducive to nausea (e.g., rapid position change).
   H. Avoiding contact with the uvula or posterior pharynx during treatments.
   I. Discouraging or restricting the ingestion of food when there is unusual emotional or physical stress (e.g., pain, severe anxiety, labor).
   J. Being aware of possible emotional components and giving supportive care accordingly.
   K. Alleviating pain as much as possible.
   L. Eliminating or minimizing unpleasant sights, sounds, odors or tastes.
   M. Administering anti-emetic and/or sedative drugs as ordered.

6. Diarrhea may be prevented or limited by:
   A. Avoiding ingestion of foods or substances that are known to cause diarrhea in patient (e.g., fatty foods, spicy foods).
   B. Avoiding ingestion of high roughage foods that stimulate the intestinal tract.
   C. Eating and drinking only small amounts at a time.

    D. Providing physical and emotional rest, particularly before, during and after meals.

    E. Being aware of possible emotional components and giving supportive care accordingly.

    F. Administering antidiarrheal or sedative drugs as ordered.

7. In general, when a patient's digestion and absorption processes are impaired because of inflammation of the gastrointestinal tract or accessory structures:

    A. Motility of the tract and secretion of digestive juices should be reduced.

        [1] Frequent feedings of food tolerated by the patient are desirable.

        [2] Foods that stimulate secretion of gastric juices should be avoided (e.g., caffeine, black pepper, alcohol, meat extracts).

        [3] Anticholinergic drugs should be administered as needed and prescribed.

        [4] Physical and emotional rest should be encouraged.

        [5] Stress-producing situations (physical and emotional) should be prevented or controlled as possible.

        [6] Smoking should be discouraged.

    B. Antacids may be administered to neutralize the hydrochloric acid.

    C. Gradual increases in the quantity, quality and consistency of foods should be made, according to toleration.

    D. Emotional support should be consistent.

    E. Possible emotional components should be identified and reported/recorded appropriately.

8. When a patient has peptic ulcer disease:

    A. Excessive hydrochloric acid may be neutralized by:

        [1] Providing frequent regular feedings with adequate amounts of protein and fat foods.

        [2] Administering antacid drugs as needed and prescribed.

    B. Close observations should be made for symptoms and signs of perforation and/or hemorrhage.

9. When symptoms and signs of perforation of the gastrointestinal tract occur:

    A. This is a medical emergency.

    B. Food and fluids should be withheld.

    C. Equipment for starting gastric suction should be ready.

    D. The patient should be placed in low Fowler's position (to promote collection of escaping contents in the lower abdominal cavity), unless this position is contraindicated because of circulatory shock.

    E. Emotional support should be consistent.

    F. Preparations should be made for prompt surgical intervention.

10. When there are symptoms and signs of obstruction within the gastrointestinal tract:

    A. This may be a medical emergency, depending upon the site and degree of obstruction.

    B. Food and fluids should be withheld pending medical orders.

    C. Equipment for starting gastric or intestinal suction should be ready.

    D. Positioning should be determined by comfort or any respiratory distress.

    E. Any bowel movements or sounds should be noted and reported/recorded.

11. When there is interference with the production or storage of bile or with its trans-

port into the small intestine (e.g., liver damage, inflamed gall bladder, obstructing stones):

A. The intake of fatty foods should be restricted.

B. Observations should be made for jaundice.

12. When there are symptoms of hypoglycemia, a ready source of glucose (e.g., corn syrup, orange juice, hard candies) should be given promptly. If oral administration is not possible, preparations should be made for intravenous administration of glucose as ordered.

13. When a patient has diabetes mellitus:

A. Medical supervision is essential.

B. All orders pertaining to diet, urine testing, insulin administration (or administration of hypoglycemic drugs) and exercise must be followed exactly.

[1] Meals should not be skipped; food that is served should be eaten. Substitutes should be provided as needed.

[2] Adequate amounts of protein and fat are necessary in the diet to maintain the blood glucose level after the carbohydrate has been broken down for energy.

C. Close observations should be made for symptoms and signs of hypoglycemia and diabetic acidosis.

14. When there is injury to the liver (e.g., viral hepatitis):

A. The diet should be highly nutritious and low in fat.

B. Alterations may be made in amounts of protein in the diet (e.g., with hepatitis, protein should be increased; in hepatic coma, protein should be restricted).

C. More than usual sleep and rest should be provided/encouraged, to reduce metabolic rate.

D. Close observations should be made for symptoms and signs of jaundice, ascites or other edema, and mental changes.

Chapter 4

Fluid Balance

Definite amounts of water are essential to maintain the fluid balance of the body.

Anatomy and Physiology

FLUID BALANCE IN THE BODY

1. Water is the principal constituent of all active living organisms. Adult bodies consist of 45 percent to 60 percent water; the newborn's body is about 80 percent water.
2. Slightly more than half of the body water is in the intracellular compartment (within the cells); the remainder is in the extracellular compartment.
   A. In the healthy, average-size adult there are approximately 42 liters of water, approximately 23 liters in the intracellular compartment and 19 liters in the extracellular compartment.
   B. Extracellular fluids include:
   [1] Interstitial fluid.
   [2] Plasma (or intravascular fluid).
   [3] Cerebrospinal fluid.
   [4] Fluid in the gastrointestinal tract.
   [5] Fluid in potential spaces in the body. Potential spaces include the peritoneal and pleural cavities.
   C. Plasma is a complex mixture of water and many substances, including proteins, inorganic salts, lipids, glucose, waste products of metabolism, vitamins, gases, enzymes, hormones and antibodies. With the exception of proteins, all these substances are able to freely diffuse through the blood capillary walls into the interstitial fluid and from the interstitial fluid into the blood capillaries.

112

  D. There is almost no water in body fat.

3. In health, water intake is balanced against water loss, and the many forces that influence the movement of water between compartments operate to maintain the amount of water necessary in each compartment.

  A. The amount of intravascular water and interstitial water can vary to a limited extent, but the amount of water required in the cells is definite and even minor changes can impair cellular activities and cause cell damage.

  B. The constant movement of water between compartments depends primarily upon two forces: the osmotic pressure created by electrolytes and plasma proteins and the hydrostatic pressure of the blood that is provided largely by force exerted by the heart.

   [1] The total osmolality of the interstitial fluid, plasma and intracellular fluid is almost exactly the same. That of the plasma is slightly greater because of the colloid osmotic effect of the plasma proteins (mainly albumin).

   [2] The transfer of water through cell membranes by osmosis occurs very quickly to maintain osmotic equilibrium.

      a. When water is added to extracellular fluid (e.g., by ingestion and absorption or by infusion), the extracellular fluid becomes hypo-osmolar (or hypotonic) in relation to the intracellular fluid, and water passes into the cells until osmotic equilibrium is reached.

      b. When water is lost from the extracellular fluid (e.g., through evaporation from the skin or in dilute urine), the extracellular fluid becomes hyperosmolar (or hypertonic), and water passes from the cells into the extracellular fluid. This results in dehydration.

   [3] The osmolality (or isotonicity) of body fluids is maintained largely by the retention or the elimination of water and certain electrolytes (primarily sodium and potassium), which is regulated by kidney function.

      a. A loss of sodium is followed by a loss of water.

      b. The ingestion of sodium is followed by water retention.

      c. The state of hydration of cells depends primarily upon the concentration of sodium ions in the extracellular fluid.

      d. Changes in the sodium serum level reflect water imbalances.

   [4] The osmotic equilibria of body fluids may be upset when intravenous solutions are administered, unless the solutions are iso-osmolar (or isotonic) with body fluids or are administered very slowly to allow for reestablishment of equilibria.

  C. Under normal conditions the forces tending to move fluid from the capillaries into the interstitial fluid are:

   [1] The mean capillary pressure.

   [2] The slightly negative interstitial pressure.

   [3] The colloid osmotic pressure of the interstitial fluid.

  D. The force tending to move fluid from the interstitial fluid into the plasma is the plasma colloid osmotic pressure.

  E. Normally there is slightly more movement of fluid into the interstitial spaces than reabsorption into the blood capillaries. The small amounts of extra fluid are returned to the circulation through the lymphatics.

  F. The amount of water in the interstitial fluid varies with:

[1] The movement of water from the arterial capillaries into the interstitial fluid. This movement varies in relation to:
   a. The rate of blood flow (inverse relationship).
   b. The pressure of blood in the capillaries (direct relationship).
   c. Capillary dilatation (direct relationship).
   d. The colloid osmotic pressure of the blood (inverse relationship).
   e. The concentration of sodium ions in the interstitial fluid (direct relationship).
[2] The reabsorption of water from the interstitial fluid into the venous capillaries. Reabsorption varies in relation to:
   a. The flow of excess interstitial fluid into the lymphatics (direct relationship).
   b. The concentration of sodium ions in the blood (inverse relationship).
   c. The colloid osmotic pressure of the blood (inverse relationship).
   d. The concentration of proteins in the interstitial fluid (inverse relationship). (Although an increase in the concentration of protein in the interstitial fluid decreases reabsorption of water, normally the excess interstitial fluid causes an increased flow of lymph which carries the proteins back into the circulating blood.)
[3] Reabsorption into the venous capillaries and the flow of interstitial fluid into the lymphatic capillaries normally does not allow for the accumulation of any excess fluid in the interstitial spaces. Excess interstitial fluid interferes with the normal exchange between the blood and the cells of nutrients, gases, metabolites, etc.

G. The plasma proteins serve to maintain the colloid osmotic pressure of the plasma.
   [1] These proteins are produced mainly in the liver.
   [2] Albumin exerts the greatest force.
   [3] Because albumin has the smallest molecular weight, it is the first plasma protein able to pass through a capillary that is injured or has become more permeable.
   [4] The normal total serum protein is 7.0–7.5 Gm. percent.
   [5] The normal serum albumin is 3.5–5.5 Gm. percent.

H. When the volume of fluid in the extracellular compartment becomes abnormally high, the blood volume is increased. The increased blood volume increases cardiac output which increases the arterial blood pressure. The increased blood pressure, in turn, causes the kidneys to excrete the excess water. The return of the volume of extracellular fluid to normal depends upon efficient cardiac and kidney function.

I. When the volume of fluid in the extracellular compartment becomes abnormally low (e.g., with hemorrhage), the body attempts to maintain normal blood volume by the retention of fluids (primarily by the kidney) and by the movement of water from other extracellular fluids into the blood. The loss of water from the interstitial fluid causes the interstitial fluid to become hyperosmolar to the intracellular fluid, and water moves out of the cells, causing dehydration.

4. The amount of water in the body is determined by the balance between the intake and output each day.

A. Water is normally taken into the body by drinking liquids and eating foods (many of which are very high in water content). Small amounts of water are synthesized from the oxidation of hydrogen in food or body tissues. (The metabolism of 1 Gm. of fat yields approximately 1 ml. of water, while the metabolism of 1 Gm. of starch or protein yields approximately 0.5 ml. of water.)

[1] Small infants require up to 150 ml. of water per kilogram of body weight every 24 hours.

[2] Older children and adults require from 1,500 to 3,000 ml. every 24 hours (average is 2,400 ml.).

[3] Thirst generally gives indication of the need to increase the intake of water.
    a. Thirst is the conscious desire for water and the major regulator of fluid intake.
    b. The thirst (or drinking) center, located within the hypothalamus, is directly affected by the state of dehydration (including circulatory failure).
    c. Dryness of the oral and pharyngeal mucosa also cause the sensation of thirst.
    d. Thirst can generally be relieved rather quickly by drinking fluids (even though it may take up to an hour for ingested water to be absorbed into the extracellular fluid).

B. Water is normally lost from the body through the lungs (vapor), the skin (insensitive perspiration and sweat), the kidneys (urine), and the gastrointestinal tract (feces).

[1] In a temperate climate the water loss for an adult with moderate exercise in a 24–hour period would probably be:

Insensible loss from the lungs	350 ml.
Insensible loss from the skin	350 ml.
Sweat	100 ml.
Urine	1,400 ml.
Feces	200 ml.
Total	2,400 ml.

[2] Insensible losses from the lungs and skin are sometimes referred to as "obligatory." These amounts are lost daily regardless of other factors.

[3] In hot weather water loss through sweat may increase up to 1,400 ml., in which case water loss through the kidneys decreases.

[4] With prolonged and heavy exercise water loss through sweat may increase up to 5,000 ml. daily.

[5] Usually there is increased secretion of sweat when there is need for loss of heat from the body.

[6] The amount of water lost through the kidneys varies inversely with the amount lost through other routes.

[7] Normally, almost all the water in the gastrointestinal fluids is reabsorbed in the small intestines. Some water is absorbed in the colon. Hypermotility of the gastrointestinal tract (which may be caused by excessive stimulation of the parasympathetic nervous system or by inflammatory processes) decreases the time available for normal reabsorption.

[8] No appreciable amount of interstitial fluid is lost through the normal skin because of the continuous layers of keratinized epithelium.

THE PRODUCTION OF URINE

1. The kidneys play a key role in fluid balance, electrolyte balance, acid-base balance and the excretion of wastes.
2. There are two kidneys in the human body. They lie in the posterior abdomen, behind the peritoneum, and are held in place by surrounding pads of adipose tissue and by blood vessels that enter and leave the kidneys.
3. The nephron is the working unit of the kidney; it is composed of the glomerulus, Bowman's capsule and the renal tubule.
   A. There are approximately 1,000,000 nephrons in each kidney.
   B. With a normal intake of proteins and salts, the kidneys can carry on their excretory functions adequately with only 25 percent of available nephrons.
4. A difference in blood pressure between the afferent and efferent arterioles (leading into and away from the glomerulus) causes fluid to be forced from the glomerulus into the Bowman's capsule.
5. The resulting glomerular filtrate is essentially an aqueous solution of all the constituents of plasma except protein. The glomerular filtrate in the normal adult is approximately 120 ml. each minute (or 170 L. each 24 hours).
6. The cells of the renal tubules select those substances that the body needs from the glomerular filtrate, and these are reabsorbed (actively or passively) into the blood. The remainder is eliminated as urine.
   A. Under normal conditions close to 99 percent of the filtrate is reabsorbed.
   B. All but about 1.5 L. of water is reabsorbed.
   C. Passive reabsorption involves the diffusion of substances back into the circulating blood because of concentration or electrical differences. For example, water and urea diffuse from the tubules into the blood capillaries.
   D. Active reabsorption requires work by the tubular cells, as substances must be transported from an area of lesser concentration to an area of greater concentration. Sodium, glucose, amino acids, calcium and phosphate ions are examples of substances that are actively transported by the tubular cells. Energy and specific enzymes are required for active transport.
   E. When the absorptive ability of the tubules for each individual substance (e.g., glucose) is exceeded, these substances spill over into the urine, and proportionate amounts of water also are not reabsorbed. This increases the amount of water lost in the urine.
   F. Normally, glucose, amino acids and vitamins are completely (or almost completely) reabsorbed by active processes.
7. The epithelial cells of the tubules and collecting ducts continually synthesize ammonia, and this diffuses into the tubules. The ammonia reacts with hydrogen ions to form ammonium ions that are then excreted in the urine, mostly as ammonium chloride. (This function is important in acid-base balance; see Chapter 6.)
8. The total volume of urine produced varies with the amount of glomerular filtration and the amount of tubular reabsorption.
   A. The amount of glomerular filtration varies directly with:
      [1] The amount of available filtering surface.
      [2] The blood pressure in the glomeruli. (A fall in arterial blood pressure, as occurs in circulatory shock, decreases glomerular filtration markedly.)
      [3] The amount of renal blood flow. (Strong sympathetic stimulation can con-

strict the arterioles to the extent that there is almost no glomerular blood flow.)

      [4] The rate of tubular reabsorption.

  B. The amount of glomerular filtration varies inversely with the colloid osmotic pressure exerted by the plasma proteins.

  C. The amount of tubular reabsorption of water varies directly with:

      [1] The amount of water in the blood.

      [2] The amount of antidiuretic hormone in the blood.

      [3] The amount of aldosterone in the blood.

  D. The amount of tubular reabsorption varies inversely with:

      [1] The rate of blood flow in the efferent capillaries.

      [2] The concentration of threshold substances (e.g., glucose) in the blood.

9. Water loss in the urine is regulated by osmoreceptors and the antidiuretic hormone system.

  A. Osmoreceptors in the hypothalamus are sensitive to changes in the osmolality of the extracellular fluids, and impulses are relayed to the posterior pituitary gland (neurohypophysis) to release antidiuretic hormone (ADH).

  B. Specialized hypothalamic nuclei secrete ADH, which is stored in the posterior pituitary gland.

  C. Normally integration of the thirst mechanism and of the release of ADH into the blood maintains normal water content and osmolality of the body fluids.

  D. In the absence of ADH almost no water is absorbed from the distal tubules and collecting ducts. Large amounts of dilute urine are excreted.

  E. If large amounts of ADH are secreted and released, only a small amount of very concentrated urine is produced.

10. Aldosterone, the major mineralocorticoid hormone produced by the adrenal cortex, is one of the factors that causes the kidney to increase the retention of sodium (and, consequently, water). Retention of salt and water increases the volume of extracellular fluid. In the absence of this hormone, water and sodium are lost in the urine, and this reduces the volume of extracellular fluid.

11. A definite amount of water is necessary for the excretion of nitrogenous waste products by the kidneys and for maintaining the various threshold substances in solution (e.g., glucose, calcium).

12. The kidneys produce urine continuously, at an average rate of 60 to 120 ml. per hour. Variations from 30 ml. per hour to 500 ml. per hour may be considered just within safe limits. The newborn should start voiding within 24–36 hours after birth.

13. The volume of urine produced is influenced by:

  A. The amount of fluid intake.

  B. The amount of water lost through other routes. (When more water is lost through sweat, less will be lost through urine.)

  C. Emotional stress. (Changes in the systemic arterial blood pressure affect urine production.)

  D. Pain. (The presence of severe pain may reduce urine production.)

  E. Age. (Infants, for their weight, produce several times more urine than adults.)

  F. Diuretics. (Some chemical substances increase urine production by increasing the filtration rate or by decreasing tubular reabsorption.)

14. The urine produced in the nephrons collects in collecting tubules that lead to the

calyces; it then empties into the pelvis of the kidney. The urine travels from the kidney pelvis to the urinary bladder through the ureters, both by gravity and the peristaltic action of smooth muscle in the ureteral wall.

15. Urine, freshly voided, is usually pale yellow to light amber and clear, with no sediment. Concentrated urine is dark and odorous.

16. Normally about 90–95 percent of urine is water. The specific gravity may vary, normally, from 1.003 to 1.040. Usually the specific gravity lessens as the volume of urine increases.

17. In the aging process degenerative changes take place in the kidneys. Circulation may be impaired; the kidneys may become atrophied. Some of the nephrons may not function properly or at all. There may be fibrosis. These changes result in impaired kidney function.

THE LYMPHATICS

1. Almost all body tissues have lymphatic channels that drain excess fluid from the interstitial spaces and return it to the circulating blood. Excess interstitial fluid in the brain flows through tiny interstitial channels and into the cerebrospinal fluid.

2. Lymphatic capillaries merge into larger and larger channels that eventually form two main ducts (the thoracic duct and the right lymph duct) that empty into the large veins of the neck.

3. Lymph enters the lymphatic capillaries when the pressure of the interstitial fluid rises. Lymph flows through the lymphatic channels because of compression (mainly by muscle contractions) and gravity and with the help of intrinsic valves.

4. The lymphatics can carry proteins and other larger-size particles that blood capillaries are unable to absorb.

THE SWEAT GLANDS

1. Sweat glands are distributed over the entire body. They produce sweat, a weak solution of sodium and other salts in water with small amounts of organic wastes (e.g., urea). As the rate of sweat secretion increases, the concentration of sodium chloride in the sweat increases. However, when there is increased sweat production over time (e.g., weeks) the concentration of sodium chloride decreases as the body acts to conserve salt.

2. The secretion of sweat is primarily a heat-regulating mechanism, but it may occur as a result of emotional stress (e.g., in anxiety states).

3. Sweat glands are stimulated to secrete by the sympathetic division of the autonomic nervous system.

Physics

1. Gravity is the force of attraction between two objects (e.g., the earth and an object on or near the earth).

2. Pressure is the force exerted on a unit area.

3. Liquids at rest exert pressure. The pressure exerted by a column of liquid in a container is equal to the height of the liquid times its weight per unit volume.

4. Fluids flow from an area of higher pressure to one of lower pressure, and the rate of volume flow is directly related to the pressure gradient.

5. Specific gravity is the weight of a substance compared with the weight of an equal volume of water. Specific gravity can be determined by dividing the weight of 1.0 ml. of fluid by the weight of 1.0 ml. of water—which is 1.0 Gm. A urinometer is used in determining the specific gravity of urine.

Chemistry

1. A true solution is a liquid mixture of ions, atoms, or molecules of 2 or more substances in which there is apparent homogeneity.
   A. Water is by far the commonest and most useful solvent.
   B. The amounts of constituents in a solution may vary within certain limits.
2. Diffusion is a process in which, because of molecular motion, 2 or more substances (gases, liquids or solids) become perfectly mixed.
3. Osmosis is the process whereby the molecules of a solvent pass through a semipermeable membrane from the area of lesser concentration to the area of greater concentration of the solute.
   A. A semipermeable membrane is one that shows selective action with regard to the passage of different substances through it.
   B. Solvent molecules pass through the semipermeable membrane, because of osmosis, until the pressure exerted on the side of the formerly stronger solution is great enough to establish a state of equilibrium. The amount of pressure necessary to prevent the flow of solvent molecules across the membrane is called the osmotic pressure of the solution. (The greater the difference between the concentrations of the solutions on either side of the membrane, the greater the osmotic pressure will be.)
   C. The osmotic effect of a substance in solution depends only on the number of particles dissolved (e.g., if a molecule in solution dissociates into 2 particles, the osmotic pressure is doubled). Units of osmotic force are expressed as osmoles and milliosmoles.
   D. An isotonic or iso-osmolar solution is one that exerts the same osmotic pressure as a solution on the other side of a semipermeable membrane.
      [1] A hypotonic or hypo-osmolar solution has less osmotic pressure, so the solvent passes through the membrane to the more concentrated solution on the opposite side.
      [2] A hypertonic or hyperosmolar solution has a higher osmotic pressure, so the solvent of the less concentrated solution passes through the membrane to the hypertonic side.
      [3] Physiological saline solution (isotonic with body fluids) is approximately a 0.9 percent aqueous solution of sodium chloride.

Pathology

SYMPTOMS AND SIGNS

1. Symptoms and signs of fluid imbalance include those related to dehydration, edema and water intoxication.
2. Symptoms and signs related to dehydration may include:
   A. Thirst, which may be excessive.

    B. Dry skin and mucous membranes, thick secretions, dysphagia.

    C. Poor skin turgor.

    D. Loss of weight.

    E. Oliguria, with highly concentrated urine.

    F. Fever.

    G. Constipation.

    H. Weakness, faintness, exhaustion and collapse.

    I. Symptoms and signs of circulatory shock. (See Chapter 1.)

    J. Mental changes; including disorientation and drowsiness which may progress to coma.

3. Symptoms and signs related to edema may include:

    A. Weight gain.

    B. Swelling of subcutaneous tissues (generalized, dependent, may be pitting).

    C. Swelling of abdomen (ascites).

    D. Symptoms and signs related to pulmonary edema. (See Chapter 2.)

    E. Symptoms and signs related to cerebral edema (caused by increased intracranial pressure, may include headache, behavioral changes, convulsions, changes in vital signs).

    F. Symptoms and signs of dehydration—if edema is very severe.

4. Symptoms and signs of water intoxication are similar to those for sodium deficiency, including:

    A. Headache.

    B. Muscle cramps.

    C. Nausea and vomiting.

    D. Excessive perspiration.

    E. Mental changes such as confusion and drowsiness which may progress to coma.

5. Symptoms and signs of renal disease may include those of edema and/or dehydration, plus:

    A. Anorexia, nausea and vomiting.

    B. Weakness, pallor.

    C. Hematuria, pyuria, abnormal specific gravities of urine.

    D. Nocturia, oliguria and anuria.

    E. Symptoms and signs of electrolyte imbalances, acid-base imbalance and uremia. (See Chapters 5, 6 and 7.)

DEHYDRATION

1. Dehydration is a condition in which fluid loss exceeds fluid intake (negative fluid balance), with a resultant decrease in the volume of body fluids.

    A. Changes in fluid volumes (intracellular and extracellular) are closely associated with changes in electrolyte balance.

    B. Concentrations of electrolytes are increased when there is a reduction in fluid intake or when water is lost from the body faster than electrolytes.

    C. Concentrations of electrolytes are decreased when water and electrolytes are lost simultaneously (e.g., as occurs when gastrointestinal secretions are not reabsorbed properly).

2. Possible causes of dehydration include:

A. Inadequate fluid intake. (Fluid intake may be reduced because fluids are un-available, because of problems with swallowing, or perhaps because of nausea and vomiting.)

B. Excessive loss of body fluids.

[1] Abnormal amounts of water may be lost from the gastrointestinal tract through vomiting, diarrhea, aspiration of gastric or intestinal contents, drainage from an ileostomy or fistulae.

[2] Abnormal amounts of water may be lost by excessive sweating, which may occur as a result of the body's attempt to increase heat loss (e.g., with fever or when there is a high environmental temperature).

[3] Abnormal amounts of water may be lost via the kidneys.

a. Diabetes insipidus is a syndrome that results from failure of the hypo-thalamic-neurohypophyseal system to secrete or release enough anti-diuretic hormone to effect the normal tubular reabsorption of water. Severe diuresis occurs in uncontrolled diabetes insipidus, with losses as high as 10 to 15 liters of water daily. There may be electrolyte im-balance.

b. Addison's disease is caused by insufficient secretion of adrenal cortical hormones. A deficiency in aldosterone results in the excessive loss of sodium and water in the urine.

c. Polyuria occurs in uncontrolled diabetes mellitus because of the hyper-glycemia with resultant glycosuria. Large amounts of water may be lost because the tubular reabsorption of water decreases as the excess glu-cose spills over into the urine.

d. Renal disease may result in excessive loss of water in the urine.

[4] Abnormal amounts of water may be lost because of hemorrhage, loss of plasma or draining wounds. (In severe burns tissue fluid leaks into the in-jured area, and plasma escapes from injured capillaries. If burns are exten-sive, large amounts of plasma may be lost from the blood, and this leads to hemoconcentration and hypotension. Severe burns may be caused by heat, radiation, electricity and certain chemicals.)

3. Intracellular dehydration impairs cellular function.

4. Abnormal loss of water from the blood results in problems related to inadequate volume and pressure of circulating blood. (See Chapter 1.)

5. When there is not enough water for the formation of urine, toxic substances formed in the body cannot be properly eliminated from the body. (See Chapter 7.)

EDEMA

1. Edema is the excessive accumulation of freely moving interstitial fluid in the inter-stitial spaces.

A. Edema may be generalized or local; occurring in loose areolar tissue, in the lungs, in the brain, in the abdominal cavity and so forth. Dependent edema is an effect of gravity.

B. Edema helps to dilute toxins in the interstitial fluid and protects the cells from electrolyte imbalance.

C. The problems caused by edema depend upon the extent of fluid loss from the plasma, the location of the edema, and the amount of edema.

    D. Because of safety factors that normally prevent the accumulation of excess fluid, edema does not usually occur until abnormalities are fairly severe.

  2. Possible causes of edema include:

    A. Increased capillary pressure, which forces water into the interstitial spaces. (Capillary pressure may be increased when there is venous obstruction or congestive heart failure. See Chapter 1.)

    B. A decreased concentration of plasma proteins, which decreases the colloid osmotic pressure of the plasma and allows more water to flow into the interstitial spaces. (The concentration of plasma proteins is reduced when there is protein deficiency, in liver disease and when plasma proteins—mostly albumin—are lost in the urine because of renal disease.)

    C. An accumulation of interstitial fluid (and increased concentration of interstitial fluid protein), due to obstruction of lymphatic drainage.

        [1] Lymphedema involves the accumulation of lymph in the subcutaneous tissue because of obstruction of the lymphatic channels. The obstruction is usually acquired and may be caused by abnormal growths, surgical procedures, parasites and inflammatory reactions that involve scarring.

        [2] Filariasis is a parasitic infestation in which the adult round worms present in lymph channels block the flow of lymph. When the worms die they become calcified and may cause permanent blockage.

        [3] Elephantiasis may develop if the majority of lymph channels in a lower extremity are affected.

    D. Increased capillary permeability, which may be due to hypoxia, inflammatory response, trauma or nutritional deficiencies. (Inflammatory response results in increased capillary permeability, which allows the escape of plasma proteins. The resultant decrease in the colloid osmotic pressure in the capillaries plus any increase in hydrostatic pressure due to hyperemia lead to edema.)

    E. Retention of fluid by the kidney is frequently associated with sodium retention.

  3. Ascites, the accumulation of interstitial fluid in the abdominal cavity, may occur when there is generalized edema or as a direct result of conditions such as cirrhosis of the liver. When there is cirrhosis of the liver:

    A. The filtration pressure in the capillaries increases because of the portal venous congestion.

    B. There is retention of sodium and water due to the liver dysfunction.

    C. There is a decrease in the colloid osmotic pressure because of a decrease in the production of plasma proteins.

  4. Myxedema occurs when there is a prolonged deficiency of thyroid hormones. Cellular metabolism is altered, and an increase in the osmotic pressure of the interstitial fluid results in a shift of water from the plasma into the interstitial spaces. The resulting edema is usually not severe.

  5. Excess fluid in the interstitial spaces interferes with the transfer of substances (nutrients, metabolites, gases, etc.) between the blood and the cells.

WATER INTOXICATION

  1. Water intoxication is a condition in which there is an excessive amount of water in the body.

  2. Water intoxication may be caused by the continued intake of water without ade-

quate excretion by the kidneys or by the increased intake of water without an adequate intake of salt. Effects are similar to those of sodium deficiency.

RENAL DISEASE

1. Renal disease may result in fluid imbalance, electrolyte imbalance, acid-base imbalance and uremia.
2. Renal failure may be due to:
   A. Nephron damage, which may be caused by:
      [1] Infections.
      [2] Mechanical obstructions of ureters or renal pelvis.
      [3] Cyst formations.
      [4] Certain poisons, toxins (e.g., resulting from hemolysis when blood transfusion is incompatible).
      [5] Certain drugs that are excreted by the kidney.
   B. An inadequate blood supply, which may be caused by:
      [1] Nephrosclerosis.
      [2] Thrombi, emboli.
      [3] Hypotension.
      [4] Problems related to toxemias of pregnancy.
      [5] Circulatory failure.
3. Acute glomerular nephritis is an infection of the glomeruli in which the glomeruli become blocked by white blood cells and proliferating epithelial cells. The affected glomeruli are sometimes completely blocked; others may become permeable to plasma protein and red blood cells.
   A. Kidney function may become so impaired that renal shutdown results.
   B. The inflammation and damage appear to be caused by antibodies that are formed in response to beta hemolytic streptococcus infections. The acute stage may last 1 to 2 weeks.
   C. Chronic glomerular nephritis may follow, with occasional acute episodes that cause increasing nephron damage, leading to renal failure.
4. Pyelitis and pyelonephritis are inflammatory processes usually caused by microorganisms (frequently *Streptococcus* and *Escherichia coli*). The inflammation can cause local congestion, swelling production of exudates, tissue destruction and fibrosis.
5. Hydronephrosis is a condition in which there is dilatation of the kidney pelvis. It is caused by an obstruction in the upper urinary tract that causes an accumulation of urine in the kidney pelvis. Tissues are stretched and injured, and there is hyperperistalsis of the smooth muscle of the ureter. Obstructions may be caused by calculi, abnormal growths, ureteral constriction and nephroptosis.
6. Polycystic kidney is a familial disease in which there is multiple cyst formation in both kidneys. These compress the nephrons, interfere with normal function and cause renal insufficiency.
7. Nephrosclerosis is a condition in which there is narrowing of the renal arterial blood vessels. Decreased blood flow interferes with normal kidney function. When severe it results in necrosis of kidney tissue with various degrees of renal insufficiency.
8. Persons with renal disease may develop nephrotic syndrome, characterized by the

loss of large amounts of plasma proteins in the urine because of the abnormal permeability of the glomerular membrane. When severe, 30–40 Gm. of plasma protein may be lost daily. The plasma colloid osmotic pressure falls, causing generalized edema, with excessive fluid accumulation in the potential extracellular spaces.

9. The toxemias of pregnancy are characterized by generalized and dependent edema. Several factors seem to be involved, including:
   A. An elevated systemic blood pressure, with increased filtration pressure in the general circulation and in the pelvic area in particular.
   B. Loss of albumin in the urine, with a resultant decrease in plasma colloid osmotic pressure.
   C. Renal retention of sodium (probably due to effect of adrenal cortical hormones).
10. Hereditary disorders may cause various problems with tubular reabsorption. Deficiencies in appropriate enzymes (or carriers) can impair the transport of particular substances (or groups of substances) across tubular membrane (e.g., in renal glycosuria, glucose is lost in the urine because the tubules are unable to reabsorb it from the glomerular filtrate; proportionate amounts of water are lost with the glucose).

Nursing Care

Nursing care should be directed toward assisting the patient to retain or regain fluid balance.

COLLECTION, EVALUATION AND COMMUNICATION OF DATA

1. Patients should be interviewed and observed to identify excessive or inadequate oral intake of fluids.
2. Patients should be interviewed and observed to identify abnormal loss of fluid from the body (e.g., in vomiting, diarrhea, sweat, polyuria).
3. Patients should be interviewed, observed and examined to identify symptoms and signs of fluid imbalance.
   A. Dehydration may be indicated by:
      [1] Unusual thirst.
      [2] Abnormal dryness of skin, mucous membranes; poor skin turgor.
      [3] Oliguria, with highly concentrated urine.
      [4] Fever.
      [5] Constipation.
      [6] Rapid weight loss (e.g., one pound—about 0.5 kg.—in 24 hours).
      [7] Weakness, exhaustion, collapse.
      [8] Symptoms and signs of circulatory shock.
      [9] Mental changes such as confusion, loss of consciousness.
   B. Edema may be indicated by:
      [1] Tissue swelling that may be generalized, dependent, pitting.
      [2] Rapid weight gain (e.g., one pound—about 0.5 kg.—in 24 hours).
      [3] Abdominal distention (ascites).
      [4] Symptoms and signs of pulmonary edema or cerebral edema.

4. Patients should be interviewed, observed and examined to identify symptoms and signs of renal problems. Renal problems may be indicated by:
   A.   Symptoms and signs of fluid imbalance.
   B.   Abnormalities in urine and urinary output.
   C.   Symptoms and signs of electrolyte imbalance, acid-base imbalance and/or uremia.

5. Systematic patient evaluation is of especial importance when the patient:
   A.   Has a condition that prevents normal fluid intake by mouth.
   B.   Has a condition in which there is abnormal loss of fluid from the body.
   C.   Has a condition in which the volume and pressure of circulating blood are not within normal limits.
   D.   Has diagnosed renal disease.
   E.   Has diagnosed liver disease.
   F.   Has a hormonal imbalance that directly or indirectly affects fluid and/or electrolyte balance (e.g., antidiuretic hormone or adrenocortical hormones).
   G.   Is receiving fluids parenterally.
   H.   Is receiving diuretic drugs.
   I.   Is pregnant.
   J.   Is at extremes of age.

6. Whenever a patient has symptoms and signs indicating actual or potential fluid imbalance:
   A.   Fluid intake and fluid output should be systematically measured and recorded.
   B.   Measurements of body weight should be made regularly and frequently (e.g., daily or q.o.d.).
   C.   Any indications of electrolyte imbalance should be reported promptly.

7. Data collected should be evaluated not only on the basis of a single deviation from normal (e.g., unusual thirst) but also on the basis of combinations of symptoms and signs that tend to occur when there is fluid imbalance (e.g., symptoms and signs associated with dehydration).
   A.   A patient's daily fluid intake should be evaluated in relation to:
   [1]   The total fluid output.
   [2]   Age of patient.
   [3]   The state of hydration.
   [4]   The diagnosed disease condition.
   B.   Whenever a patient complains of thirst despite adequate ingestion of water or when actual water deficit does not seem to exist, the patient should be observed closely for indications of hemorrhage and/or circulatory shock. (See Chapter 1.)
   C.   A patient's urinary output should be evaluated in relation to:
   [1]   The quantity of urine the kidneys normally excrete within a given period of time.
   [2]   The total fluid intake.
   [3]   The state of hydration.
   [4]   Amount of fluid loss via other routes.
   [5]   The emotional state.
   [6]   The frequency and volume of each urinary elimination.
   [7]   The diagnosed disease condition.
   [8]   Any diuretic drugs that the patient has received.

D. A patient's urine should be evaluated in relation to:
[1] Volume.
[2] Color and transparency.
[3] Odor.
[4] Presence of sediment.
[5] Presence of abnormal substances (e.g., blood, pus). (When the urine appears to be abnormally dilute or concentrated, the specific gravity should be measured and recorded/reported.)
8. How, when and what data are communicated to the physician and/or other nursing personnel depend upon:
A. Any immediate threat to the patient's life processes (e.g., anuria).
B. Any potential threat to the patient's life and well-being (e.g., excessive loss of body fluids).
C. Any particular implications for the physician in relation to:
[1] The patient's progress or lack of progress toward recovery (e.g., change in urine production).
[2] Making a diagnosis (e.g., new objective or subjective data).
[3] The patient's physical and emotional responses to specific diagnostic procedures or therapeutic measures.
D. Any particular implications for nursing care (e.g., regulation of fluid intake).

PROMOTION OF HEALTH AND PREVENTION OF DISEASE/INJURY

1. Health teaching to promote fluid balance should be concerned with:
A. Importance of:
[1] Adequate fluid intake throughout the life cycle. (Thirst is the normal indicator of the body's need for fluid.)
[2] Increasing intake of sodium chloride along with increased fluid intake when there is excessive loss of water through sweating.
[3] Avoiding use of cathartics, especially repeated use of saline cathartics.
B. Importance of:
[1] Periodic health evaluations.
[2] Prompt medical attention when:
a. There are problems in which fluid intake is reduced and/or there is loss of large amounts of fluid from the body.
b. There are early symptoms and signs of possible renal problems (e.g., abnormal urinary output, abnormal urine, back pain).
c. There is tissue swelling, unusual thirst, rapid weight gain or loss.
[3] Proper medical treatment of acute infections.
[4] Proper obstetrical care.
2. An adequate fluid intake should be provided (within medical orders and according to individual needs) during waking hours. (Unless contraindicated, persons who are ill should be encouraged to have an oral intake of 2,000–3,000 ml. daily.)
3. Parenteral fluids should be administered exactly as prescribed—in relation to the quantity of solution, the type of solution, the rate of flow, the time of administration, and so forth.

4. Any observed abnormalities in relation to fluid intake or fluid loss should be reported/recorded appropriately.
5. When a patient has a tube draining fluid from the body into a container, the drainage should be measured and reported/recorded appropriately.
6. Accurate measurements (whenever possible) and estimated descriptions (as necessary) of fluid loss (e.g., sweat, vomitus, stools, wound drainage, etc.) should be made and reported/recorded appropriately.
7. Unless contraindicated by such conditions as nausea and vomiting or impaired kidney or heart function, oral fluids should be encouraged when there has been or is excessive loss of body fluid.
8. Injury to the kidneys should be prevented.
   A. Circulatory failure should be identified and treated as quickly as possible.
   B. Transfusion reactions should be prevented. (See Chapter 1.)
   C. All nursing procedures involving the urethra, bladder, ureters and/or kidneys must be carried out with surgical aseptic techniques.
   D. When patients are inactive, bedridden or immobilized, stasis of urine and formation of renal calculi should be prevented by such means as:
      [1] Providing and encouraging an ample intake of fluid.
      [2] Assisting with frequent position changes.
      [3] Encouraging and assisting with an exercise regime each day.

CARE OF PATIENTS WITH SPECIFIC
FLUID IMBALANCE PROBLEMS

1. When a patient has a problem involving fluid imbalance:
   A. All fluid intake and fluid output should be measured accurately and reported/recorded appropriately.
   B. All medical orders pertaining to fluid intake (oral and parenteral) and salt intake must be followed exactly.
   C. Close observations should be made for indications of electrolyte imbalance.
2. When a patient has dehydration (negative fluid balance), the oral intake of fluids should be encouraged (within medical orders and unless contraindicated by other factors). Intake should be regulated in relation to amount and time.
3. When a patient has edema:
   A. The prescribed amount of oral fluid intake should be distributed through the patient's waking hours.
   B. Dietary orders must be followed exactly.
   C. Accurate measurement of body weight should be made daily or as ordered. Weighing should be done under essentially the same conditions each time.
   D. Diuretics should be administered exactly as prescribed, and accurate measurements of urinary output must be made.
   E. Careful observations should be made for indications of cerebral edema and pulmonary edema.
      [1] Cerebral edema represents a medical emergency. Equipment for the prompt administration of appropriate diuretic drugs should be ready.
      [2] Pulmonary edema represents a medical emergency. (See Chapters 1 and 2.)
4. When a patient has impaired renal function:

A. All medical orders pertaining to fluid intake, salt intake, protein and carbohydrate intake must be followed exactly.

B. Fluid intake and fluid output should be measured accurately and reported/recorded appropriately.

C. More than usual sleep and rest should be encouraged and provided to limit demands made on the kidneys.

D. Close observations should be made for:

    [1] Abnormalities of the urine.

    [2] Symptoms and signs of fluid, electrolyte and acid-base imbalances.

Chapter 5

Electrolyte Balance

All the cells of the body require definite amounts of certain electrolytes for efficient functioning.

Anatomy and Physiology

1. Electrolytes play an essential role in metabolic processes, by:
   A. Contributing to proper osmotic pressure relationships.
   B. Providing buffer systems and mechanisms for regulating acid-base balance. (Chapter 6 covers acid-base balance.)
   C. Providing proper ionic balance for normal neuromuscular irritability and cellular function.
   D. Often serving as enzyme activators.
2. Electrolytes are distributed in all the body fluids.
   A. Proper concentrations of electrolytes must be maintained intracellularly and extracellularly for efficient cell functioning.
   B. The numbers of cations and anions must be equal, to maintain electrochemical neutrality.
   C. The body fluids normally maintain an osmotic pressure of about 0.9 percent sodium chloride. The total plasma osmolality is approximately 300 milliosmoles.
3. The primary cations are sodium (Na^+), potassium (K^+), calcium (Ca^{++}) and magnesium (Mg^{++}).
   A. A well-balanced diet provides adequate amounts of these electrolytes.
   B. Sodium is the primary extracellular cation, representing about 90 percent of the cations in extracellular fluids.

[1] The normal concentrations of sodium are:
   a. 138–142 mEq/liter of plasma.
   b. 2–10 mEq/liter of intracellular water.
[2] Sodium is necessary for the normal functioning of nerve and muscle cells.
C. Potassium is the primary intracellular cation.
   [1] The normal concentrations of potassium are:
      a. 3.8–5.0 mEq/liter of plasma.
      b. 135–155 mEq/liter of intracellular water.
   [2] Potassium is essential for the normal functioning of nerve and muscle cells.
   [3] Potassium is found in the gastrointestinal secretions.
D. Slightly more calcium is found extracellularly than intracellularly.
   [1] The normal concentrations of calcium are:
      a. 5 mEq/liter of plasma.
      b. 2–4 mEq/liter of intracellular water.
   [2] Proper concentration of calcium is essential to bone metabolism, normal nueromuscular irritability, normal membrane permeability, normal cardiac rhythmicity and blood coagulation.
E. Magnesium is the second major intracellular cation.
   [1] The normal concentrations of magnesium are:
      a. 5 mEq/liter of plasma.
      b. 25–30 mEq/liter of intracellular water.
   [2] Magnesium is an important catalyst for intracellular enzyme systems and plays an important role in neuromuscular activity, protein synthesis and formation of bones and teeth.
F. The kidneys play a key role in the regulation of these cations.
   [1] Under normal conditions most of the sodium and potassium lost from the body are lost in the urine. Some sodium and potassium are lost in the feces. Sodium is also lost in sweat.
   [2] The amount of sodium reabsorbed in the kidney tubules is determined mainly by the concentration of aldosterone (an adrenocortical hormone) in the body fluids. An increased concentration of aldosterone increases reabsorption.
   [3] Potassium ion concentration is regulated by aldosterone and by the tubular excretion of potassium. When sodium reabsorption is increased, there is increased excretion of potassium, so that the appropriate ratio between sodium and potassium in the extracellular fluids is maintained.
   [4] Under normal conditions most of the calcium and magnesium that is lost from the body is lost in the feces, although some is lost in the urine.
   [5] Calcium ion concentration is regulated largely by parathyroid hormone, but there is some control by the kidney tubules. If the concentration of calcium ions in the body fluids is decreased, parathyroid hormone causes the withdrawal of calcium from the bones and increases reabsorption from the kidney tubules and from the intestinal tract.
4. The primary anions are chloride (Cl^-), bicarbonate (HCO_3^-), dihydrogen phosphate ($HPO_4^=$), phosphate ($PO_4^=$) and protein$^{(-)}$.
   A. A well-balanced diet provides adequate amounts of these electrolytes.

B. Chloride is a primary extracellular anion.
   [1] The normal concentrations of chloride are:
        a. 95–105 mEq/liter of plasma.
        b. 4–10 mEq/liter of intracellular water.
   [2] Chloride ions combine with hydrogen ions to form hydrochloric acid, which is secreted by gastric glands.
   [3] The transport of carbon dioxide in the form of bicarbonate ions involves the diffusion of chloride ions from the plasma into red blood cells (chloride shift).
C. Bicarbonate is an important intracellular and extracellular anion.
   [1] The normal concentrations of bicarbonate are:
        a. 24–28 mEq/liter of plasma.
        b. 31 mEq/liter of intracellular water.
   [2] Bicarbonate provides an important buffer system for acid-base balance.
   [3] Pancreatic juices contain large amounts of bicarbonate, which act to neutralize the highly acidic chyme entering the duodenum.
D. Phosphate is the primary intracellular anion and is also important in maintaining normal acid-base balance.
   [1] Both dihydrogen phosphate and phosphate ions are found in the plasma.
        a. The normal concentration of dihydrogen phosphate is 1 mEq/liter.
        b. The normal concentration of phosphate is 2 mEq/liter.
   [2] Intracellular phosphate is essential for energy-producing activities within the cells. The normal intracellular concentration in muscle is 95 mEq/ kilogram of water.
E. Protein ions are found primarily intracellularly.
   [1] The normal concentrations of protein are:
        a. 13 mEq/liter of plasma.
        b. 40–60 mEq/liter of intracellular water.
   [2] Protein ions provide one of the body's buffer systems for acid-base balance.
F. The same mechanisms that regulate reabsorption of cations cause the reabsorption of anions, maintaining electrical neutrality.
   [1] The ratio between chloride and bicarbonate in the extracellular fluid is extremely important in maintaining acid-base balance.
   [2] If the intracellular fluids become acidic the reabsorption of bicarbonate ions is increased (to shift the pH of the buffer systems back to normal), and the reabsorption of chloride ions is decreased.
   [3] The concentration of phosphate ions is controlled mainly by the kidney tubules. When the plasma concentration exceeds the renal threshold value, phosphate spills over into the urine.
   [4] There is a reciprocal relationship between calcium and phosphorus in the extracellular fluids. If the concentration of one increases, the other decreases. Parathyroid hormone increases the reabsorption of calcium and decreases reabsorption of phosphates.
5. Proper concentrations of intracellular potassium and extracellular sodium are essential to fluid balance and acid-base balance.
6. Kidney function plays a key role in electrolyte balance through:
   A. The retention or elimination of water.

    B.   The tubular reabsorption of electrolytes.

    C.   The tubular excretion of potassium.

    D.   The substitution of ammonium ion for sodium ion when sodium is needed by the body.

Chemistry

1. An ion is a charged atom or group of atoms, caused by gain or loss of electrons.
    A. Strongly electropositive elements form positive ions (e.g., potassium, sodium, calcium, magnesium).
    B. Strongly electronegative elements form negative ions (e.g., oxygen and chlorine).
2. Electrolytes are electrovalent compounds that, in solution, form ions and conduct electricity.
    A. Positively charged ions are attracted to the negative pole (cathode), and are called cations.
    B. Negatively charged ions are attracted to the positive pole (anode), and are called anions.
    C. Electrolytes combine with each other in proportion to their ionic valence. They combine equivalent for equivalent.
        [1] One milliequivalent (mEq) of an electrolyte means there is one cation or anion available to combine with one cation or anion of another substance.
        [2] The number of milliequivalents of an electrolyte per liter of solution (mEq/liter) is computed by:
            a. Dividing the number of milligrams contained in 100 ml. of solution by the element's atomic weight; then
            b. Multiplying this number by the valence; then
            c. Multiplying by 10.
3. Osmosis is the process whereby the molecules of a solvent pass through a semipermeable membrane from the area of lesser to the area of greater concentration of the solute.
    A. A semipermeable membrane is one that shows selective action with regard to the passage of different substances through it.
    B. Solvent molecules pass through the semipermeable membrane because of osmosis until the pressure exerted on the side of the formerly more concentrated solution is great enough to establish a state of equilibrium. The amount of pressure necessary to prevent the flow of solvent molecules across the membrane is called the osmotic pressure of the solution (e.g., the greater the difference between the concentrations of the solutions on either side of the membrane, the greater the osmotic pressure).
    C. The osmotic effect of a substance in solution depends only on the number of particles dissolved. If a molecule in solution dissociates into 2 particles, the osmotic pressure is doubled; if it dissociates into 3 particles, the pressure is tripled; etc. Units of osmotic force are expressed as osmoles and milliosmoles.
    D. In the body, colloid osmotic pressure (or oncotic pressure) is the osmotic force exerted by plasma proteins.
    E. An iso-osmolar (or isotonic) solution is one that exerts the same osmotic pressure as a solution on the other side of a semipermeable membrane.

[1] A hypo-osmolar (or hypotonic) solution has less osmotic pressure, so the solvent passes through the membrane to the more concentrated solution on the opposite side.

[2] A hyperosmolar (or hypertonic) solution has a higher osmotic pressure, so the solvent of the less concentrated solution passes through the membrane to the hyperosmolar solution.

[3] Physiological saline solution (isotonic with body fluids) is approximately a 0.9 percent aqueous solution of sodium chloride.

Pathology

SYMPTOMS AND SIGNS

1. Symptoms and signs of electrolyte imbalance generally are related to abnormal neuromuscular function.
2. Symptoms and signs of sodium deficiency include:
   A. Weakness, headache, hypotension (related to dehydration).
   B. Vomiting and diarrhea.
   C. Muscle cramping, muscle spasms, convulsions.
3. Symptoms and signs of excess sodium are those associated with edema. (See Chapter 4.)
4. Symptoms and signs of potassium deficiency include:
   A. General skeletal muscle weakness, which may progress to paralysis (including the respiratory muscles).
   B. Cardiac arrythmias and symptoms and signs of impaired cardiac function. (See Chapter 1.)
   C. Abdominal distention, vomiting, constipation.
   D. Apathy, mental confusion.
5. Symptoms and signs of excess potassium include:
   A. Symptoms and signs of impaired heart action.
   B. Numbness of extremities.
   C. Abdominal cramping, diarrhea.
   D. Apathy, mental confusion.
6. Symptoms and signs of calcium deficiency include:
   A. Neuromuscular hyperirritability, with muscle twitchings, painful tonic spasms and possibly convulsions.
   B. Numbness in the extremities.
7. Symptoms and signs of excess calcium may include:
   A. General muscle weakness.
   B. Polyuria and corresponding thirst.

ELECTROLYTE IMBALANCE

1. Fluid imbalance and electrolyte imbalance are interrelated.
   A. Because water in the body is in solution, shifts of water between fluid compartments or loss of water are accompanied by shifts or loss of electrolytes.
   B. Because electrolytes are in aqueous solution, shifts of electrolytes between fluid compartments or loss of electrolytes are accompanied by shifts or loss of water.

2. Sodium deficiency (hyponatremia) may occur when there is:
   A. Inadequate dietary intake to replace daily sodium loss. This may be due to a prescribed low sodium diet or an inadequate diet.
   B. Excessive loss of sodium from the body which may be caused by:
      [1] Excessive sweating (may occur with high environmental temperature or with fever).
      [2] Excessive loss of gastrointestinal secretions (e.g., from vomiting, diarrhea or continued aspiration of gastrointestinal contents).
      [3] Decreased secretion of aldosterone by the adrenal cortex, so that sodium is not reabsorbed properly.
      [4] Renal disease that prevents normal reabsorption of sodium in the tubules.
      [5] Excessive loss of blood or plasma (e.g., with hemorrhage or burns).
3. Hyponatremia may cause:
   A. Dehydration, as the kidneys excrete more water to maintain normal osmotic pressure in the extracellular fluids.
   B. Abnormal neuromuscular functioning, with cramping, spasms and convulsions.
   C. Abnormal gastrointestinal functioning (nausea, vomiting, diarrhea), related to increased motility of the tract.
4. Sodium excess (hypernatremia) may occur when there is:
   A. Excessive intake of sodium (by ingestion or infusion).
   B. Decreased excretion of sodium, which may be caused by:
      [1] Increased secretion of aldosterone by adrenal cortex or therapeutic administration of the hormone.
      [2] Renal disease in which there is increased reabsorption of sodium.
5. Hypernatremia causes edema. Water retention decreases urinary output. (See Chapter 4.)
6. Potassium deficiency (hypokalemia) may occur when there is:
   A. Inadequate dietary intake (unlikely unless there is starvation) or when there is inadequate absorption from the gastrointestinal tract due to intestinal disorders.
   B. Excessive loss of potassium from the body, which may be caused by:
      [1] Excessive loss of gastrointestinal secretions.
      [2] Increased secretion of aldosterone, which increases the excretion of potassium.
      [3] Renal disease in which tubules fail to reabsorb potassium properly.
7. An inadequate amount of potassium in the body results in impaired functioning of muscle tissues (skeletal, cardiac and smooth):
   A. There is general skeletal muscular weakness which may progress to paralysis.
   B. There may be cardiac arrhythmias, and cardiac muscle contractions may become inefficient, leading to dilatation of the heart and eventual cardiac failure.
   C. There is decreased motility of the gastrointestinal tract, leading to distention, vomiting, constipation.
8. A decreased concentration of potassium in the extracellular fluids causes potassium to leave the cells. In the body's attempt to maintain electrical neutrality, sodium and hydrogen ions remain in the cells. Not only is cellular function greatly impaired, but electrolyte and acid-base imbalance result.

9. Potassium excess (hyperkalemia) may occur when there is:
   A. Excessive intake of potassium (by ingestion—possibly of medications—or by infusion).
   B. Decreased excretion of potassium, which may be caused by:
      [1] Decrease in urinary output (e.g., with renal disease or with circulatory shock).
      [2] Decreased secretion of aldosterone, which increases the reabsorption of potassium by renal tubules.
   C. Excessive tissue destruction (e.g., burns), with release of potassium into the extracellular fluids.
10. Hyperkalemia results in mental changes (confusion, apathy), numbness in the extremities, changes in cardiac action and increased motility of the gastrointestinal tract (with abdominal cramping and diarrhea).
11. Calcium deficiency of the extracellular fluids (hypocalcemia) may occur when there is:
    A. Inadequate dietary intake or inadequate absorption from the gastrointestinal tract. (Vitamin D is needed for optimal calcium absorption.)
    B. Decreased secretion of parathyroid hormone in the parathyroid glands. (See Chapter 8.)
    C. Renal disease in which tubules fail to reabsorb calcium properly.
12. A deficiency of calcium in the extracellular fluids causes increased neuromuscular irritability (tetany).
    A. Depending upon the degree of deficit, there may be muscle twitchings, painful tonic muscle spasms or convulsions.
    B. If the laryngeal muscles or respiratory muscles are involved, breathing will be impaired.
13. An excess of calcium in the extracellular fluids may occur when there is:
    A. Excessive intake of Vitamin D.
    B. Increased secretion of parathyroid hormone by the parathyroid glands.
    C. Abnormal breakdown of bone tissue, which may be due to bone disease (e.g., tumor growth) or to prolonged immobilization.
    D. Renal disease with failure to excrete calcium.
14. An abnormally high concentration of calcium in the extracellular fluids may cause muscle weakness, anorexia, nausea and vomiting. If abnormal amounts of calcium are being excreted by the kidney there may be polyuria, as the kidney tries to maintain the calcium in solution. Excessive amounts of calcium in the urine sometimes leads to the development of renal and/or bladder calculi.
15. Pathology related to chlorides and bicarbonate is covered in Chapter 6.

Nursing Care

Nursing care should be directed toward assisting the patient to retain or regain electrolyte balance.

COLLECTION, EVALUATION AND COMMUNICATION OF DATA
1. Patients should be interviewed and observed to identify abnormal intake or loss of fluid from the body.

2. Patients should be interviewed, observed and examined to identify symptoms and signs of electrolyte imbalance. Electrolyte imbalance may be indicated by:
   A. Abnormalities in neuromuscular function (smooth muscle, skeletal muscle, cardiac muscle).
   B. Numbness, tingling in extremities.
   C. Symptoms and signs of fluid imbalance. (See Chapter 4.)
   D. Mental changes, including apathy, confusion and loss of consciousness.
3. Systematic patient evaluation is of especial importance when the patient:
   A. Has actual or potential fluid imbalance.
   B. Has malnutrition.
   C. Has a diagnosed disorder involving:
      [1] Renal function.
      [2] Secretion of adrenocortical hormones.
      [3] Secretion of parathyroid hormone.
   D. Is receiving medication containing electrolytes (e.g., potassium).
   E. Is receiving extended intravenous therapy involving administration of electrolytes.
   F. Is receiving adrenocortical hormone therapy.
4. Data collected should be evaluated not only on the basis of a single deviation from normal (e.g., mental confusion), but also on the basis of combinations of symptoms and signs that tend to occur when there is electrolyte imbalance (i.e., symptoms and signs associated with deficiencies and excesses of specific electrolytes).
5. How, when and what data are communicated to the physician and/or other nursing personnel depend upon:
   A. Any immediate threat to the patient's life processes (e.g., cardiac arrhythmias).
   B. Any potential threat to the patient's life and well-being (e.g., neuromuscular hyperirritability).
   C. Any particular implications for the physician in relation to:
      [1] The patient's progress or lack of progress toward recovery (e.g., change in mental alertness or change in muscle tone).
      [2] Making a diagnosis (e.g., new objective or subjective data).
      [3] The patient's physical and emotional responses to specific diagnostic procedures and therapeutic measures.
   D. Any particular implications for nursing (e.g., regulation of fluid intake).

PROMOTION OF HEALTH AND PREVENTION OF DISEASE/INJURY

1. Health teaching to promote electrolyte balance should be concerned with:
   A. The importance of:
      [1] A balanced, nutritious diet throughout the life cycle.
      [2] An adequate fluid intake.
      [3] Increasing intake of sodium chloride along with increased fluid intake when there is excessive loss of water through sweating.
      [4] Avoiding overdosage of Vitamin D.
   B. The importance of:
      [1] Periodic health evaluations.
      [2] Prompt medical consultation when:

    a. There are problems in which fluid intake is greatly reduced and/or there is abnormal loss of fluid from the body.

    b. There are indications of possible kidney problems.

    c. There is tissue swelling, unusual thirst, rapid gain or loss of weight.

    d. There are abnormalities in muscle functioning (e.g., spasms or weakness).

2. A proper dietary intake should be provided and encouraged. (See Chapter 3.)

3. Fluid balance should be promoted and imbalance prevented. (See Chapter 4.)

4. Parenteral fluids should be administered exactly as prescribed, in relation to the quantity of solution, the type of solution, the rate of flow, the time of administration and so forth. Particular care must be taken in administration of solutions containing potassium so that patients do not receive too much potassium too rapidly.

5. Unless otherwise ordered, isomolar (or isotonic) solutions should be used in performing treatments such as irrigations.

6. When gastric contents are being continuously aspirated, the oral intake of fluid should be restricted to prevent increased loss of chloride.

7. When a patient has a condition in which there is or may be decreased secretion of parathyroid hormone, with resulting hypocalcemia:

    A. Close observations should be made for indications of neuromuscular hyperirritability, and these should be reported promptly.

    B. Appropriate preparations of calcium should be ready for immediate administration.

CARE OF PATIENTS WITH ELECTROLYTE IMBALANCE

1. It is essential that medical orders relative to diet and fluid intake be followed exactly.

2. Accurate measurements (time and amount) of fluid intake and fluid loss must be made, evaluated and reported/recorded appropriately.

3. Actual dietary intake should be observed closely, evaluated and reported/recorded appropriately.

4. Symptoms and signs of fluid imbalance, more advanced electrolyte imbalance and/or acid-base imbalance should be reported promptly.

Chapter 6

Acid-Base Balance

All the cells of the body require a definite pH environment.

Anatomy and Physiology

1. Normal cellular functioning requires an environment with a pH value of 7.4.
   A. Variations of even a few tenths of one percent may be fatal.
   B. To maintain this nearly neutral pH, the acid and base elements of the body fluids must be balanced.
      [1] Acid-base balance is achieved by regulation of the hydrogen ion concentration in the body fluids.
      [2] Most of the carbohydrates and fats that are metabolized are oxidized completely, to form carbon dioxide and water. No excess hydrogen ions are produced from the volatile carbonic acid as long as carbon dioxide is properly eliminated by the lungs.
      [3] Other acid end products of metabolism are organic acids (formed by incomplete oxidation of carbohydrates and fats); sulfuric acid (formed from the oxidation of some amino acids); and phosphoric acid (formed from phosphoprotein substances).
   C. The normal pH of arterial blood is 7.4. Plasma is slightly alkaline because it contains fairly strong bases, including bicarbonate, diphosphate and protein ions.
2. The proper pH of body fluids is maintained by:
   A. The elimination of carbon dioxide in the lungs.
   B. The elimination or retention of certain electrolytes by the kidneys.
   C. The buffering action of various buffer systems, such as those composed of bicarbonate, phosphate and protein.

[1] The bicarbonate buffer system (carbonic acid and bicarbonate) is the most important. The concentration of each compound can be regulated by the respiratory system (carbon dioxide) and the kidneys (bicarbonate).

[2] The phosphate buffer system (acid phosphate and alkaline phosphate) provides important buffering in the kidney tubules as well as intracellularly.

[3] The protein buffer system is especially important in intracellular buffering and may operate either as an acidic or as a basic buffering system.

3. The pH of the plasma depends upon the ratio between the concentration of carbonic acid and the concentration of bicarbonate. Rapid adjustment of this ratio may be brought about by changes in the rate and depth of respiration, by certain compensatory chemical shifts in the blood and by the elimination or retention of certain electrolytes (e.g., bicarbonate, chlorides) by the kidneys.

A. The rate of alveolar ventilation affects the hydrogen ion concentration of the body fluids (by the retention or elimination of carbon dioxide), and the hydrogen ion concentration of the body fluids affects the rate of alveolar ventilation.

[1] The normal partial pressure of carbon dioxide is maintained by the balance achieved between the rate at which carbon dioxide is produced in the tissues and the rate at which the lungs eliminate it from the body.

[2] The rate of pulmonary ventilation is regulated by the respiratory center, to keep the partial pressure of carbon dioxide at approximately 40 mm. of Hg.

    a. An increase in the arterial pressure of carbon dioxide to 50 mm. of Hg can increase ventilation as much as 4 times.

    b. If the pressure of carbon dioxide falls below the normal value, the rate of ventilation can be decreased as much as 50 percent.

B. The kidneys regulate hydrogen concentration primarily by regulating the concentration of bicarbonate in the body fluids.

[1] Regulation is accomplished by the kidney tubules through the secretion of hydrogen ions and ammonia and the reabsorption of sodium.

[2] In regulating acid-base balance, the kidneys may excrete urine at a pH as low as 4.5 or as high as 8.0.

C. The ratio of bicarbonate ions to dissolved carbon molecules increases as the pH rises above 7.4. Normally this causes increased excretion of bicarbonate, which decreases the bicarbonate portion of the bicarbonate buffer system. This shifts the pH of the body fluids toward the acid side.

D. The ratio of carbon dioxide molecules to bicarbonate ions increases as the pH falls below 7.4. Normally this causes increased excretion of hydrogen ions and decreased excretion of bicarbonate ions. This increases the bicarbonate portion of the bicarbonate buffer system, and there is a shift of the pH in the alkaline direction. Excess hydrogen ions are eliminated in the urine, in combination with phosphates and ammonia which is secreted by the renal tubules. (Ammonium ions combine with chloride to form ammonium chloride.)

4. The alkali reserve in the blood represents the amount of base in the blood that is available for the neutralization of fixed acids (e.g., sulphuric acid, lactic acid, hydrochloric acid).

A. Practically all estimations of acid-base balance are based upon the analysis of the bicarbonate buffer system.

B.   The normal carbon dioxide combining power of plasma (essentially a measure of plasma bicarbonate) is 28 millimoles per liter.
5. Hydrochloric acid is produced by gastric glands.
6. The intestinal digestive juices (succus entericus, pancreatic juice and bile) are all highly alkaline.

Chemistry

1. The pH of a solution is equal to the negative logarithm of the hydrogen ion concentration. The pH of 7.0 is neutral; a pH above 7.0 is alkaline; a pH below 7.0 is acidic.
2. An acid-base buffer is a solution of 2 or more chemical compounds (generally a weak acid and the salt of that acid) which prevents any marked change in its hydrogen ion concentration when small amounts of an acid or a base are added to it.

Pathology

SYMPTOMS AND SIGNS

1. Symptoms and signs of respiratory acidosis (or acute hypercapnia) include a progressive loss of consciousness and, possibly, tremors.
2. Symptoms and signs of respiratory alkalosis (or hypocapnia) are most frequently related to symptoms and signs of hyperventilation and include:
   A.   Numbness of the extremities.
   B.   Tonic muscle spasm; possibly, convulsions.
   C.   Sensation of light-headedness, nervousness.
   D.   Loss of consciousness.
3. Symptoms and signs of metabolic acidosis depend largely upon the cause of the acidosis.
   A.   General symptoms and signs of metabolic acidosis are:
       [1] Deep and rapid respirations (forced breathing, sometimes referred to as Kussmaul breathing).
       [2] Increased urinary output.
       [3] Progressive loss of consciousness.
   B.   When the acidosis is associated with uncontrolled diabetes mellitus, acetone appears in the urine and is also eliminated through the lungs. It has a typical odor.
4. Symptoms and signs of metabolic alkalosis depend primarily upon the cause of the alkalosis. Frequently, there are symptoms and signs associated with hypokalemia, including:
   A.   Muscle weakness or paralysis.
   B.   Abdominal distention.
   C.   Cardiac arrhythmias.

ACIDOSIS

1. Acidosis (or acidemia) is a condition in which the pH of the arterial blood falls below 7.4.
   A.   In very severe cases, the pH may fall as low as 7.0. A pH of 6.8 is incompatible with life.
   B.   Acidosis that is related to carbon dioxide is referred to as respiratory; acidosis that is not related to carbon dioxide is referred to as metabolic.
2. Any factor that decreases the rate of pulmonary ventilation, leading to an increased

concentration of carbonic acid in the blood and an increase in hydrogen ions in the extracellular fluids, can be a cause of respiratory acidosis.

  A. Causes of respiratory acidosis include:
    [1] Pulmonary disease (e.g., emphysema).
    [2] Depression of the respiratory center (e.g., by drugs).
    [3] Injury to the respiratory center.
    [4] Disorders of the respiratory muscles.
    [5] Airway obstruction.
  B. Hypercapnia causes depression of the central nervous system. There is drowsiness and progressive loss of consciousness.
  C. Voluntary breath-holding can cause the arterial pH to fall as low as 7.1—temporarily.

3. Metabolic acidosis occurs when there are increased hydrogen ions in the extracellular fluids or a reduced pH due to acids other than carbonic acid.

  A. Possible causes of metabolic acidosis include:
    [1] Diabetic ketoacidosis. (When it is necessary for fatty acids to be oxidized for energy [instead of glucose], acetoacetic acid, beta-hydroxybutyric acid and acetone are formed. The more acids that are produced, the more neutralization required. This reduces the alkaline reserve. Acetone is eliminated both in the urine and through the lungs.)
    [2] Renal insufficiency which causes an accumulation of nitrogenous waste products in the blood (azotemic renal failure).
    [3] Lactic acidosis (usually associated with hypoxia).
    [4] Drug intoxication (e.g., salicylates, methyl alcohol, paraldehyde).
    [5] Excessive loss of alkaline fluids from the gastrointestinal tract (e.g., through diarrhea or draining fistulae).
  B. Effects of metabolic acidosis include:
    [1] Excretion of a more acidic urine (pH of less than 5.0), as chlorides and other acid substances are eliminated.
    [2] A reduction in the concentration of plasma bicarbonate (because it is used to neutralize acidic substances and then eliminated in the urine).
    [3] The loss of sodium in the urine, which causes disturbance in electrolyte balance.
    [4] Diuresis, which occurs as a direct result of increased requirements for elimination and the loss of sodium.
    [5] Stimulation of the respiratory center, due to the changed ratio between carbonic acid and bicarbonate in the plasma. (Deep and rapid respirations result as the body attempts to rid itself of carbon dioxide and reestablish a balance between carbonic acid and bicarbonate.)
    [6] Depression of the central nervous system as the pH falls.

ALKALOSIS

1. Alkalosis (or alkalemia) is a condition in which there is increased alkalinity of the blood, above a pH of 7.45.
  A. In severe cases the pH may rise as high as 7.8. Such an extreme variation in pH almost always causes death.
  B. Alkalosis that is related to carbon dioxide is referred to as respiratory; alkalosis that is not related to carbon dioxide is referred to as metabolic.

2. Any factor that increases pulmonary ventilation, leading to a decreased concentration of carbonic acid and hydrogen ions in the extracellular fluids, can be a cause of respiratory alkalosis.
   A. Possible causes of respiratory alkalosis include:
      [1] Hypoxia (e.g., due to right or left shunts in congenital heart disease or to congestive heart failure).
      [2] Psychogenic hyperventilation (e.g., in hysteria, anxiety states).
      [3] Hypermetabolic states (e.g., fever, thyrotoxicosis).
      [4] Injury of the respiratory center.
   B. Overbreathing can cause a temporary increase in pH as high as 7.8.
   C. Possible effects of respiratory alkalosis include:
      [1] Dizziness.
      [2] Increased neuromuscular irritability.
3. Metabolic alkalosis occurs when there is an elevation of the plasma bicarbonate concentration and an alkaline arterial pH.
   A. Possible causes of metabolic alkalosis include:
      [1] Loss of hydrochloric acid from the stomach (e.g., through vomiting or gastric aspiration).
      [2] Chloride depletion, which may result from:
         a. Loss of chlorides from the gastrointestinal tract.
         b. Diuretic therapy.
      [3] Excessive intake of alkaline foods or drugs (e.g., sodium bicarbonate for gastric disturbances).
   B. Effects of metabolic alkalosis include:
      [1] Excretion of an alkaline urine (pH above 7.4), as the kidney excretes more bicarbonate.
      [2] Loss of sodium and potassium in the urine, causing additional disturbance in electrolyte balance.
      [3] Diuresis, which occurs with the increased excretion of sodium.
      [4] Loss of potassium, which causes symptoms and signs of hypokalemia. (See Chapter 5.)
      [5] A changed ratio between carbonic acid and bicarbonate in the blood that depresses the respiratory center and causes slow, shallow respirations. There may be periods of apnea and then hyperpnea, depending upon the concentration of carbonic acid.
      [6] Loss of consciousness results when the increase in blood alkalinity is enough to cause injury to the brain cells.

Nursing Care

Nursing care should be directed toward assisting the patient to retain or regain acid-base balance.

COLLECTION, EVALUATION AND COMMUNICATION OF DATA
1. Patients should be interviewed, observed and examined to identify symptoms and signs of acid-base imbalance. Imbalance may be indicated by:
   A. Abnormal breathing patterns.
   B. Loss of consciousness.

   C. Symptoms and signs associated with potassium deficiency or excess. (See Chapter 5.)
2. Systematic patient evaluation is of critical importance when the patient:
   A. Has impaired respiratory and/or circulatory function with resultant hypoxia.
   B. Has impaired respiratory function resulting in inadequate alveolar ventilation.
   C. Has excessive loss of fluids from the gastrointestinal tract.
   D. Has uncontrolled diabetes mellitus.
   E. Has renal insufficiency.
3. Data collected should be evaluated not only on the basis of a single deviation from normal (e.g., abnormal breathing pattern) but also on the basis of combinations of symptoms and signs that tend to occur when there is acid-base imbalance (e.g., symptoms and signs associated with diabetic acidosis).
4. How, when and what data are communicated to the physician and/or other nursing personnel depend upon:
   A. Any immediate threat to the patient's life processes (e.g., progressive loss of consciousness).
   B. Any potential threat to the patient's life and well-being (e.g., polyuria).
   C. Any particular implications for the physician in relation to:
      [1] The patient's progress or lack of progress toward recovery (e.g., change in character of respirations).
      [2] Making a diagnosis (e.g., new objective or subjective data).
      [3] The patient's physical and emotional responses to specific diagnostic procedures or therapeutic measures.
   D. Any particular implications for nursing care (e.g., need for accurate record of fluid intake and fluid loss).

PROMOTION OF HEALTH AND PREVENTION
OF DISEASE/INJURY

1. Health teaching to promote acid-base balance should be concerned with:
   A. The importance of:
      [1] A nutritious, balanced diet throughout the life cycle.
      [2] Avoiding continued or excessive use of sodium bicarbonate for gastric distress.
   B. The avoidance of hyperventilation.
   C. The importance of prompt medical consultation when:
      [1] There is abnormal loss of fluid from vomiting and/or diarrhea.
      [2] There are indications of possible kidney problems.
      [3] There are persistent gastric disturbances.
2. A nutritious, balanced dietary intake should be provided and encouraged. An inadequate dietary intake should be reported appropriately.
3. Fluid and electrolyte imbalances should be prevented. (See Chapters 4 and 5.)
4. The best possible cardiac function should be promoted. (See Chapter 1.)
5. The best possible respiratory function should be promoted. (See Chapter 2.)
6. Parenteral fluids should be administered exactly as prescribed—in relation to the quantity of solution, the type of solution, the rate of flow, the time of administration and so forth. Particular care must be taken in administration of solutions containing ammonium chloride, so a patient does not receive too much of this acidic drug too fast.

7. Patients should be assisted to control their breathing so as to prevent hyperventilation or hypoventilation.
8. Patients with diabetes mellitus or renal insufficiency should be properly counselled in relation to:
    A. The importance of adhering conscientiously to medical orders relative to diet, medications, fluid intake, urine testing, exercise and so forth.
    B. The importance of obtaining prompt medical consultation when problems with any of the above arise or when there are traumatic injuries, infections or other stress-producing conditions.
9. When gastric contents are being continuously aspirated, the oral intake of fluid should be restricted to prevent increased loss of chloride and hydrogen ions.

CARE OF PATIENTS WITH ACID-BASE IMBALANCE

1. When a patient has acid-base imbalance:
    A. This represents a medical emergency.
        [1] Equipment for intravenous administration of appropriate parenteral fluids (acidic, alkaline, electrolytes) should be ready.
        [2] It is essential that requested laboratory tests be performed and reported with all possible haste.
        [3] Nursing care should be provided in relation to the basic cause(s) of the imbalance (e.g., uncontrolled diabetes mellitus, hypoxia, chronic pulmonary obstruction, severe diarrhea).
    B. It is essential that medical orders relative to diet and fluid and electrolyte intake be followed exactly.
    C. Accurate measurements (of time and amount) of fluid intake and fluid loss must be made, evaluated and reported/recorded appropriately.
    D. Urine testing (pH, sugar, acetone) should be performed precisely and reported/recorded appropriately.
    E. Systematic evaluation should be made for indications of fluid imbalance, electrolyte imbalance and more advanced acidosis or alkalosis, and these should be reported appropriately.
2. When a patient has symptoms of respiratory alkalosis, breathing exhaled air from a paper bag for a very brief period may be helpful in increasing the concentration of carbon dioxide in the blood. Carbon dioxide should be available for inhalation as prescribed.

Chapter 7

Elimination

Efficient body functioning requires that food residues and gases be eliminated from the gastrointestinal tract, that urine be eliminated and that toxic substances formed in the body be rendered harmless and/or eliminated.

Anatomy and Physiology

GASTROINTESTINAL ELIMINATION

1. The large intestine is a musculomembranous tube that extends up the right side of the abdominal cavity from the ileocecal valve, across the abdomen and down the left side to end with the anal canal.
   A. The rectum, in the adult, is about 6 to 8 inches long. It extends from the sigmoid flexure to the anus.
   B. The anal canal, approximately an inch in length, has two sphincter muscles. The internal sphincter is smooth muscle; the external sphincter is striated muscle.
2. The functions of the large intestine (colon) are:
   A. Absorption of water and electrolytes from the chyme that enters the colon through the ileocecal valve.
   B. Storage of feces until evacuation occurs.
3. Normally about 450 ml. of chyme enter the cecum daily. All but about 100 ml. is absorbed into the capillaries of the large intestine.
   A. If the body is dehydrated, water absorption in the colon increases.
   B. Retention of feces allows for increased water absorption.
   C. Increased intestinal motility decreases the amount of water absorption.
4. There are 2 types of movements of the colon: mixing movements (that facilitate

absorption) and propulsive or mass movements (that propel the intestinal contents toward the anus).

   A. Movements of the colon are much slower than those of the small intestine.

   B. Movements of the colon are stimulated by:

      [1] Parasympathetic stimulation. (Sympathetic stimulation decreases peristalsis.)

      [2] Local reflex stimulation, caused by factors such as distention, mechanical irritation or chemical irritation. (The effects of different foodstuffs upon motility varies with individuals.)

   C. Normally, mass movements occur only a few times daily. They tend to occur within a short time after eating breakfast or after eating anytime when the stomach has been empty for a prolonged period. They result from reflex actions originating mainly in the duodenum (duodenocolic reflex) but also to some extent in the stomach (gastrocolic reflex).

   D. There may be some atony of the smooth muscle of the large colon:

      [1] In old age.

      [2] When fecal bulk is retained repeatedly.

      [3] When the muscles have been repeatedly overstimulated (e.g., due to mechanical irritation by high-fiber foods or to the chemical irritation of laxatives).

5. The feces normally contain bacteria (mostly dead), sloughed-off epithelial cells, food residues, bile pigments, some mucus and some inorganic salts.

   A. The volume of feces is increased by the intake of indigestible material such as cellulose.

   B. Lack of food intake causes the bulk of feces to be greatly reduced.

   C. Bile pigment gives the feces a brown color.

   D. The color, consistency and odor of feces vary to some extent with the type of food eaten.

      [1] Feces are normally soft and shaped in the cylindrical form of the rectum.

      [2] The odor of feces is due primarily to gases formed in the large intestine by protein putrefaction.

   E. Although some food residues are evacuated within 24 hours after ingestion, most are gradually disposed of over several days.

   F. Meconium is a greenish tarry substance in the intestines of the newborn. It is normally eliminated completely within 2 to 3 days following delivery.

6. The sudden passage of feces into the rectum (due to mass movements) initiates the defecation reflex.

   A. Sensory impulses are relayed to the spinal cord, and peristaltic movement is stimulated by motor nerves.

   B. The internal sphincter relaxes, and (after voluntary control is developed) the external sphincter is relaxed voluntarily.

   C. The contraction of the levator ani muscles pulls the anal canal up over the feces.

   D. Downward pressure can be exerted by contracting the abdominal muscles and the diaphragm against the abdominal organs.

      [1] Flexion of the thighs on the abdomen facilitates the expulsion of feces.

      [2] Downward pressure against the rectum is increased in the sitting position.

E.   A relatively weak defecation reflex may be initiated by using the abdominal muscles and diaphragm to push feces into the rectum.

7. The act of defecation can usually be inhibited by voluntarily constricting the external anal sphincter.
   A.   A child usually has enough neuromuscular development by the age of two to learn to voluntarily control defecation. This development may occur earlier in some children, later in others.
   B.   When defecation is voluntarily prevented, the defecation reflex may disappear after a few minutes and generally does not occur again for many hours.
   C.   The most common cause of constipation is irregular bowel habits, due to continued inhibition of natural defecation reflexes.
8. Bowel movements may normally occur as frequently as several times a day or as infrequently as 2 or 3 times a week.
9. Sensory nerve endings for pain and pressure in the bowel wall are stimulated by smooth muscle spasms and by distention. Prolonged internal pressure exerted against the walls of the rectum may cause headache and lethargy.
10. The gases found in the gastrointestinal tract include:
    A.   Swallowed air (mostly nitrogen and oxygen).
    B.   Gases formed by bacterial action on foodstuffs in the large intestine.
         [1] Putrefaction and fermentation produce carbon dioxide, methane and hydrogen.
         [2] When these gases become mixed with oxygen from swallowed air they can actually become explosive in nature.
         [3] Some foods tend to contribute to gas formation.
    C.   Gases that diffuse from the blood into the gastrointestinal tract.
11. Most of the swallowed air is expelled from the stomach by belching; small amounts may enter the small intestine.
12. In the adult with a normal dietary intake, from 7 to 10 liters of gases are formed in the large intestine each 24 hours. Normally, all but about 0.5 liter is absorbed into the intestinal capillaries.
13. The expelling of large quantities of flatus may indicate:
    A.   An excessive intake of gas-forming foods.
    B.   Increased motility of the large intestine, which decreases the time available for absorption.

RENAL ELIMINATION OF NITROGENOUS WASTES AND OTHER TOXIC SUBSTANCES

1. The kidneys eliminate most of the nitrogenous wastes of cellular metabolism.
   A.   Nitrogenous wastes come from protein metabolism and include organic and inorganic compounds.
        [1] The organic compounds include urea, uric acid and creatinine.
             a. The liver plays a predominant role in the formation of urea.
             b. Sweat contains small amounts of urea.
        [2] The most abundant inorganic compound is ammonia, which is eliminated in ammonium salts.
   B.   Kidney function normally keeps the blood urea nitrogen level below 20 mg. percent.

2. The kidneys also eliminate any excessive ketone bodies formed in the body (associated with oxidation of fatty acids for energy) and excessive amounts of electrolytes.
3. See Chapter 4 for anatomy and physiology related to the kidneys.

ELIMINATION OF URINE
1. Urine, continuously produced by the kidneys (at the rate of 30–50 ml. per hour in the adult), is transported to the urinary bladder by 2 ureters. Gravity and periodic contractions of the ureters serve to move urine into the bladder.
2. The urinary bladder is a musculomembranous sac in which urine is stored before being eliminated from the body.
   A. The bladder is located in the pelvic cavity. It is anterior to the uterus and upper vagina in the female, anterior to the rectum in the male.
   B. The region of the bladder through which both the ureters and urethra pass is called the trigone.
   C. The body of the bladder expands upward as the bladder fills with urine, and the detrusor muscle (the lower main portion of the bladder) contracts to empty the bladder.
   D. The internal sphincter is the trigonal muscle that keeps urine in the bladder until the micturition reflex is initiated.
3. The urethra extends from the bladder to the urinary meatus and transports urine from the bladder to the outside. Surrounding the urethra just below the bladder is a ring of voluntary skeletal muscle called the external sphincter. This muscle normally remains contracted. It can be relaxed through reflex action or voluntarily.
4. The mucous membrane lining of the urinary tract is continuous from the kidney pelvis to the urinary meatus, making possible ascending infections of urinary tract.
5. Micturition (urination) involves the contraction of the detrusor muscle and the opening of the internal and external sphincters.
   A. The bladder wall contains sensory receptors that respond to the rise in pressure exerted on them as the bladder fills. When the volume of urine reaches a point at which the pressure excites the stretch receptors, the micturition reflex is elicited.
      [1] Sensory stimuli travel to the voiding reflex center in the spinal cord.
      [2] Parasympathetic nerves cause contraction of the detrusor muscle and the relaxation of the internal sphincter.
      [3] In the infant or small child the external sphincter is relaxed by involuntary action, and voiding occurs whenever the micturition reflex is initiated.
      [4] After the age of 2 to 3 years neuromuscular development has progressed to the point where higher centers in the cortex are able to control voiding.
         a. The spinal reflex responsible for detrusor contraction and relaxation of the internal sphincter can be inhibited or facilitated by nerve impulses from higher centers.
         b. The external sphincter can be powerfully closed even when the internal sphincter is relaxed and the detrusor muscle contracts.
   B. Once the micturition reflex is initiated it will occur more frequently and more powerfully as the bladder becomes increasingly filled.

C. Voluntary control of micturition requires:
   [1] Perception of the desire to void.
   [2] Ability to inhibit or postpone voiding.
   [3] Ability to initiate micturition voluntarily.
6. Awareness of the need to void normally occurs in the adult when the bladder contains 300–500 ml. of urine. The desire to void may be increased greatly when external pressure is exerted on the bladder or if the bladder or urethra is irritated.
7. A distended bladder can be palpated above the symphysis pubis.
   A. Bladders can be greatly distended. Some adult bladders can hold up to 3,000–4,000 ml. of fluid before the bladder wall begins to tear. Other bladders can contain much less than this.
   B. Continued bladder distention causes loss of bladder tone. Recovery of tone is more likely to occur if excessive internal pressure is reduced gradually.
8. An overflow of urine from the bladder may occur when the pressure caused by the accumulated urine is sufficient to overcome the normal tone of the sphincters. Dribbling of small amounts of urine will continue until the pressure has been decreased enough for sphincter control to be resumed.
9. The prostate gland is a firm body located just below the internal urethral orifice and around the proximal portion of the urethra in the male. The gland produces secretions important in male reproductive functions. This gland may become enlarged in later life, causing difficulty in micturition.

HEPATIC EXCRETION OF BILE AND DETOXIFICATION
1. The liver excretes bile continually. Approximately 600–700 ml. are produced daily. In addition to secreting or excreting bile salts, cholesterol, water and electrolytes in the bile, the liver excretes bilirubin. (The biliary system is covered in Chapter 3.)
   A. Bilirubin is the pigment formed from the heme portion of erythrocytes when they undergo disintegration.
   B. Bile pigment eliminated by the gastrointestinal tract is responsible for the normal brown color of feces.
   C. Small amounts of bile pigment are also eliminated in urine, giving urine a pale yellow color.
2. The liver deaminizes protein substances (e.g., from the globin portion of disintegrated erythrocytes and from cellular breakdown) and converts the amine radical (NH_2) to urea, which is excreted by the kidneys.
3. Kupffer's cells, in the liver, detoxify the toxic substances that are formed from protein putrefaction in the large intestine and absorbed into the blood.

ELIMINATION OF CARBON DIOXIDE
1. Carbon dioxide, a waste product of carbohydrate metabolism, is carried to the lungs by the plasma and red blood cells as bicarbonate, as carbonic acid, and in combined form with hemoglobin.
2. Under normal conditions the partial pressure of carbon dioxide in the alveoli of the lungs is less than that in the venous blood. The carbon dioxide is released from the various compounds and diffuses into the alveoli. It is exhaled during the expiratory phase of respiration.

Physics

1. Pressure is the force exerted on a unit area.
2. Fluids flow from an area of higher pressure to one of lower pressure, and the rate of volume flow is directly related to the pressure gradient.

Chemistry

1. The human digestive system does not have appropriate enzymes for the digestion of cellulose.
2. Fermentation is a chemical process in which carbohydrates are decomposed by the action of microorganisms. Carbon dioxide and hydrogen are formed in the process.
3. Putrefaction is a chemical process in which proteins are decomposed by the action of microorganisms; several gaseous products are produced (e.g., hydrogen sulfide).
4. The chemical breakdown of hemoglobin in the formation of bile pigment involves the breakdown of heme to bilirubin (red), which can be oxidized to biliverdin (green), which can, in turn, be reduced to sterobilin (brown). Sterobilin gives the normal brown color to feces.

Pathology

INADEQUATE GASTROINTESTINAL ELIMINATION

1. Symptoms and signs of inadequate elimination of gases and food residues from the gastrointestinal tract include:
   A. Headache, general malaise, anorexia.
   B. Abdominal pain, cramping (which may be severe).
   C. Feeling of rectal fullness.
   D. Abdominal distention.
   E. Elimination of small amounts of dry, hard feces or absence of defecation.
   F. Stools of very narrow caliber.
   G. Elimination of small amounts of liquid feces.
   H. Symptoms and signs of large intestine obstruction (complete constipation, cramping abdominal pain, increasing abdominal distention, vomiting of fecal material and indications of fluid and electrolyte imbalance).
2. Constipation may be chronic or acute and is characterized by the absence of defecation or the passage of hard, dry stools. It may be caused by:
   A. Problems involving the nervous control of evacuation.
      [1] Imbalance between parasympathetic and sympathetic stimulation, frequently associated with emotional stress, may cause excessive tonus of the colon. The colon may be referred to as being spastic or irritable; smooth muscle spasms prevent normal movements of the tract.
      [2] Retention of feces may be related to:
         a. Psychic disturbances, possibly from bowel training in childhood.
         b. Time pressures of daily living, which cause persons to ignore natural defecation reflexes.
         c. Voluntary retention because of pain associated with defecation (e.g., due to hemorrhoids, anal fissure, recent rectal surgery).

[3] There may be injury to the afferent or efferent nerves involved in defecation (e.g., due to spinal cord tumors or various degenerative disorders involving the brain, spinal cord or peripheral nerves).

[4] Megacolon is a congenital anomaly which may cause constipation. Parasympathetic ganglia are absent in a section of the bowel, and this prevents normal motility. Fecal content is retained, and there is bowel distention.

[5] Mental depression may result in decreased motility.

[6] Certain drugs (e.g., opiates, anticholinergics) depress motility of the gastrointestinal tract by decreasing nervous stimulation.

B. Problems interfering with normal local reflex stimulation of movements of the colon.

[1] An inadequate intake of food and/or inadequate fiber in the diet prevents normal mechanical stimulation.

[2] Overstimulation of the colon by mechanical or chemical irritation can result in loss of normal bowel bone (e.g., excessive intake of bran or repeated use of laxatives).

[3] Injury of the abdominal or pelvic viscera (e.g., due to trauma or infections) may result in loss of normal motility of the intestinal tract.

C. Inadequate fluid intake. (See Chapter 4.)

D. Blocking. Movement of fecal contents through the colon and defecation may be blocked by:

[1] Compression of the colon by abnormal growths, ascites, pregnant uterus.

[2] Inflammatory response of intestinal walls, resulting in edema, smooth muscle spasm, scarring.

[3] Abnormal growths within the lumen.

[4] Accumulation of gas in pockets.

[5] Strangulated hernias, volvulus.

[6] Fecal impactions.

[7] Rectoceles.

[8] Imperforate anus.

E. Problems interfering with effective use of voluntary muscles used in normal defecation, including:

[1] General physical weakness.

[2] Lack of proper exercise.

[3] Paralysis.

[4] Ascites.

[5] Pregnancy.

[6] Abdominal, pelvic or perineal surgery.

F. Problems resulting in weakness of smooth muscle contractions within the gut wall.

[1] Potassium deficiency decreases neuromuscular function of the intestinal tract. (See Chapter 5.)

[2] Degenerative changes in smooth muscle that are associated with the aging process may cause weakening of muscle contractions.

[3] Distention of the tract, due to accumulation of fecal contents and gases, prevents effective muscle contractions.

3. Hemorrhoids are dilated, congested and sometimes thrombosed hemorrhoidal

veins. They may occur internally or externally. They may be a result of many factors such as poor venous return (e.g., during pregnancy), straining with defecation or congenital weakness of the veins. They may cause itching or rectal discomfort and may become extremely painful, especially during and following defecation.

4. An anal fissure is an ulceration of the anal wall. It is irritating, painful and often becomes infected, leading to abscess formation. This, in turn, may lead to the formation of an anal fistula.

5. A fecal impaction is a large hard mass of feces that fills and obstructs the rectal vault. Sometimes small amounts of liquid feces seep around the impaction and are expelled.

6. A rectocele is an outpouching of the rectum and vaginal wall into the vagina. The condition is frequently associated with muscle injury sustained during childbirth.

7. Excessive swallowing of air may occur when there is nausea, sipping of fluids or chewing of gum.

RENAL FAILURE AND UREMIA

1. Symptoms and signs of renal failure and associated uremia include:
   A. Oliguria with low specific gravity (an adult output of less than 500 ml. in a 24–hour period).
   B. Anuria (an adult output of less than 300 ml. in a 24–hour period).
   C. Presence of uremic "frost" (crystals of urea) and odor of urine on the skin.
   D. Loss of consciousness.
   E. Symptoms and signs of fluid, electrolyte and acid-base imbalances. (See Chapters 4, 5 and 6.)

2. Uremia is a clinical syndrome in which there is a marked elevation of nitrogenous waste products (primarily urea) in the blood. The condition accompanies renal failure.
   A. The increased concentration of waste products becomes toxic to body cells. There is loss of consciousness, which is related to the accompanying electrolyte and acid-base imbalance and probably is related to some extent to the uremic state.
   B. Because urea cannot be eliminated by the kidneys, increased amounts are excreted in sweat. Urea crystals can sometimes be observed as tiny white particles on the skin, and there is an odor of urine.

URINE RETENTION

1. Symptoms and signs of urine retention include:
   A. Absence of voiding, voiding frequently in small amounts (possible nocturia) and slowing of urinary stream.
   B. Palpable bladder.
   C. Discomfort in bladder area, possibly severe pain.
   D. Restlessness.
   E. Symptoms and signs of urinary infection, which may result from urinary stasis and retention (e.g., burning sensation during and after voiding, urgency, frequency, lower back pain).

2. Possible causes of urinary retention include:
   A. Ureteral or urethral strictures, which may be acquired or congenital. Strictures

may be acquired through injury (e.g., trauma or infection) that results in scarring.

B. Urinary calculi.

    [1] Stasis of urine predisposes to calculi formation.

    [2] Mineral substances excreted in the urine may tend to precipitate in a particular pH environment (e.g., calcium tends to precipitate in alkaline urine).

    [3] Hypercalcemia, which may be caused by excessive mobilization of calcium from the bone, leads to an increased loss of calcium in the urine.

        a. Hypercalcemia may occur because of immobilization or hyperparathyroidism or may be due to fractures.

        b. An increased concentration of calcium in the urine plus urinary stasis predispose to the formation of calcium calculi.

    [4] Small renal calculi may not cause symptoms, but ureteral calculi cause severe pain and there may be hematuria due to traumatic injury to the ureteral wall.

    [5] Calculi may form in the bladder due to bladder infections or retention of urine.

C. Compression of the urinary tract (e.g., by prostatic enlargement in males).

D. Inflammatory edema or abnormal growths within the tract.

E. Local injuries to the bladder wall or to muscles involved with micturition (e.g., may occur in relation to childbirth or gynecologic surgery).

F. Injury to sensory and/or motor nerves that are involved in micturition (e.g., spinal cord injury).

3. Enlargement of the prostate gland may be due to:

A. Inflammatory edema.

B. Benign hypertrophy (which may occur in the aging process).

C. Tumor growth.

4. A cystocele is a downward displacement of the bladder and vaginal wall into the vagina. It may be caused by injuries related to childbirth. Bladder function is impaired.

5. Accumulation of urine in the kidney causes a condition of hydronephrosis. The kidney tubules, calyces and pelvis are distended, and the compression causes damage to renal tissue.

IMPAIRED LIVER FUNCTION AND JAUNDICE

1. Symptoms and signs of impaired liver function includes those related to:

A. Inadequate nutrition. (See Chapter 3.)

B. Fluid and electrolyte imbalance. (See Chapters 4 and 5.)

C. Impaired blood clotting. (See Chapter 1.)

D. Jaundice.

    [1] Yellowing of sclera, skin and mucous membranes.

    [2] Clay-colored stools.

    [3] Dark brown urine.

E. Mental changes, with progressive loss of consciousness. (This may be caused by injury to brain cells from increased concentration of nitrogenous metabolites in the blood).

2. Jaundice is a condition in which bile pigments accumulate in body tissues and fluids. This accumulation may be due to an excessive breakdown of erythrocytes, impaired excretion of bile pigment or obstruction in the biliary system.
   A. Reduced excretion of bile pigment may be caused by liver disease.
   B. Inadequate elimination of bile pigment through the gastrointestinal tract may be due to obstruction in the biliary system. Obstruction may be caused by gallstones, parasites, neoplasms, strictures, spasms, inflammatory edema or adhesions.
   C. The back pressure of bile within the liver can result in impairment of liver function and damage to hepatic cells.

INADEQUATE ELIMINATION OF CARBON DIOXIDE
1. Inadequate elimination of carbon dioxide in the lungs causes respiratory acidosis.
2. See Chapter 6 for pathology related to respiratory acidosis.

Nursing Care

Nursing care should be directed toward assisting the patient to attain, retain or regain:
- **proper elimination of food residues and gases from the gastrointestinal tract.**
- **proper elimination of urine.**
- **the best possible respiratory, renal and hepatic functions.**

(Nursing Care in this chapter has been subdivided into 3 separate sections, according to the 3 nursing care goals indicated above.)

PROPER GASTROINTESTINAL ELIMINATION
Collection, Evaluation and Communication of Data

1. Patients should be interviewed, observed and examined to identify symptoms and signs of inadequate elimination from the gastrointestinal tract. Elimination problems may be indicated by:
   A. Symptoms and signs of constipation.
   B. Symptoms and signs of obstruction of the large intestine.
2. Systematic patient evaluation is of especial importance when the patient:
   A. Has a diagnosed disorder that involves or may affect bowel function.
   B. Has a disorder involving or affecting the muscles used for normal defecation.
   C. Has had abdominal, pelvic or perineal surgery.
   D. Has been or is receiving drugs that decrease motility of the intestinal tract.
   E. Has a restricted dietary and/or fluid intake.
   F. Has a condition resulting in immobility.
   G. Is dependent upon others for physical care (e.g., because of loss of consciousness, psychic disorders, mental retardation).
   H. Has a history of chronic constipation.
   I. Is an infant (especially newborn), a small child or elderly.
3. The elimination of feces should be evaluated in relation to:

A.   The individual's usual pattern for bowel evacuation.

B.   The amount and type of diet.

C.   The state of fluid balance.

D.   Indications of possible constipation (e.g., passage of only small amounts of liquid feces).

4.   Feces should be evaluated in relation to consistency, number of stools, color, odor and presence of abnormal constituents.

A.   Specimens of abnormal stools should be saved for inspection.

B.   Stool abnormalities should be evaluated on the basis of:

[1]   The patient's diagnosed disorder (e.g., a patient with biliary obstruction would not be expected to have brown feces).

[2]   Dietary intake (amount and type).

[3]   Any drugs that might cause a change in the character of feces.

5.   Flatus should be observed in relation to the amount and odor. Excessive amounts of flatus and/or particularly foul-smelling flatus should be reported.

6.   Data collected should be evaluated not only on the basis of a single deviation from normal (e.g., passage of small amounts of liquid feces) but also on the basis of combinations of symptoms and signs that tend to occur when there is inadequate elimination of feces and gases from the gastrointestinal tract.

7.   How, when and what data are communicated to the physician and/or other nursing personnel depend upon:

A.   Any potential threat to the patient's life and well-being (e.g., indications of lower intestinal obstruction).

B.   Any particular implications for the physician in relation to:

[1]   The patient's progress or lack of progress toward recovery (e.g., passage of flatus).

[2]   Making a diagnosis (e.g., new objective or subjective data).

[3]   The patient's physical and emotional responses to specific diagnostic procedures and therapeutic measures.

C.   Any particular implications for nursing (e.g., special bowel training).

Promotion of Health and Prevention of Disease/Injury

1.   Health teaching to promote efficient elimination from the gastrointestinal tract should be concerned with:

A.   The importance of:

[1]   A balanced dietary intake that provides ample fiber content.

[2]   Regular mealtimes.

[3]   Establishing and maintaining a regular time for elimination, utilizing natural defecation reflexes and providing enough time for complete evacuation.

[4]   An adequate fluid intake.

[5]   A balanced program of exercise throughout the life cycle.

[6]   Avoiding prolonged emotional stress.

[7]   Learning to cope with unavoidable emotional stress.

[8]   Avoiding a diet excessively high in roughage (e.g., overuse of bran).

[9]   Avoiding use of any harsh laxative or repeated use of laxatives or enemas.

B.   Normal variations in bowel patterns.
C.   Significance of the relationship between bowel training in early childhood and development of proper bowel habits.
D.   Safe and effective methods of administering enemas.
E.   The importance of:
[1]   Periodic health evaluations.
[2]   Proper obstetrical care.
[3]   Prompt medical attention if constipation occurs frequently or occurs suddenly.
2. A nutritious, balanced dietary intake with ample fiber should be provided and encouraged, within medical orders. Dietary orders relative to fiber content or residue of diet should be carefully followed.
3. An adequate fluid intake should be provided and encouraged.
4. Regularity of bowel habits should be promoted. This may include a carefully planned and implemented program of bowel training.
5. Every effort should be made to assist patients with bowel elimination promptly when the urge to defecate is felt.
A.   Patients may need to be encouraged to ask for assistance when the reflex occurs.
B.   Patients should be helped (within medical orders) into a position as close to sitting as possible.
6. Patients should be provided adequate time for evacuation.
7. Patients should be provided as much emotional comfort as possible in relation to defecation, to promote relaxation and prevent tension. (Provision of privacy and positive attitudes on the part of the nurse may be very important in preventing embarrassment and anxiety.)
8. Physical discomforts should be relieved as much as possible. This is especially important when the patient has a disorder involving the rectum or anus or has had abdominal, pelvic or perineal surgery.
9. Physical exercise should be encouraged and provided within medical orders.
10. Flatulence may be prevented by:
A.   Encouraging and providing a well-balanced diet, including adequate fiber content.
B.   Restricting intake of food that is known to be particularly gas-forming.
C.   Discouraging drinking of carbonated beverages.
D.   Discouraging the swallowing of air (e.g., from sipping fluids, gum-chewing or excessive belching).
E.   Helping an infant to bring up swallowed air during and after feedings.

Care of Patients with Specific Gastrointestinal Problems

1. When constipation occurs:
A.   Foods that tend to have a laxative effect for the individual may be encouraged (within dietary orders).
B.   Fluids should be encouraged (within medical orders).
C.   Possible emotional components should be recognized, handled with appropriate nursing measures and reported appropriately.

D. Enemas should be administered effectively as frequently as ordered and needed.

2. Flatulence may be decreased by:
   A. Encouraging the voluntary expelling of gas through the rectum, unless this is contraindicated by certain types of surgeries or treatments.
   B. Providing optimal position for expelling of gas (e.g., sitting position for belching of gas and expelling of flatus, possibly knee-chest position for expelling of flatus).
   C. Increasing physical activity, as possible.
   D. Changing positions frequently (within medical orders).
   E. The effective use of rectal tube or enemas as prescribed and needed.

3. When a patient has a colostomy and irrigations are ordered:
   A. These should be done as close to the same time each day as possible.
   B. The irrigations should be done as effectively as possible to provide for proper emptying of the colon. Factors that affect effectiveness include: amount of fluid injected, the rate and force of injection and time allowed for drainage.

4. When gastric or intestinal suction is used:
   A. Appropriate suction must be maintained.
   B. Drainage must be evaluated systematically, and any abnormalities (e.g., amount or character) should be reported promptly.
   C. No food or fluids should be given by mouth unless there are specific medical orders.

5. Care of patients with intestinal obstruction is included in Chapter 3.

PROPER ELIMINATION OF URINE
Collection, Evaluation and Communication of Data

1. Patients should be interviewed, observed and examined to identify symptoms and signs of urine retention.
2. Systematic patient evaluation is of especial importance when the patient:
   A. Has a diagnosed disorder involving:
      [1] The ureters, bladder or urethra (e.g., infections, obstructions).
      [2] The neuromuscular control of micturition (e.g., spinal cord injury).
   B. Has sustained injury (or possible injury) to ureters, bladder, urethra, or voluntary muscles important for proper micturition.
   C. Is immobilized.
   D. Is a newborn.
   E. Is a male over 50 years of age.
   F. Is dependent upon others for physical care (e.g., because of age, loss of consciousness, psychic disorders, mental retardation).
   G. Has a ureteral catheter or indwelling urethral catheter.
3. Data collected should be evaluated not only on the basis of a single deviation from normal (e.g., frequent voiding of small amounts of urine) but also on the basis of combinations of symptoms and signs that tend to occur when there is urinary retention.
4. How, when and what data are communicated to the physician and/or other nursing personnel depend upon:
   A. Any potential threat to the patient's life and well-being (e.g., indications of acute urinary retention).

   B. Any particular implications for the physician in relation to:
      [1] The patient's progress or lack of progress toward normal urination.
      [2] The patient's physical and emotional responses to specific diagnostic procedures and therapeutic measures.
   C. Any particular implications for nursing (e.g., special rehabilitative needs).

Promotion of Health and Prevention of Disease/Injury

1. Health teaching to promote proper elimination of urine should be concerned with the importance of:
   A. Periodic health evaluations.
   B. Proper obstetrical care.
   C. Prompt medical consultation when there are abnormalities in urination. (Especially important for men over age of 50 years.)
2. An adequate fluid intake should be provided and encouraged.
3. Micturition may be facilitated by:
   A. Providing for as close to normal voiding position as possible.
   B. Providing physical comfort which promotes muscle relaxation (e.g., by proper positioning with support).
   C. Providing emotional comfort which promotes muscle relaxation (e.g., by providing privacy and demonstrating a positive, reassuring attitude.)
   D. Promoting relaxation of perineal muscles (in the female) by local application of heat (e.g., a sitz bath, if allowed).
   E. Having the patient listen to the sound of running water.
4. Catheterization should be performed promptly when ordered and needed.
   A. Surgical aseptic technique must be maintained.
   B. A distended bladder should be emptied gradually and should not be emptied completely at once if it has been greatly distended.
5. When a patient is immobilized, has sustained fractures or has hyperparathyroidism, the formation of urinary calculi may be prevented by:
   A. Providing and encouraging a large, fluid intake to dilute the urine (within medical orders).
   B. Providing and encouraging an upright position as much as possible and/or frequent position changes to prevent urine stasis (within medical orders).
   C. Providing and encouraging a regular program of exercise to limit mobilization of calcium from bone.
   D. Providing and encouraging an acid-ash diet to decrease the pH of urine.
6. When a patient has a tube draining urine from the urinary tract, it is essential that the tube be kept patent.
   A. Any problem with drainage should be investigated and dealt with promptly.
   B. Urethral catheters should not be clamped without specific orders to do so.
      [1] Orders should include the frequency and period of time the catheter can be clamped.
      [2] When a urethral catheter is clamped, this fact should be known by persons caring for that patient.
      [3] If a urethral catheter is clamped, the patient should be watched closely fo indications of urinary retention.

C.   Fluid intake and urinary output should be measured accurately and reported/recorded appropriately.

Care of Patients with Acute Urinary Retention

1.   When a patient has acute urinary retention, this is a medical emergency.
2.   Preparation should be made for immediate catheterization.

BEST POSSIBLE RESPIRATORY, RENAL
AND HEPATIC FUNCTIONS

1.   See Nursing Care in Chapter 2 in regard to respiratory function.
2.   See Nursing Care in Chapter 3 in regard to hepatic function.
3.   See Nursing Care in Chapters 4, 5 and 6 in regard to renal function.
4.   The following nursing care is in addition to the care identified in the above chapters.

Care of Patients with Specific Respiratory, Renal and Hepatic Problems

1.   The care of patients with respiratory acidosis is identified in Chapter 6.
2.   When a patient has uremia:
     A.   Fluid output must be measured accurately and reported/recorded properly.
     B.   Systematic patient evaluation should be made for indications of changes in fluid, electrolyte, and acid-base imbalances (including changes in level of consciousness).
3.   When a patient has impaired hepatic function, and toxic substances are not being properly detoxified:
     A.   Dietary orders pertaining to protein intake must be followed exactly.
     B.   Physical and emotional rest should be provided and encouraged, to decrease the metabolic rate.
     C.   Some drugs may be definitely contraindicated.

Chapter 8

Enzymes and Hormones

Normal body functioning depends upon the presence of certain enzymes and hormones.

Anatomy and Physiology

ENZYMES

1. Enzymes are organic catalysts produced by a living organism. The production of enzymes depends upon proper nutrition and metabolic processes. (See Chapter 3.)
2. Enzyme systems play essential roles in catalyzing biochemical reactions involved in such processes as:
   A. The digestion and absorption of foodstuffs.
   B. The metabolism of carbohydrates, fats and proteins.
   C. Active transport through cell membranes.
   D. Transmission of nerve impulses.
   E. Muscle contractions.
   F. Blood clotting.

HORMONES

1. Hormones are chemical regulators, secreted by a cell or a group of cells (endocrine glands), that affect the functioning of other body cells. Hormones are secreted into the body fluids and are carried by the blood to the tissues they affect.
2. The hypophysis, or pituitary gland, lies in the sella turcica of the sphenoid bone, at the base of the brain. It is connected with the hypothalamus by the hypophyseal or pituitary stalk. The gland has two distinct portions.
   A. The anterior gland (adenohypophysis) produces six important hormones and several others that are of lesser significance.

[1] These hormones play major roles in the regulation of metabolic activities. All but one control the secretion of other endocrine glands.

[2] The growth hormone (somatotropin) acts directly on all—or nearly all—body tissues.

    a. Somatotropin promotes increased cell growth, in number and size.

    b. Somatotropin causes an increase in the rate of protein synthesis, conservation of carbohydrates and utilization of fats for energy.

[3] Corticotropin (adrenocorticotropic hormone, ACTH) controls the secretion of some of the adrenocortical hormones that affect the metabolism of glucose, proteins and fat.

[4] Thyrotropin controls the secretion of thyroxine by the thyroid gland and so affects the body's metabolic rate.

[5] Three gonadotropic hormones (follicle-stimulating hormone or FSH; luteinizing hormone or LH; and luteotropic hormone or LTH) control the growth and reproductive functions of the gonads. (See Chapter 19.)

B. The posterior gland (neurohypophysis) contains many terminal nerve fibers and terminal nerve endings of tracts originating in the hypothalamus. The 2 neurohypophyseal hormones are secreted in nuclei located in the hypothalamus and transported by nerve fibers to the gland.

[1] Antidiuretic hormone (ADH), or vasopressin, increases reabsorption of water in the kidney tubules. (See Chapter 4.)

    a. Large amounts of ADH have a slight pressor effect in the circulatory system. Secretion of this hormone is stimulated by excessive blood loss.

    b. ADH secretion may be stimulated when the body sustains severe trauma, during anxiety states and when there is severe pain. Some drugs stimulate secretion. Water retention is followed by diuresis when the factor or factors causing the increased secretion are removed.

    c. ADH secretion may be inhibited by the presence of alcohol in the blood, which partly accounts for the diuresis that occurs with ingestion of alcohol.

[2] Oxytocin causes contractions of the pregnant uterus, especially near the end of gestation. It may play a part in effecting normal labor and delivery.

    a. The hormone oxytocin plays a role in lactation, causing milk produced in the mammary lobes to enter the lactiferous ducts, from which it can be suckled.

    b. Sensory stimuli caused by suckling causes the release of oxytocin, which not only allows milk to flow but also stimulates uterine contractions. This promotes involution of the uterus.

[3] ADH and oxytocin are not released into the blood stream continuously; their release is under nervous system control.

C. One of the less important hormones produced in small amounts in the pars intermedia (which lies between the anterior and posterior portions of the hypophysis) is melanocyte-stimulating hormone. This hormone stimulates cells that contain the black pigment, melanin. An excessive amount of this hormone, which may occur when there is pathology of the adrenal cortex, can cause darkening of the skin.

3. The thyroid gland, located anterior to and just below the trachea, secretes thyroxine

and small amounts of other iodine-containing hormones, all of which affect the body's metabolic rate.

A. Thyroid hormones are necessary for normal growth and development in childhood.

B. Approximately 1 mg. of iodine is needed per week to produce normal amounts of thyroxine.

C. Thyrotropin (secreted by the adenohypophysis) stimulates all activities of the thyroid gland and controls the release of thyroxine into the body fluids. Thyrotropic hormone secretion may be increased by:

   [1] Prolonged exposure to cold.

   [2] Prolonged emotional states, such as anxiety.

D. Normally, thyrotropic hormone secretion is regulated by the concentration of thyroxine in the body fluids (a feedback mechanism).

4. The parathyroid glands are imbedded in the posterior of the thyroid gland. Usually there are 4, but there may be more. They secrete parathyroid hormone.

A. Parathyroid hormone is the prime regulator of calcium ion concentration in the blood.

   [1] A constant concentration of calcium in the extracellular fluids is essential to normal neuromuscular functioning.

   [2] Parathyroid hormone increases bone absorption (the dissolution of bone with release of calcium, phosphate and the end products of digestion of the organic matrix into the extracellular fluids).

   [3] Parathyroid hormone causes increased reabsorption of calcium by the kidney tubules and in the gastrointestinal tract, while it increases excretion of phosphate.

B. Normally, the calcium ion concentration in the extracellular fluids controls parathyroid secretion. When the concentration is elevated, secretion is reduced; when reduced, secretion is increased.

C. The parathyroid glands become enlarged, and secretion is increased during pregnancy and lactation.

5. There is an adrenal gland located on the top of each kidney. The outer portion is called the cortex; it secretes hormones that are called adrenocortical hormones or corticosteroids, some of which are essential to life. The adrenal medulla (the inner portion) secretes epinephrine and norepinephrine in response to sympathetic stimulation.

A. The adrenocortical hormones include:

   [1] The mineralocortocoids (aldosterone; corticosterone, which has some glucocorticoid effects; and desoxycorticosterone).

     a. Aldosterone is responsible for most of the mineralocortocoid activity.

     b. Mineralocorticoids act to increase renal tubular reabsorption of sodium (and chloride, secondarily) and to increase renal excretion of potassium.

     c. A decrease in aldosterone secretion causes a decrease in the reabsorption of salt and water. Extracellular fluid volume is reduced. Cardiac output is reduced, and the blood pressure falls.

     d. An increase in the secretion of aldosterone causes increased reabsorption of salt and water and can result in generalized edema.

     e. There is a normal increase in the secretion of mineralocorticoids when there is physical stress and when there is a low concentration of sodium in the extracellular fluids.

[2] The glucocorticoids (cortisol, also known as hydrocortisone; corticosterone; and cortisone).

    a. Cortisol is responsible for most of the glucocorticoid activity.

    b. Glucocorticoids stimulate the liver to form glycogen and then convert glycogen to glucose and release it into the blood stream. Amino acids are mobilized from the tissues, which increases the concentration of blood amino acids available for conversion into glycogen. Fatty acids are mobilized from adipose tissue and are utilized for energy production.

    c. Corticotropic hormone, secreted by the adenohypophysis, stimulates secretion of the glucocortocoids. Either physical or neurogenic stress will cause an increase in corticotropic hormone, and this is followed within minutes by increased secretion of cortisol. Examples of such stress include traumatic injury due to surgical procedures or accidents, severe infections, debilitating diseases or extremes of environmental temperature.

    d. Excess amounts of glucocorticoids have an anti–inflammatory process effect.

[3] Adrenal androgens. These hormones have a slight masculinizing effect.

B. Secretion of both the mineralocorticoids and the glucocorticoids is increased at times of stress.

C. Epinephrine (adrenalin) and norepinephrine (noradrenalin) are released from the adrenal medulla at times of stress (physical or emotional) and as a part of the body's alarm system when threat is perceived. They affect body tissues and processes in a manner similar to sympathetic stimulation.

[1] Epinephrine causes:

    a. Increased blood flow in the skeletal muscles and in the coronary vessels.

    b. Constriction of other peripheral vessels, with resultant elevation of blood pressure.

    c. Relaxation of the smooth muscles of the bronchioles and of the gastrointestinal tract.

    d. Increased cardiac output (heart rate and force of contractions are increased).

    e. Dilatation of the pupils.

    f. Increased conversion of glycogen to glucose in the liver, and release of glucose into the blood.

    g. Increased metabolic rate, with increased mental alertness.

[2] Norepinephrine effects a generalized vasoconstriction, which serves to elevate the blood pressure.

6. The pancreas secretes 2 hormones, insulin and glucagon.

A. Although insulin's primary effect is on carbohydrate metabolism, it also influences fat and protein metabolism.

[1] Insulin increases the rate of glucose metabolism, decreases the concentration of blood glucose and increases the storage of glycogen in body tissues.

a. The transportation of glucose through cell membranes is facilitated.
b. Storage of glycogen is enhanced because of the increased intracellular concentration of glucose.
c. Normally, secretion of insulin is regulated by the concentration of blood glucose (a feedback mechanism).
d. A proper concentration of glucose in the blood must be maintained to provide necessary nutrition to the brain and to the retina. These tissues can utilize only glucose for energy production.

[2] Lack of insulin causes an increase in the mobilization of fats, with consequent increase in the concentration of free fatty acids in the blood. The metabolism of fatty acids produces ketone acids, with resultant ketosis.

[3] Insulin increases the transport of amino acids across cell membranes. In addition, insulin can be called a "protein-sparer," as it prevents the utilization of protein for energy because of its effects on carbohydrate metabolism.

B. Glucagon causes the conversion of glycogen to glucose in the liver and release of glucose into the blood. This hormone serves to prevent hypoglycemia.

Pathology

PITUITARY GLAND DISORDERS

1. Symptoms and signs of abnormal hormone secretion by the pituitary gland depend upon which lobe is involved, whether the pathology causes hyposecretion or hypersecretion and which particular cells are affected. Symptoms and signs may include:
   A. Abnormal growth patterns.
   B. Symptoms and signs of hyposecretion or hypersecretion of target glands: thyroid, adrenal cortex and gonads.
   C. Symptoms and signs of diabetes insipidus. (See Chapter 4.)

2. Disorders of the pituitary gland may be caused by pathologic changes within the gland (e.g., due to tumor growth or impaired circulation) or by compression of the gland, with resultant cellular damage.
   A. Hyposecretion of the growth hormone before adolescence causes dwarfism.
   B. Hypersecretion of the growth hormone before adolescence causes gigantism (or giantism).
      [1] All body cells grow rapidly, and as the epiphyses of the long bones have not yet fused with the shaft, there is rapid growth of the long bones.
      [2] Gigantism is usually accompanied by hyperglycemia. Diabetes mellitus often develops, due to degeneration of the islet cells of the pancreas.
   C. Hypersecretion of the growth hormone after adolescence causes acromegaly, a condition in which there is thickening of the bones transversely. This can be noted mainly in the mandible and the bones of the hands and feet.
   D. Hyposecretion of all adenohypophyseal hormones occurs in Simmonds' disease. There is a deficiency in hormone secretion in the target glands.

THYROID GLAND DISORDERS
1. Symptoms and signs of abnormal hormone secretion by the thyroid gland may include:
   A. Enlargement of the thyroid gland.
   B. Those symptoms and signs related to hyposecretion (hypothyroidism) and caused by a decrease in the metabolic rate.
      [1] Weight gain.
      [2] Retarded physical growth and mental development (in childhood).
      [3] Mental dullness, slowness of response, much time spent sleeping.
      [4] Retarded sexual development, when occurring before adolescence.
      [5] Loss of sexual drive, menstrual disorders (e.g., amenorrhea), when occurring after adolescence.
      [6] Depressed muscle activity, weakness and fatigue.
      [7] Depressed circulatory and respiratory function.
      [8] Subnormal body temperature, cool and dry skin and increasing sensitivity to cold.
      [9] Poor appetite and constipation.
      [10] Thick tongue.
      [11] Small amount of generalized edema.
   C. Those symptoms and signs related to hypersecretion (hyperthyroidism) and caused by an increase in the metabolic rate.
      [1] Some enlargement of the thyroid gland.
      [2] Mild to severe weight loss.
      [3] Rapid skeletal growth in children.
      [4] Unusual muscular vigor (until muscles become weakened with the excessive catabolism of protein).
      [5] Fine tremors of the hands.
      [6] Increased mental activity, with resulting excitability and nervousnesss, possible anxiety and even paranoia.
      [7] Menstrual disorders (e.g., scanty menses or amenorrhea).
      [8] Fatigue, yet inability to relax and sleep.
      [9] Increased motility of the gastrointestinal tract, possibly causing diarrhea.
      [10] Increased demands on circulatory and respiratory functions. There is usually tachycardia, and there may be dyspnea upon exertion, due to oxygen deficiency.
      [11] Hot, moist skin, with hypersensitivity to heat.
      [12] Exophthalmos (protrusion of the eyeballs, with retraction of the superior eyelids).
2. Disorders of the thyroid gland may be caused by pathologic changes within the gland (e.g., inflammatory process, tumor growth), by iodine deficiency or by abnormal secretion of thyrotropic hormone.
   A. Iodine deficiency causes hypertrophy of the thyroid gland, as the glandular cells attempt to produce sufficient hormone. This type of goiter is sometimes called endemic, simple or nontoxic. Water and soil in areas distant from sea water may be deficient in iodine.

B. Lack of thyroid secretion may cause the basal metabolic rate to fall to -40 to -60, while excessive secretion can raise the rate as high as $+60$ to $+100$.

C. Hypothyroidism in the child is called cretinism. If the condition persists over time, hormone replacement therapy cannot bring about improvement of either the physical or mental development.

D. Hypothyroidism after adolescence is called myxedema. Abnormal deposits of mucopolysaccharides in the subcutaneous tissues retain water, causing a small amount of general edema.

E. Hyperthyroidism is sometimes referred to as thyrotoxicosis, toxic goiter or Graves' disease. There is usually some enlargement of the gland.

    [1] If exophthalmos exists it may be called exophthalmic goiter. The exophthalmos is caused by edema and fibrosis of the retro-orbital tissues and is thought to be caused by a chemical substance produced in association with the excessive thyrotropic secretion.

    [2] Young adult women tend to develop this condition, and it tends to follow periods of severe physical and/or emotional stress. The cause is probably excessive secretion of thyrotropic hormone in the adenohypophysis.

DISORDERS OF THE PARATHYROID GLANDS

1. Symptoms and signs of abnormal hormone production by the parathyroid glands include:

    A. Those related to hyposecretion. Symptoms and signs of hypocalcemia, caused by hyposecretion, include:

        [1] Numbness and tingling of extremities.

        [2] Carpopedal spasms, muscle twitchings.

        [3] Tetany, with laryngeal spasms.

    B. Those related to hypersecretion. Symptoms and signs of hypercalcemia and increased bone absorption, both caused by hypersecretion, include:

        [1] Depression of neuromuscular function, with anorexia, constipation and muscular weakness.

        [2] Increased urinary output and possibly formation of urinary calculi.

        [3] Tenderness and pain in the bones, especially with weight-bearing.

        [4] Development of bone deformities and/or pathologic fractures.

2. Disorders involving parathyroid secretion may be caused by pathological changes within the glands (e.g., due to tumor growth, impaired circulation) or by traumatic injury to the glands or even by accidental removal of them in relation to thyroid surgery.

    A. Hypoparathyroidism causes hypocalcemia. When the blood calcium level falls to 7 mg. percent, hypocalcemic tetany develops. The laryngeal muscles are particularly susceptible to hypocalcemia, and laryngeal spasms can cause airway obstruction.

    B. Hyperparathyroidism causes an increased concentration of calcium in the extracellular fluids.

        [1] There is an abnormal absorption of bone, which weakens the bone structure. Deformities and/or pathologic fractures may occur.

        [2] Increased excretion of calcium results in increased urinary output, as the

kidneys attempt to keep the excess calcium in solution. When this is not possible, urinary calculi may occur.

[3] The increased concentration of calcium in the body fluids causes some depression of neuromuscular function.

[4] Hyperparathyroidism tends to occur more frequently in adult females. Pregnancy and lactation may be predisposing factors.

[5] Prolonged calcium and phosphate deficiency (often related to lack of Vitamin D rather than to inadequate intake of minerals) causes increased parathyroid secretion and a subsequent increase in bone absorption. Proper calcification of bone cannot occur.

DISORDERS OF THE ADRENAL GLANDS

1. Symptoms and signs of abnormal hormone secretion by the adrenal cortex include:
   A. Those related to hyposecretion.
      [1] Symptoms and signs of hyponatremia, hyperkalemia and dehydration (see Chapters 4 and 5). In cases of sudden and severe insufficiency, hypotension may progress rapidly to circulatory shock.
      [2] Bronzing of the skin.
      [3] Poor response to stress (physical or emotional), increased susceptibility to infections.
      [4] Possibly some degree of feminism in the male.
   B. Those related to hypersecretion.
      [1] Symptoms and signs of hypernatremia, hypokalemia and water retention. (See Chapters 4 and 5.)
      [2] Obesity or abnormal fat distribution (e.g., moon face, girdle of fat).
      [3] Increased susceptibility to infections.
      [4] Virilism in the female, perhaps precocious puberty in the male.
2. Disorders involving adrenal cortex hormone secretion may be caused by pathologic changes within the gland (e.g., tumor growth), by abnormalities of adrenocorticotropin secretion by the pituitary gland or by surgical removal of adrenals.
   A. Mental changes sometimes accompany disorders of the adrenal cortex. There may be frequent mood changes, depression or hyperirritability, and psychoses may develop.
   B. Hyposecretion of the adrenal cortex causes clinical manifestations related to deficiencies of mineralocorticoids, glucocorticoids and adrenal androgens. Therefore, the symptoms and signs are associated with fluid and electrolyte imbalances and with problems involving carbohydrate metabolism (especially in relation to stress).
      [1] Hyposecretion of adrenocortical hormones is sometimes referred to as Addison's disease.
      [2] When Addison's disease suddenly becomes acute, it is called Addisonian crisis. Crises may be precipitated by physical and/or emotional stress. Complete circulatory collapse can occur rapidly.
   C. Hypersecretion of the adrenal cortex causes clinical manifestations related to excesses of mineralocorticoids, glucocorticoids and adrenal androgens. Therefore, the symptoms and signs are associated with fluid and electrolyte imbal-

ances and disorders of carbohydrate, fat and protein metabolism. There is increased susceptibility to infection. Excess androgen secretion may cause masculinization in the female and may cause precocious sexual development in the male prior to puberty. The condition of hypersecretion is referred to sometimes as Cushing's syndrome.

3. Hyperfunction of the adrenal medulla may be caused by a neoplasm, pheochromocytoma. The primary symptom is hypertension, which may occur intermittently or continuously. (See Chapter 1.)

DISORDERS OF THE PANCREAS

1. Symptoms and signs of abnormal secretion of insulin in the islets of Langerhans include:
   A. Those related to hyposecretion.
      [1] Hyperglycemia and glycosuria.
      [2] Polyuria and excessive thirst.
      [3] Weakness and easy fatigue.
      [4] Weight loss.
   B. Those related to hypersecretion.
      [1] Sweating.
      [2] Muscular tremors.
      [3] Apprehension.
      [4] Hunger.
      [5] Weakness, dizziness, fainting.
      [6] Muscular twitchings, uncoordinated movements.
      [7] Progressive loss of consciousness.
2. Diabetes mellitus is a prevalent, chronic disorder caused by either hyposecretion of insulin or ineffectiveness of the insulin that is secreted. Carbohydrate metabolism is impaired, and there is hyperglycemia.
   A. Predisposition to the development of primary diabetes mellitus is inherited.
   B. Most adults who develop diabetes are obese or have a history of obesity.
   C. Hyposecretion of insulin that is due to degeneration of the secreting (beta) cells is called secondary diabetes mellitus.
      [1] Hormones such as somatotropin, the glucocorticoids and glucagon may be causative factors in the degenerative process, because they promote hyperglycemia which stimulates insulin secretion.
      [2] Degeneration may be caused by injury to the pancreas (e.g., traumatic injury, infections or tumor growth).
   D. Insulin antagonists may block the effectiveness of insulin.
   E. Hyperglycemia causes glycosuria.
      [1] The high glucose content of the urine may predispose to infections of the vulva in the female. Pruritus is a symptom.
      [2] Glycosuria causes polyuria, which may lead to dehydration. (See Chapter 4.)
   F. Impaired carbohydrate metabolism over time causes:
      [1] Increased utilization of protein for energy production, and this results in loss of weight.

[2] Increased utilization of fatty acids for energy production, with production of ketone bodies. Excessive amounts of ketone bodies in the blood cause metabolic acidosis. (See Chapter 6.)

G. Diabetes mellitus almost always causes some degenerative changes in blood vessels. Atherosclerosis and thickening of capillary walls develops most often in the retina, the lower extremities, the kidneys and the heart. (See Chapter 1.)

3. Hypersecretion of insulin by the islets of Langerhans occurs only rarely and may be caused by tumor growth or by overactivity of the insulin-producing cells from undetermined causes. Symptoms and signs are related to hypoglycemia. (See Chapter 3.) Brain cells may be permanently damaged by periodic or continuous lack of glucose.

Nursing Care

Nursing care should be directed toward assisting the patient to attain, retain or regain the best possible chemical regulation of body functioning.

COLLECTION, EVALUATION AND COMMUNICATION OF DATA

1. Patients should be interviewed, observed and examined to identify symptoms and signs of endocrine problems.
   A. Endocrine problems may be indicated by:
      [1] Abnormalities in growth and development, both physical and mental.
      [2] Symptoms and signs of:
         a. Improper nutrition.
         b. Fluid and electrolyte imbalance.
         c. Acid-base imbalance.
      [3] Abnormal neuromuscular function.
      [4] Abnormalities in sleep patterns.
      [5] Abnormalities in body temperature.
      [6] Changes in sexuality and/or reproductive functioning.
      [7] Abnormalities in bone structure and function.
      [8] Changes in mental status.
      [9] Poor response to stress, increased susceptibility to infections.
      [10] Goiter, exophthalmos.
   B. Systematic patient evaluation is of especial importance when the patient:
      [1] Has a diagnosed endocrine disorder.
      [2] Has sustained injury (e.g., surgery) that involves or may affect an endocrine gland.
      [3] Is receiving hormone replacement therapy.
      [4] Is obese, has a history of obesity or a family history of diabetes mellitus.
   C. Data collected should be evaluated not only on the basis of a single deviation from normal (e.g., polyuria) but also on the basis of combinations of symptoms and signs that are commonly associated with specific endocrine disorders.
2. How, when and what data are communicated to the physician and/or other nursing personnel depend upon:

A. Any immediate threat to the patient's life processes (e.g., symptoms and signs of diabetic ketosis).

B. Any potential threat to the patient's life and well-being (e.g., symptoms and signs of hyperthyroidism).

C. Any particular implications for the physician in relation to:

[1] The patient's progress or lack of progress toward recovery (e.g., changes in neuromuscular irritability in a patient with hypoparathyroidism).

[2] Making a diagnosis (e.g., new objective and subjective data).

[3] The patient's physical and emotional responses to specific diagnostic procedures and therapeutic measures.

D. Any particular implications for nursing care (e.g., special counselling needs).

PROMOTION OF HEALTH AND PREVENTION
OF DISEASE/INJURY

1. Health teaching to promote proper chemical regulation of body functions should be concerned with:

A. Normal growth and development patterns.

B. The importance of:

[1] A balanced, nutritious diet throughout the life cycle, with:

a. Avoidance of an excess of calories.

b. An adequate intake of iodine.

[2] Weight reduction under medical supervision, when there is a condition of overweight.

2. The patient should be taught the importance of:

A. Periodic health evaluations (especially important for persons who have family histories of diabetes mellitus).

B. Prompt medical consultation when there are early indications of possible endocrine disorders, including:

[1] Variations from normal growth and development patterns.

[2] Abnormal muscle movements, such as tremors.

[3] Muscle weakness, unusual fatigue.

[4] Excessive urination, excessive thirst, excessive eating.

[5] Unusual weight loss or weight gain.

[6] Changes in sexuality or reproductive functions.

CARE OF PATIENTS WITH SPECIFIC ENDOCRINE PROBLEMS
Pituitary Gland Disorders

1. When a patient has giantism or acromegaly:

A. It is very important that dietary orders be followed. A high caloric diet may be indicated.

B. Emotional support should be consistent.

C. Close observations should be made for indications of diabetes mellitus, abnormal thyroid function, abnormal adrenal cortical function and abnormal gonadal function.

2. When a patient has Simmonds' disease, nursing care should be related to problems resulting from hyposecretion of the thyroid gland, the adrenal cortex and the gonads.

Thyroid Gland Disorders

1. Patients with goiters should be observed for difficulty with swallowing and/or breathing.
2. Patients with thyroid disorders should be under medical supervision.
3. When a patient has hypothyroidism:
    A. It is essential that medical orders for thyroid preparations be followed exactly. Symptoms and signs of excess thyroid hormone should be reported promptly.
    B. Emotional support should be consistent.
    C. Prescribed central nervous system depressants should be administered with great caution. The patient should be observed closely for depression of respiratory function.
4. When a patient has hyperthyroidism:
    A. It is essential that medical orders for any antithyroid drugs be followed exactly.
    B. The dietary intake should provide ample amounts of nutrients.
    C. Body weight should be measured frequently and reported/recorded appropriately.
    D. The metabolic rate should be reduced as possible.
        [1] Sleep and rest should be provided and encouraged.
        [2] Stress-producing situations, both physical and emotional, should be prevented as possible. It may be necessary to restrict physical activity.
        [3] Commonly used stimulants, such as coffee, tea and tobacco, should be restricted.
    E. The vital signs should be evaluated frequently and abnormalities reported/recorded appropriately. (See Chapters 1, 2, 9.)

Disorders of the Parathyroid Glands

1. When a patient has hypoparathyroidism:
    A. It is essential that medical orders for the administration of parathyroid hormone, calcium and Vitamin D be followed exactly.
    B. Emotional support should be consistent.
    C. If tetany occurs:
        [1] This is a medical emergency.
        [2] Equipment should be ready for prompt intravenous administration of calcium.
        [3] External stimuli should be limited (e.g., providing a quiet environment).
2. When a patient has hyperparathyroidism:
    A. Dietary orders for calcium restriction should be carefully followed.
    B. The daily fluid intake should be increased up to 3,000–4,000 ml., unless this is contraindicated by some other problem.
    C. Symptoms and signs of urinary calculi should be reported promptly.

Adrenal Cortex Disorders

1. Patients with disorders of the adrenal cortex should be under medical supervision.
2. When a patient has Addison's disease:
    A. It is essential that medical orders for administration of adrenal cortical hormones be followed exactly.

B.   It is very important that medical orders pertaining to fluid and dietary intake be followed exactly. Daily sodium intake should be prescribed.
C.   Stress-producing situations (physical and emotional) should be prevented as possible. It is extremely important that the patient be protected from infection. (See Chapter 20.)
D.   Emotional support should be consistent.
E.   If symptoms and signs of Addisonian crisis occur (including symptoms and signs of hypoglycemia and hypotension):
     [1]   This is a medical emergency.
     [2]   Appropriate intravenous solutions and cortisol should be ready for immediate administration.
     [3]   Appropriate nursing actions should be taken in relation to the hypotension. (See Chapter 1.)
F.   The patient should be counselled to obtain medical attention promptly:
     [1]   When there is infection.
     [2]   When there are symptoms of hypoglycemia and hypotension.
   3. When a patient has Cushing's syndrome, systematic evaluation should be made for indications of fluid, electrolyte and acid-base imbalances. (See Chapters 4, 5 and 6.)

Disorders of the Pancreas

   1. When a patient has diabetes mellitus:
A.   He should be under medical supervision.
B.   It is essential that medical orders related to diet be followed exactly. Any vomiting or diarrhea should be reported promptly.
C.   It is essential that medical orders related to the administration of insulin or other hypoglycemic drugs be followed exactly. Symptoms and signs of hypoglycemia should be reported appropriately and treated promptly.
D.   It is very important that medical orders relating to a program of physical exercise be followed.
E.   Urine testing must be performed accurately and at proper times and be reported/recorded appropriately.
F.   It is especially important that the patient be protected from infections. (See Chapter 20.)
G.   Symptoms and signs of hyperglycemia, dehydration and developing ketosis should be reported promptly.
     [1]   Systematic patient evaluation is of critical importance when the patient has an infection or is experiencing other types of stress, such as pregnancy or surgery.
     [2]   Symptoms and signs of diabetic acidosis represent a medical emergency. Insulin and appropriate intravenous solutions should be ready for immediate administration. (See Chapters 4, 5 and 6, in relation to care of patients with dehydration and metabolic acidosis.)
H.   Patients and their families should be helped to understand the importance of:
     [1]   Controlling diabetes through all prescribed measures.
     [2]   Obtaining prompt medical consultation when:
           a.   There is infection or traumatic injury.
           b.   There are gastrointestinal problems involving vomiting and/or diarrhea.

    c. There are indications of hyperglycemia, dehydration and/or metabolic acidosis.

2. When a patient has symptoms and signs of hypoglycemia:

   A. This may be a medical emergency.

   B. A concentrated form of sugar should be administered promptly by mouth. If oral administration is not possible, preparations should be made for immediate intravenous administration of glucose.

Chapter 9

Temperature Regulation

A definite body temperature range is required for efficient cellular functioning and proper enzymatic activity.

Anatomy and Physiology

1. The optimal temperature for normal activity of enzymes falls within the normal body temperature range of 36° C. to 38° C. (97° F. to 100.4° F.), with an average of 37° C. (98.6° F.).
2. Body cells vary in their abilities to function when their temperature is below 34.4° C. (94° F.) or above 40° C. (104° F.).
   A. Local hemorrhaging and cellular degeneration usually begin when the temperature rises above 41° C. (106° F.).
      [1] If the cells of the central nervous system are damaged, nervous regulation of body functions is impaired.
      [2] Hyperthermia can cause permanent brain damage, as destroyed neuronal cells cannot be replaced.
   B. Hypothermia causes depression of all metabolic processes.
      [1] Depression of circulatory function may cause cardiac arrhythmias (including cardiac arrest).
      [2] Severe and/or prolonged depression of metabolic activities results in cellular death.
   C. Body fluids freeze when exposed to freezing temperatures. Unless thawing is prompt, cellular damage is irreparable.
3. The body temperature represents a balance between heat produced in the tissues (plus a small amount which may be acquired from the external environment) and heat lost to the environment.

174

A. Heat production is due to exothermic chemical reactions.
  [1] When the body is at rest the liver produces the greatest amount of heat.
  [2] During exercise the voluntary muscles produce the greatest amount of heat. (Children often have a considerable rise in temperature with exercise.)
  [3] Thyroxine increases the metabolic rate and thus the body temperature.
  [4] The basal metabolic rate increases about 10 percent for every degree Centigrade rise in body temperature (approximately 7 percent for every degree Fahrenheit rise).
  [5] As stimulation of the sympathetic nervous system (with release of epinephrine and norepinephrine) increases the metabolic activities of nearly all body tissues, strong emotional states, such as excitement and anxiety, can increase body temperature.
  [6] An increased metabolic rate increases demands upon the cardiovascular and respiratory systems. (See Chapters 1 and 2.)
B. Heat is distributed through the body by:
  [1] Conduction through the tissues.
  [2] The circulating blood.
C. The total amount of heat in a given area in the body is influenced by the rate of blood flow within that area.
D. Heat is lost from the body through:
  [1] Conduction.
  [2] Radiation.
  [3] Convection.
  [4] Vaporization of sweat. (Approximately 0.6 calorie is required for the vaporization of 1 gram of water from the skin or mucous membrane of the respiratory tract.)
E. The amount of heat lost from the body surface by radiation and conduction varies with:
  [1] The amount of body insulation (e.g., subcutaneous fat, clothing).
  [2] The amount of skin area exposed.
  [3] The external environmental temperature.
  [4] The amount of blood flow in the peripheral capillaries.
F. The amount of heat lost from the body surface by vaporization depends upon:
  [1] The production of sweat.
  [2] The amount of skin area exposed.
  [3] The amount of blood flow in the peripheral capillaries.
  [4] The humidity of the surrounding atmosphere.
  [5] The air currents.
G. The amount of heat lost from the body surface by convection depends upon the amount of surface area exposed and the air currents.
H. There is a normal diurnal variation of body temperature. If the waking and active hours are in the day, the maximum temperature is reached in the late afternoon or early evening; the minimum is reached in the early morning.
I. Infants and children, because of a higher metabolic rate related to growth and physical activity, may have a normal temperature as much as 1 degree Fahrenheit higher than adults.

J.   In the female, there is a slight increase in body temperature (0.5 to 1.0 degree Fahrenheit) from the time of ovulation until menstruation. This elevation generally continues during the first several months of pregnancy.

4. When thermometers are kept in place for short periods of time (e.g., 2 to 3 minutes), rectal temperature measurements are higher than oral measurements, and oral measurements are higher than axillary measurements. The oral and axillary measurements are approximately the same as the rectal measurement when thermometers are kept in place for longer periods of time.

5. The physiological mechanisms for temperature regulation are controlled almost entirely by the temperature-regulating center in the hypothalamus. There are heat-sensitive neurons in the thermostatic center of the anterior hypothalamus which control body temperature.
   A.   Overheating of the heat-sensitive neurons causes an increase in heat loss.
        [1] Sympathetic nerves stimulate the sweat glands to secrete sweat. Heat is lost through vaporization.
        [2] Sympathetic centers in the posterior hypothalamus are inhibited, to allow increased blood flow in the skin. Heat loss through conduction, radiation and convection is increased.
   B.   Cooling of the heat-sensitive neurons causes an increase in the production of body heat.
        [1] Sympathetic stimulation causes vasoconstriction in the blood vessels of the skin and pilo-erection, which has an insulating effect in furry animals and causes "goosebumps" in man. Sweating is inhibited.
        [2] The primary motor center for shivering (located in the posterior hypothalamus) transmits impulses to the skeletal muscles, increasing muscle tone. When the tone rises above a certain level, muscles contract involuntarily. Shivering and shaking increase heat production.

6. Nerve receptors for heat and cold, located in the skin, also help to regulate body temperature.
   A.   Awareness of feeling too warm or too cool can result in deliberate actions to conserve body heat, produce more body heat or lose some body heat. Awareness and response vary with the level of consciousness, neuromuscular de-development, locomotor ability and mental development.
   B.   Signals from the heat and cold receptors in the skin are able to:
        [1] Modify the thermostatic settings of the heat-regulating center, so that mechanisms for heat regulation can be initiated at a slightly lower or higher temperature than is normally required for stimulation of the heat-sensitive neurons.
        [2] Initiate spinal cord reflexes that influence blood flow and sweating.

7. Heat-regulating mechanisms are generally not fully developed at birth, so there may be marked fluctuations in body temperature during the first year of life. The external temperature is a major factor in the raising or lowering of body temperature in an infant.

8. The body temperature may become elevated when the environmental temperature and humidity are high enough to prevent normal, physiologic compensations.

9. Pyrogens are chemical substances that cause the thermostatic setting in the heat-regulating center to be elevated.

A. Elevation of the thermostatic setting causes mechanisms for increasing the body temperature to come into play.

[1] Heat loss is decreased by intense peripheral vasoconstriction. There is a sensation of chilling.

[2] Shivering, which may become severe shaking, occurs as the body attempts to increase heat production.

[3] The increased heat production is followed by peripheral vasodilatation (with flushed, dry and hot skin) and an uncomfortable warm feeling.

B. Pyrogenic substances include lipopolysaccharide toxins produced by bacteria, many protein substances and the breakdown products of protein (e.g., from tissue destruction).

[1] It is thought that pyrogens are released from leukocytes, as a part of the body's inflammatory response to injury.

[2] Hemolysis that occurs with incompatible blood transfusions results in the release of pyrogenic substances from the red blood cells.

Physics

1. Heat can be defined as the kinetic energy of molecules.
2. Heat travels from a point of higher temperature to one of lower temperature.
3. Conduction is the transfer of energy (e.g., heat) from particle to particle or between objects in contact.
4. Radiation is the transmission of energy (e.g., heat) through space in the form of waves.
5. Convection involves the movement of heat by the currents of air (fluids). Warmed air moves upward as it expands and is replaced by cooler air.
6. Vaporization is the process whereby a substance in liquid state is transformed to a vapor state. Vaporization requires heat; therefore, it is a cooling process.

Chemistry

1. Exothermic chemical reactions are those in which there is a liberation of heat.

Pathology

SYMPTOMS AND SIGNS

1. Symptoms and signs of hyperthermia include:
   A. An abnormally elevated body temperature measurement.
   B. A rapid pulse, which may be full or weak.
   C. Rapid respirations.
   D. Hyperemia of the skin, which may be preceded by paleness of the skin.
   E. Profuse sweating.
   F. Hot, dry skin and mucous membranes.
   G. General uncomfortable warm feeling, possibly hypersensitive skin.
   H. Chills.
   I. Headache, general malaise, restlessness.

    J.   Delirium, loss of consciousness.

    K. Convulsions (seen fairly frequently in infants and small children).

2. Symptoms and signs of hypothermia include:
   A. An abnormally low body temperature measurement.
   B. Slow pulse rate that becomes weaker as the temperature falls.
   C. Slow respirations.
   D. "Goosebumps" on the skin.
   E. Pale skin that may become mottled in appearance.
   F. Shivering, shaking, chattering of teeth.
   G. General uncomfortable cold feeling, numbness in extremities.
   H. Loss of sensation, loss of consciousness.

FEVER

1. Fever is the elevation of body temperature that occurs in disease.
   A. Fever is "continuous" when the body temperature remains elevated through-out a 24–hour period.
   B. Fever is "intermittent" if the body temperature returns to normal at least once in a 24–hour period.
   C. Fever is "remittent" if the body temperature fluctuates but does not return to normal.
   D. "Recurrent" or "relapsing" fevers last for several days, with intervals of normal temperature in between.
2. Fever may be due to conditions that:
   A. Increase heat production.
   B. Decrease heat loss.
   C. Affect the heat-regulating center in the brain.
3. In thyrotoxicosis there is an increased metabolic rate, which causes the elevation of body temperature.
4. Conditions that decrease heat loss include:
   A. Obesity.
   B. Dehydration, which results in decreased secretion of sweat.
   C. Peripheral vasoconstriction.
   D. Congenital absence of sweat glands (rare).
5. Conditions that may affect the heat-regulating center include:
   A. Damage to the heat-regulating center, which may be caused by:
      [1] Head injury (includes brain surgery).
      [2] Cerebrovascular accidents.
      [3] Abnormally high body temperatures (e.g., in heat stroke or thyroid crisis).
   B. Tissue destruction and/or inflammatory response that involve the release of pyrogenic substances into the blood.
   C. Infectious diseases (e.g., brucellosis, malaria), in which pyrogens are released into the blood stream.
      [1] Brucellosis is a bacterial infection caused by *Brucella* organisms. After incubation periods within some of the body cells, the organisms erupt into the bloodstream; this causes chills and fever.
      [2] Malaria is a protozoan infection of the blood. The parasites enter the red blood cells, and when the schizont form develops and ruptures the cells,

the entrance of pyrogenic substances into the bloodstream causes chills and fever.

6. Heat stroke is a condition in which there is high fever and loss of consciousness. The fever may be between 40.6° C. and 43.3° C. (105° F.–110° F.). There is no sweating.

   A. Heat stroke is caused by exposure to high environmental temperature.

   B. Individuals who are elderly or have impaired cardiac function are more apt to develop this condition.

HYPOTHERMIA

1. Hypothermia may occur when there is prolonged exposure to a cold environmental temperature. If vasodilatation exists concurrently with the exposure (e.g., which may occur following the ingestion of alcohol), heat loss is accelerated.

2. Hypothermia may also occur when there is depression of the central nervous system by drugs (e.g., opiates, barbiturates).

Nursing Care

Nursing care should be directed toward assisting the patient to
attain, retain or regain optimal body temperature.

COLLECTION, EVALUATION AND COMMUNICATION OF DATA

1. Patients should be interviewed, observed and examined to identify an abnormal body temperature.

2. Systematic evaluation of body temperature is of especial importance when the patient:

   A. Has an abnormally high or low temperature.

   B. Has a disorder in which there is increased heat production or decreased heat loss (e.g., thyrotoxicosis or dehydration).

   C. Has a disorder in which the heat-regulating center is (or is likely to be) affected. Such disorders include:

      [1] Head injury, brain surgery, cerebrovascular accident.

      [2] Tissue damage, which may be caused by traumatic injury, chemical or physical agents, tumor growth.

      [3] Infectious processes that involve release of pyrogens.

   D. Is a newborn, especially if premature.

   E. Is exposed to extremes of temperature, such as induced hypothermia.

   F. Is unconscious.

3. Body temperature should be evaluated in relation to:

   A. The usual body temperature.

   B. Any diagnosed disorder and its commonly associated temperature variations.

   C. The time of day.

   D. The environmental temperature.

   E. Amount of recent physical exercise (especially with children).

   F. Phase of menstrual cycle or early months of pregnancy.

   G. Age.

   H. Emotional status.

    I.   The method of measurement (i.e., rectal, oral or skin and the time thermometer is left in place).

    J.   Safe ranges for body temperature.

4. How, when and what data are communicated to the physician and/or other nursing personnel depend upon:

    A.   Any immediate threat to the patient's life processes (e.g., body temperature measurements over 41° C. [106° F.] or below 34.4° C. [94° F.]).

    B.   Any potential threat to the patient's life and well-being (e.g., continuous high fever).

    C.   Any particular implications for the physician in relation to:

        [1] The patient's progress or lack of progress toward recovery (e.g., a drop or rise in temperature).

        [2] Making a diagnosis (e.g., sudden onset of chills and fever).

        [3] The patient's physical and emotional responses to specific therapeutic measures.

    D.   Any particular implications for nursing (e.g., measures to reduce body temperature).

PROMOTION OF HEALTH AND PREVENTION OF DISEASE/INJURY

1. Health teaching to promote optimal body temperature should be concerned with:

    A.   How to measure body temperature safely and accurately and some of the factors that normally affect temperature.

    B.   The importance of:

        [1] Protection against extremes of environmental temperature, especially with the very young and elderly, by increasing or decreasing:

            a. Insulation.

            b. Conduction, convection, vaporization.

            c. Physical exercise.

        [2] Preventing or eliminating overweight.

        [3] Lowering very elevated temperatures promptly and knowing methods of doing this at home (especially important with infants and small children).

    C.   The importance of prompt medical attention when there is fever or abnormally low temperature.

2. Patients should be protected from extremes of environmental temperatures, and this is of particular importance when the patient:

    A.   Is an infant, especially premature newborn, or is elderly.

    B.   Has impaired cardiovascular function.

    C.   Has an abnormal metabolic rate.

    D.   Is fatigued, unconscious or in a debilitated state.

    E.   Is physically very active or inactive.

    F.   Has extensive injury to the skin.

    G.   Is emaciated or obese.

3. Dehydration should be prevented. (See Chapter 4.)

4. Patients should be protected from injury due to trauma, physical agents, chemical agents and infectious agents.

CARE OF PATIENTS WITH ABNORMAL BODY TEMPERATURES

1. When a patient has a fever:
   A. It is a medical emergency if the temperature rises above 41° C. (106° F.).
   B. The body temperature may be lowered by such means as:
      [1] Adjusting the environmental temperature.
      [2] Exposing a greater expanse of skin to the air.
      [3] Increasing vaporization from the skin, by:
         a. Increasing air currents.
         b. Applying cool sponges that allow evaporation.
      [4] Cold applications (e.g., ice packs, bedding).
      [5] Providing/encouraging complete rest.
      [6] Administration of antipyretic drugs.
   C. Close observations should be made of the vital signs, and they should be reported/recorded appropriately.
2. When a patient has hypothermia:
   A. It may be a medical emergency if the temperature falls below 34.4° C. (94° F.).
   B. The body temperature may be elevated by such means as:
      [1] Warm applications.
      [2] Adjusting the environmental temperature.
      [3] Elimination of air currents.
      [4] Use of insulating materials around the body.
      [5] Ingestion of hot food and fluids.
      [6] Physical activity, friction of the skin.
   C. The body temperature should be elevated gradually, to prevent circulatory shock due to too rapid dilatation of the arterioles.
   D. Close observations should be made of the vital signs, and they should be reported/recorded appropriately.

Chapter 10

Sleep and Rest

Body cells require periods of decreased activity, during which they can restore themselves.

Anatomy and Physiology

1. To maintain optimal body functioning (physical and mental), human beings require definite amounts of sleep in extended periods.
   A. Required hours of sleep vary with each individual. Sleep requirements are influenced by:
      [1] Age.
         a. Infants generally require 14 to 18 hours sleep each day.
         b. Children generally require 10 to 14 hours sleep each day.
         c. Adolescents and adults of all ages generally require 7 to 9 hours sleep each day.
      [2] Individual physiological characteristics.
      [3] The health status (e.g., sleep needs may be increased by certain disease conditions).
      [4] The level of stress (during periods of stress, sleep needs may be increased).
      [5] The presence or absence of motivation to be awake and mentally and/or physically active.
      [6] Conditioning.
   B. Sleep appears to restore normal balance between different parts of the nervous system.
   C. The entire body is affected when there are periods of increased or decreased nervous excitability. During sleep:

[1] Sympathetic activity decreases.
    a. The arterial blood pressure drops.
    b. The heart rate drops.
    c. The blood vessels of the skin dilate.

[2] Parasympathetic activity sometimes increases (e.g., motility and secretion of gastrointestinal tract).

[3] Muscle tone is decreased; at times there is almost no muscle tone.

[4] The metabolic rate is reduced 10 to 20 percent.

2. The reticular activating system, which controls the degree of central nervous system activity, controls wakefulness and sleep.

  A. The reticular activating system is a network of nerve cells and nerve fibers which originate in the brain stem, extend upward through the mesencephalon and thalamus and then are distributed throughout the cerebral cortex.

  B. Varying degrees of wakefulness and sleep are possible because of the vast numbers of nerve pathways between the cerebral cortex and the reticular activating system and between the body's periphery and the reticular activating system.

    [1] Sleep occurs when the brain's reticular activating system becomes sufficiently depressed by the reduction of stimuli from the cerebral cortex and the periphery. During sleep the system is almost completely quiet.

    [2] Wakefulness occurs after the reticular activating system has been activated and feedback mechanisms from the cerebral cortex and the periphery maintain the stimulation.

      a. Sensory stimuli of sufficient strength and/or numbers can normally cause immediate wakefulness. These include sensations of pain, sensations of pressure, auditory or visual stimuli, visceral sensations.

      b. It is more difficult to awaken an individual from a deep sleep than from a light sleep.

  C. Biphasic sleep and wakefulness patterns develop early in life. Individuals learn to be wakeful for an extended period, then to sleep for an extended period.

  D. Sleep patterns are learned (e.g., environments conducive to sleep, conditions for falling asleep and remaining asleep, time for and length of sleep periods).

  E. The aging adult may require longer periods of time for sleep, as there is a tendency to awaken more often and to remain awake.

3. Sleep cycles have two phases: non-rapid eye movement sleep (NREM) and rapid eye movement sleep (REM).

  A. Within a 7- to 8-hour sleep period there are usually 3 to 4 periods of REM sleep. These tend to occur every 1 to 2 hours and may last for 5 minutes to 1 hour.

  B. Transition from NREM to REM sleep is generally indicated by slight involuntary muscle jerks.

  C. REM sleep varies with age. It represents approximately 50 percent of the sleep of the newborn, 20 percent of an adult's sleep and 15 percent of the elderly person's sleep.

  D. Individuals who fail to have the usual REM periods of sleep tend to develop a feeling of extreme fatigue, become hyperirritable and may demonstrate neurotic behavior.

  E. NREM sleep appears to provide for the rest and restoration of the body.

4. Physical activity during waking hours tends to promote adequate sleep periods; however, stimulating physical activity just prior to bedtime tends to interfere with falling asleep.
5. Normal fatigue is experienced after strenuous work. A period of rest or sleep normally restores the ability to do work and a general sense of well-being.
6. The higher the metabolic rate, the greater the body's demands for increased blood flow, increased oxygen, increased amounts of nutrients and the greater the need for increased elimination of waste products of cellular metabolism.
7. Total body response to serious stress can be increased if body demands are reduced to a minimal level by rest and sleep.

Pathology

1. Symptoms and signs of sleep deprivation may include:
   A. Feeling of fatigue, lassitude.
   B. Inability to concentrate, incorrect perceptions.
   C. Excessive irritability, restlessness.
   D. Muscular incoordination, dizziness.
   E. Inflamed conjunctiva, puffiness and darkened areas around eyes, glazed appearance to eyes.
   F. Progressive disorientation and hallucinations.
2. Insomnia is frequently associated with nervousness.
   A. Nervousness is a state of mental and, usually, bodily restlessness that is accompanied by a feeling of uneasiness and apprehension. There may be hyper-irritability.
   B. Nervousness may occur in relation to:
      [1] Mental or emotional conflict. (It is an early symptom of major mental disorders.)
      [2] Neurological conditions, such as traumatic brain injuries or encephalitis.
      [3] Hyperthyroidism. (See Chapter 8.)
   C. Excessive nervousness can result in a state of extreme fatigue that cannot be relieved by sleep and rest.

Nursing Care

**Nursing care should be directed toward assisting the patient to
meet his needs for rest and sleep.**

COLLECTION, EVALUATION AND COMMUNICATION OF DATA
1. Patients should be interviewed, observed and examined to determine the quantity and quality of their rest and sleep.
2. The quantity and quality of rest and sleep should be evaluated in relation to:
   A. Usual rest and/or sleep patterns.
   B. Age.
   C. Health status, physical and emotional.
   D. Current stress level.
   E. Any drugs that have been administered to promote sleep and rest.

3. Patients should be observed for indications of sleep deprivation.
   A. Observations should be made for:
      [1] Inadequate number of hours of sleep.
      [2] Wakefulness during sleep periods.
      [3] Behavioral changes (e.g., inability to concentrate, confusion, hyper-
          irritability).
      [4] Muscular incoordination.
      [5] Eyes reddened with glazed appearance, puffiness around eyes, possibly
          darkened areas under eyes.
   B. Systematic patient evaluation is of especial importance when the patient:
      [1] Is under unusual physical or emotional stress.
      [2] Is convalescing from illness or injury.
      [3] Has a high metabolic rate (e.g., with hyperthyroidism).
      [4] Has a diagnosed disorder involving the heart, respiratory system, the kid-
          neys and/or the liver.
      [5] Has a mental disorder.
      [6] Is very young or elderly.
4. How, when and what data are communicated to the physician and/or other nursing
   personnel depend upon:
   A. Any potential threat to the patient's well-being (e.g., inadequate sleep and rest
      for a cardiac patient).
   B. Any particular implications for the physician in relation to:
      [1] The patient's progress or lack of progress toward recovery (e.g., the length
          of quiet sleep for a hyperactive patient).
      [2] The patient's physical and emotional responses to sedative, tranquilizing
          or hypnotic drugs.
   C. Any particular implications for nursing (e.g., scheduling of activities and nurs-
      ing functions in relation to sleep periods).

PROMOTION OF HEALTH AND PREVENTION
OF DISEASE/INJURY

1. Health teaching to promote proper sleep and rest should be concerned with:
   A. Variations in sleep needs throughout the life cycle and normal individual
      variations.
   B. Common sleep aids.
   C. The importance of:
      [1] Meeting sleep and rest needs throughout the life cycle.
      [2] Recreation and relaxation and the avoidance of excessive and/or prolonged
          emotional stress.
      [3] Learning to cope with unavoidable emotional stress.
      [4] A balanced program of exercise throughout the life cycle.
      [5] Increased sleep and rest during illness and convalescence.
   D. The importance of medical consultation when there is persistent insomnia.
2. Sleep and rest may be encouraged by:
   A. Providing a nonstimulating environment (e.g., minimizing light and sound).
   B. Providing physical comfort (e.g., positioning, control of environmental tem-
      perature, alleviation of pain).

   C. Providing psychological comfort. (See Part III.)

   D. Providing muscle relaxation. (See Chapter 11.)

   E. Providing both physical and mental activities and varieties of each during a 24-hour period.

   F. Discouraging stimulating activities just before bedtime.

   G. Scheduling activities and performing nursing functions to allow for rest periods and for longest possible uninterrupted sleep periods.

   H. Providing helpful sleep aids for individual patients (e.g., a warm bath, a cup of hot milk, nonstimulating reading matter, soft music).

   I. Administering sedative, tranquilizing or hypnotic drugs as ordered and needed and at appropriate times.

Chapter 11

Locomotion

The neuromusculoskeletal system provides means of locomotion.

Anatomy and Physiology

THE NEUROMUSCULOSKELETAL SYSTEM IN GENERAL

1. The skeleton is composed of a definite arrangement of bones joined together by ligaments, cartilage and muscles.
   A. The skeleton provides:
      [1] A framework for the body.
      [2] Protection for soft tissues. (See Chapter 12.)
      [3] A system of levers for locomotion.
   B. Each bone has a distinctive size and shape.
   C. The bones of the skeleton are joined to one another by connective tissue structures, which permit varying degrees of movement between the adjoining bones.
      [1] The amount of motion permitted at an articulation depends upon the shapes of the adjoining bones and the arrangement of ligaments, tendons and muscles surrounding the joint.
      [2] A freely movable joint has the following characteristics:
         a. The contiguous bony surfaces are covered with hyaline cartilage.
         b. A fibrous capsule surrounds the articulation.
         c. Synovial membrane lines the capsule and secretes the lubricating synovial fluid.
         d. Some joints are divided by cartilage discs (e.g., the knee).
         e. Healthy joints move easily and freely, with no sensation other than position of joint and speed of movement.

[3] Joint movement is limited or can be lost entirely when the joint is not moved through its normal range of motion for a prolonged period of time.

   a. When the connective tissue of the joint's fibrous capsule is not stretched by normal joint motion it loses its flexibility. The joint gradually becomes immovable, as the fibrous network becomes increasingly dense.

   b. The mobility of a normal joint can be reduced after only a few days without appropriate exercise. Fibrosis progresses even more rapidly when circulation is impaired.

[4] A bursa is a small membranous sac (within fascia) that contains a film of synovial fluid. Bursae act as lubricating devices and can be found:

   a. Where tendons rub against resistive structures.

   b. In some joint cavities.

   c. Subcutaneously, over joints that undergo acute flexion or over bones subject to considerable pressure.

2. Bones are formed by a protein matrix that allows for growth and change in shape. Within this pliable organic framework, salts of calcium and phosphorus are deposited. It is the inorganic portion that gives bone its normal hardness and rigidity.

   A. The amount of inorganic substance deposited increases with age.

   B. The long bones in children are largely cartilaginous, and calcification is usually not complete until 18 to 20 years of age. Also, the epiphyses usually do not close until this time.

   C. Children's feet grow constantly and rapidly.

   D. Bone is continually being formed (by osteoblasts) and resorbed into the system (by osteoclasts). If bone is to be normal, a balance must be maintained between these two processes.

      [1] The balance between bone formation and bone resorption is maintained as long as bones are subjected to normal stresses associated with weight-bearing and movement.

      [2] When normal stresses on bones are decreased or removed entirely, resorption tends to proceed at a slightly more rapid rate than bone formation. Consequently, calcium is lost from the bone, and it becomes increasingly porous.

         a. Normal bone loses calcium after approximately 2 weeks of immobilization.

         b. If normal stresses are restored before decalcification has progressed too far, the process can be reversed.

   E. The formation of bone and its growth and repair are influenced by:

      [1] The availability of adequate amounts of protein, minerals (especially calcium and phosphorus) and vitamins (especially Vitamins C and D). (See Chapter 3.)

      [2] The presence of certain hormones (e.g., parathyroid hormone, thyroid hormone, somatotropin). (See Chapter 8.)

      [3] The quality of blood circulation.

   F. The shape and growth of bones are altered by pressure and stresses related to muscle contractions and weight-bearing. Changes in shape occur most readily prior to complete calcification of bone or when there is faulty bone structure.

G. There are three phases in the repair of a fractured bone.
  [1] When the bone is fractured, there is hemorrhage from both edges of the break. Blood collects in the periosteal sheath or adjacent tissues and forms a clot. Capillary loops, fibrocytes, phagocytes and osteoblasts from the periosteum and surrounding bone invade the blood clot. The soft fibrous tissue which is formed is sometimes referred to as the procallus. If injured it bleeds easily.
  [2] The osteoblasts produce collagen and osseomucin, which can be converted into bone and then calcified. The newly calcified bone mass is called the callus.
  [3] Osteoclasts from the periosteal sheath and surrounding bone then begin resorptive function to shape the bone.

H. The rate and quality of bone healing depend upon:
  [1] The size of the bone involved.
  [2] The alignment of the fractured parts (which may be accomplished through reduction and/or traction).
  [3] The blood supply to the part.
  [4] The quality of nutrition.
  [5] Immobilization of the involved part.
  [6] Protection from further trauma.
  [7] The absence or presence of infection.

I. Repaired bone may be even stronger than the original bone.

3. Bones are moved by the contraction of skeletal muscles.
  A. Skeletal muscles are called voluntary muscles because they are under the direct control of a conscious brain.
  B. Individual muscles are formed by bundles of muscle fibers (or cells) held together by connective tissue. Individual muscles are separated, held together and maintained in proper position by tough sheets of connective tissue called fascia.
  C. Most skeletal muscles are attached to bones, cartilage or ligaments by tendons or aponeuroses.
    [1] Other skeletal muscles attach to the skin (fascial muscles), to mucous membrane (the tongue), to a fibrous plate (eye muscles) or form circular bands (sphincters).
    [2] The attachments of the two ends of a muscle are called the origin and the insertion. The origin is considered the more fixed and proximal end.
  D. Almost every muscle that acts upon a joint is matched by another muscle that has an opposite action. Either muscle of such a pair is the antagonist of the other (e.g., flexors and extensors, abductors and adductors, supinators and pronators).
  E. Most body movements require the combined action of a number of muscles.
    [1] The muscles that bring about the desired movement are called the prime movers.
    [2] The muscles that hold the body in proper position are called fixator muscles.
  F. Different parts of the same muscle may have different actions.

4. Muscle contractions are effected by the contraction of myofibrils within the individual muscle fibers.
   A. Myosin and actin filaments contained within the myofibrils are responsible for the contraction of the myofibrils.
   B. A definite concentration of magnesium is needed for proper muscle cell excitability.
   C. A proper concentration of calcium ions in the myofibrils is necessary to initiate the contractile process.
   D. Adenosine triphosphate provides energy for muscle contractions.
5. Muscle contractions are said to be isometric when the muscle does not shorten during contraction and isotonic when the muscle shortens but the tension on the muscle remains the same.
6. Skeletal muscle contractions perform mechanical work (e.g., lifting objects or moving them against force).
   A. Performance of work requires increased amounts of oxygen, glucose and other nutrients.
   B. Approximately 70 percent of the energy produced by muscle contractions is converted into heat.
   C. Normal muscle tone (a partial tension and firmness) enables muscles to perform mechanical work.
      [1] The action potential of individual muscle fibers is probably responsible for muscle tonus.
      [2] Centers in the brain and spinal cord function in the maintenance of normal muscle tone.
7. Forceful muscle activity over time results in muscle hypertrophy.
8. When muscles are not used or used only partially they atrophy.
   A. A healthy muscle may be reduced to one-half its normal size after 2 months of disuse.
   B. Denervation of a muscle causes atrophy. Muscle fibers begin to degenerate after approximately 4 months without innervation. Fat and fibrous tissue replace the muscle tissue.
9. Continuous or frequently repeated "all-out" contractions of a muscle can injure the muscle fibers.
10. Sudden, violent muscle contractions or tension of muscles can cause tearing, stretching and rupture of muscles, tendons and blood vessels.
11. Muscle contraction is under nervous control.
12. Sensory information from all parts of the body is integrated at all levels of the nervous system and effects specific motor responses. For example, simple reflexes are effected at the spinal cord level, while exceedingly complex motor responses are effected at the level of the cerebral cortex.
13. Somatic sensations include:
    A. Mechanoreceptive somatic senses, which detect changes in the relationships of body tissues.
       [1] The kinesthetic sense determines the positions of body parts and rates of movement.
          a. Kinesthetic receptors, located in joint capsules and ligaments, are stimulated by joint movements.

b. Sensory nerve fibers for the kinesthetic sense transmit signals to the spinal cord and on to the brain very rapidly.

[2] The tactile senses include touch, pressure and vibration.

B. Thermoreceptive senses, which detect changes in temperature.

C. The pain sense, which detects tissue damage.

14. All somatic sensations are transmitted via sensory nerve fibers that enter the spinal cord through the posterior roots. Upon entering the cord these first-order neurons separate into medial and lateral divisions.

A. The medial fibers enter the dorsal columns of the cord and ascend the full length of the cord. The dorsal columns transmit touch, pressure, vibratory and kinesthetic sensations to the brain.

B. The lateral fibers synapse with other neurons that form the spinothalamic tracts that ascend the spinal cord in the ventral and lateral columns. The spino-thalamic tracts transmit crude touch and pressure sensations; pain, thermal and sexual sensations; tickle and itch sensations.

15. The sensory nerve fibers from the separate body parts are maintained in a definite spatial relationship from where they originate in the dorsal columns to the cerebral cortex.

A. Second-order neurons, originating in the medulla, cross to the opposite side before passing upward to the thalamus.

B. Third-order neurons, originating in both sides of the thalamus, project almost exclusively to the postcentral gyrus of the cerebral cortex. This area is designated as Somatic Sensory Area I. (Somatic Sensory Area II lies posteriorly and laterally to Area I, and little is known about its function.)

16. Somatic Sensory Area I enables the conscious individual to:

A. Localize sensations.

B. Discern degrees of pressure exerted against body parts.

C. Judge the weights of different objects.

D. Judge the shapes, forms and textures of objects (without the visual sense).

E. Recognize the relative positions of body parts.

F. Discriminate between slight variations in temperature.

17. Change in the position of any body part depends upon a constant series of nervous impulses, mediated by efferent nerves, which cause smooth coordinated contractions of the agonist muscles and relaxation of the antagonist muscles involved.

18. Most of the patterns of muscle movements that are necessary for posture and locomotion can be effected at the spinal cord level.

A. The neurons responsible for spinal cord reflexes are between the sensory and motor roots in the gray matter of the cord.

[1] Internuncial (or intermediate) nerve cells are located in the dorsal and anterior horns and in between. They have many interconnections among themselves, and some innervate the anteromotor neurons.

[2] Interconnections between the internuncial neurons and the anterior motor neurons provide for many integrative functions of the spinal cord.

B. The anterior motor neurons give rise to nerve fibers that leave the cord in the spinal nerves. Motor signals leave the spinal cord through the anterior roots.

C. The stretch reflex (or myotatic reflex) is initiated by muscle stretch and causes the stretched muscle to contract.

[1] The stretch can be elicited in most skeletal muscles by sharply striking either the muscle tendon or the belly of the muscle. An example is the knee jerk.

[2] The reflex controls the length of a muscle and serves to prevent jerky muscle contractions.

[3] Muscle jerks are increased by facilitory impulses from higher centers. When these impulses are reduced or eliminated, muscle jerks are decreased or entirely absent.

D. The tendon reflex controls the tension of muscles.

[1] If extreme tension is applied to the tendon of a muscle, this reflex causes the muscle to relax.

[2] It is believed that higher centers are able to set the tension levels to be maintained by different muscle groups while certain muscle movements are being performed.

E. The flexor reflex (or withdrawal reflex) causes muscle contractions that move a limb or other body part away from a stimulus, often a painful stimulus. The arms and legs have highly developed flexor reflexes.

F. Sudden transection of the spinal cord causes spinal shock, involving complete loss of motor, sensory, autonomic and reflex activity below the injury.

[1] Skeletal muscle reflexes are completely blocked because normal facilitory impulses from the higher centers are absent.

[2] Although sacral reflexes for bladder and bowel evacuation may return to normal within several weeks, reflexes concerned with posture and locomotion rarely return to normal.

19. Muscle spasms are sudden, strong involuntary muscle contractions.

A. Rapid and repeated muscle contraction and relaxation caused by repeated synchronous activation of many motor units are called clonic muscle spasms (or clonus).

B. A muscle contraction that persists is called a tonic muscle spasm (or muscle cramp).

20. Muscle spasms caused by spinal cord reflexes may indicate injury to muscle tissue due to:

A. Fractures. (Spasm provides physiologic splinting.)

B. Overexercise.

C. Inadequate blood flow (sometimes related to vasoconstriction due to sudden chilling).

D. Inflammation of adjacent tissues (e.g., irritation of the parietal peritoneum causes spasms of the abdominal muscles).

21. There are reflex mechanisms governing the orientation of the head in space, the relation of the head to the trunk, and the appropriate adjustments of the limbs to the position of the head.

A. Sensory nerve endings in the inner ear; the retina; and the skeletal muscles, tendons and joints all receive stimuli. Impulses are transmitted to the spinal cord, the midbrain and the cerebellum. Motor nerves cause appropriate postural adjustments.

B. There are centers in the brain stem that function to maintain postural tone and provide equilibrium reflexes.

[1] Most of the reticular formation is excitatory. Stimulation of the bulbo-

reticular facilitory area causes a general increase in muscle tone, which may be generalized or local.

[2] Impulses from the reticular formation and the vestibular nuclei cause the contraction of extensor muscles that support body parts against gravity. The tonus of antigravity muscles (e.g., the jaw extensors) is markedly decreased during sleep or when the central nervous system is depressed (e.g., by CNS depressants).

[3] The vestibular apparatus (composed of the utricle and the semicircular canals in the inner ear) detects sensations concerned with equilibrium.

    a. Signals are transmitted by the vestibular nerves to nuclei in the brain stem which control facilitation and inhibition of the extensor muscles.

    b. Vestibular signals also pass into the cerebellum.

    c. Normally functioning semicircular canals provide for prediction of the loss of equilibrium. Signals transmitted to the equilibrium centers cause appropriate adjustments in muscle contractions so that equilibrium can be maintained.

    d. Nystagmus is the process that occurs automatically when a person rotates his head. The eyes rotate far to the opposite side as they are fixed on an object, then suddenly they jump in the direction of the head rotation and fix on a new object. The eye movements are caused by centers located in the brain stem and occur normally when the semicircular canals are stimulated by rotation of the head.

    e. When the vestibular apparatus is not functioning properly visual mechanisms can serve to provide for equilibrium, as long as body movements are slow.

22. The motor areas of the cortex initiate muscular activity and control the sequences of muscle contractions, providing purposefulness and progression in locomotion.

  A. The primary motor cortex is located immediately in front of the central sulcus. Because it contains vast numbers of pyramid-shaped cells it is sometimes referred to as the pyramidal area.

  B. There is a spatial organization of the motor cortex that corresponds with different muscle groups in the body (i.e., the fingers, the arm, the shoulder).

  C. The corticospinal (or pyramidal) tract is a major pathway, by which motor signals are transmitted from the motor area to the anteromotor neurons of the spinal cord.

    [1] Before the corticospinal tract leaves the brain many collateral nerve fibers branch off to:

      a. Other cortical areas.

      b. The basal ganglia. (The basal ganglia lie between the thalamus and the white matter of each cerebral hemisphere and include the caudate nucleus, the lentiform nucleus, the claustrum and the amygdaloid body.)

      c. The reticular substance of the brain stem.

      d. The cerebellum.

    [2] Motor pathways pass directly or indirectly (through subcortical integration centers, such as those in the basal ganglia system) to the medulla, where up to 85 percent of the fibers cross before entering the spinal cord.

    D. All other tracts that transmit motor signals from the brain to the spinal cord are called extracorticospinal (or extrapyramidal).

    E. Most of the corticospinal nerve fibers descend the cord in lateral or ventral tracts and synapse with internuncial cells. Impulses are transmitted by the internuncial cells to the anterior motor neurons.

        [1] The internuncial system and the motor neurons provide the final integration of motor signals from all areas.

        [2] The anterior motor neurons actually effect the contraction of individual skeletal muscles.

        [3] The individual muscles innervated by the motor nerves lie either at the same level or slightly below the level of origin of the anteromotor neurons in the ventral horns of the spinal cord.

23. Some of the structures that are part of the basal ganglia system are concerned with muscle activity. They function to:

    A. Inhibit muscle tone.

    B. Control gross voluntary movements that may be carried out at the unconscious level.

    C. Provide for muscle contractions that serve to stabilize body parts in specific positions.

24. The cerebellum lies between the brain stem and the occipital lobes of the cerebrum.

    A. The cerebellum is attached to the brain stem.

        [1] There are afferent pathways to the cerebellum from the:

            a. Motor cortex.

            b. Basal ganglia.

            c. Vestibular system.

            d. Brain stem.

            e. Body proprioceptors.

        [2] There are efferent tracts from the cerebellum to the:

            a. Motor cortex and basal ganglia.

            b. Brain stem.

    B. The cerebellum functions to:

        [1] Prevent errors (e.g., overaction) in body movements initiated by the motor cortex.

        [2] Predict the future positions of moving body parts.

        [3] Predict loss of equilibrium.

        [4] Coordinate voluntary movement (especially important when body movement is rapid).

25. The peripheral nerves provide communicating pathways that connect the central nervous system (brain and spinal cord) with the periphery of the body.

    A. The peripheral nerves consist of 12 pairs of cranial nerves and 31 pairs of spinal nerves.

    B. The spinal nerves arise at different segmental levels of the spinal cord.

        [1] There are 8 pairs of cervical nerves, 12 pairs of thoracic nerves, 5 pairs of lumbar nerves, 5 pairs of sacral nerves and 1 pair of coccygeal nerves.

        [2] Because the spinal cord terminates at the highest part of the lumbar region, the nerves from the lower part of the spinal cord must pass downward through the spinal canal before passing through the spinal foramina.

C. The spinal nerves that supply the upper extremities and those that supply the lower extremities divide, recombine and divide again in complicated patterns to form two nerve plexuses.

    [1] The brachial plexuses are located between the neck and the axilla in each shoulder; the nerves supply all the muscles of the upper extremities.

    [2] The lumbosacral plexuses are located in the lower back; the nerves supply all the muscles of the lower extremities.

D. Peripheral nerves (branches from spinal nerves), which run very superficially in the extremities, include:

    [1] The ulnar, along the medial upper arm and down the ulna side of the forearm.

    [2] The radial, around the back of the humerus and down the radial side of the forearm.

    [3] The sciatic, in the hip and down the back of the thigh.

    [4] The peroneal, in the popliteal space.

SPECIFIC BONES, MUSCLES AND JOINTS
INVOLVED IN LOCOMOTION

1. The bones of the upper extremity include those of the shoulder girdle (clavicle and scapula), the upper arm (humerus), the lower arm (radius and ulna), the wrist (8 carpal bones), and the hand (5 metacarpal bones and 14 phalanges).

2. The shoulder joint, formed by the articulation of the head of the humerus with the scapula, is of the ball and socket type.

    A. The socket is shallow.

    B. The ligaments surrounding the joint are relatively loose.

    C. The shoulder joint allows movement of the humerus in all directions.

    D. The scapula is connected to the trunk by muscles only.

3. Muscles that originate on the trunk and insert on the shoulder girdle (acting singly or in combinations) act to adduct, abduct, elevate, depress and rotate the shoulder girdle. (For complete abduction of the shoulder, the humerus must be outwardly rotated after the first 90° of motion.)

4. Muscles that originate on the trunk and shoulder girdle and insert on the humerus (acting singly or in combinations) act to adduct, abduct, flex, extend and rotate the humerus.

5. The elbow joint comprises three different portions: the joints between the ulna and humerus, between the radius and humerus, and between the radius and the ulna.

    A. The joint between the ulna and the humerus is a simple hinge joint.

    B. Muscles that originate on the shoulder girdle and/or the humerus and insert on the radius or ulna act to flex and to extend the forearm.

    C. Muscles that originate and insert on the ulna and radius act to supinate and to promote the forearm.

6. The wrist joint proper, formed by the articulations of several carpal bones and the distal end of the radius, is of the gliding type.

    A. Muscles of the posterior aspect of the forearm act to extend the hand.

    B. Muscles of the anterior aspect of the forearm act to flex the hand.

    C. The flexors and extensors acting in different groupings also abduct, adduct and circumduct the hand.

7. The joints between the metacarpal and the carpal bones are of the gliding type, and have limited motion, with the exception of the first metacarpal, which is a saddle joint and allows for abduction, adduction, circumduction and opposition of the thumb.

8. The joints between the metacarpal and phalangeal bones are of the condyloid type and allow flexion, extension, limited abduction and adduction and circumduction of the fingers. (Flexion of the fingers can best be accomplished when the wrist is in hyperextension; the flexion should allow for the natural deviation of the fingers toward the thumb side of the palm.)

9. The joints between the phalanges of each digit are of the hinge type and allow for flexion and extension.

10. The vertebral column is composed of individual vertebrae, the bodies of which are separated by fibrocartilaginous discs; and all are bound together by numerous ligaments that pass from one bone to another.

   A. The intervetebral discs absorb shock and permit a slight degree of movement.

   B. The vertebral column articulates with the skull and with the iliac bones of the pelvic girdle.

11. At birth and until a baby is able to hold up his head, the primary curve of the vertebral column is posteriorly convex. After the baby's muscles have developed enough so that he can hold up his head and stand and walk, the secondary curves of the vertebral column appear.

   A. The cervical curve is anteriorly convex.

   B. The thoracic curve is posteriorly convex.

   C. The lumbar curve is anteriorly convex.

   D. The natural curves of the vertebral column give resilience and help to absorb shock.

   E. The natural curves may be changed by prolonged postural changes, variations in walking, and pregnancy.

   F. In walking or sitting the pelvic girdle normally provides support for the vertebral column.

   G. Normal variations in the depth and length of the curves of the vertebral column are related to age, sex, race, height and weight.

12. Muscles of the back that essentially attach vertebrae to vertebrae or vertebrae to ribs act to extend the spine and assist in rotation of the spine. (These muscles are fixator muscles and are arranged primarily for the purpose of support, not for the performance of work.)

13. Muscles that originate on the pelvic girdle and insert on the ribs act to flex the spine.

14. Muscles that originate on the vertebrae or shoulder girdle and insert on the posterior skull act to extend the head.

15. Muscles that originate on the temporal bone or cervical vertebrae and insert on the clavicle or rib cage act to flex the head.

16. The bones of the lower extremity include those of the pelvic girdle (hip bones, sacrum and coccyx), the thigh (femur), the leg (tibia, fibula and patella), the ankle (7 tarsal bones) and the foot (5 metatarsal bones and 14 phalanges).

A.   The hip bone consists of three parts: the ileum, the ischium and the pubis. The hip bones articulate anteriorly at the symphysis pubis.

B.   During pregnancy there is some relaxation of the ligaments of the pelvic girdle.

17.   The hip joint, formed by the articulation of the head of the femur fitting into the acetabulum of the hip bone, is of the ball and socket type.

18.   Muscles that originate on the vertebrae or pelvic girdle and insert on the femur (acting singly or in combinations) act to flex, extend, abduct, adduct and rotate the femur.

19.   The knee joint, formed by the articulation of the distal femur and the tibia, is both condyloid and gliding.

A.   The knee movements are closely related to movements of the hip joint (e.g., flexion of femur and flexion of lower leg).

B.   The patella is a flat bone located in the tendon on the quadriceps femoris in front of the knee joint; it articulates with the femur. (It helps to protect the knee joint, especially in kneeling.)

C.   Menisci (small crescents of fibrocartilage) lie between the tibia and the femur and help to adapt the surfaces of these bones and prevent jarring.

20.   Muscles that originate on the pelvic girdle or femur and insert on the tibia (acting singly or in combinations) act to extend, flex and (in certain positions) rotate, medially and laterally, the lower leg.

21.   The ankle joint, formed by the articulation of the distal ends of the tibia and fibula and one of the tarsal bones, is both hinge and condyloid in type.

A.   Muscles that originate on the tibia and fibula and insert on the medial or lateral aspects of the tarsal or metatarsal bones act either to invert or evert the foot.

B.   Muscles that originate on the anterior aspects of the tibia and fibula and insert on the tarsal bones act to dorsiflex the foot.

C.   Muscles that originate on the posterior aspects of the femur, tibia and fibula and insert on the tarsal bones act to plantar-flex the foot. (The major muscles that act to plantar-flex the foot insert in the tendon of Achilles.)

22.   The tarsal and metatarsal articulations allow limited gliding motions.

23.   The metatarsal and phalangeal articulations allow some flexion, extension, abduction and adduction.

24.   The interphalangeal joints permit flexion and limited extension.

25.   The foot has a longitudinal arch and a series of transverse arches formed by the arrangement of the tarsal and metatarsal bones and the ligaments that bind them together. (When the body is raised on the ball of one foot, the stress on the longitudinal arch is increased fourfold.)

26.   The major muscle groups may be considered to include:

A.   Flexors and extensors of the toes and fingers.

B.   Flexors, extensors and rotators of the feet and hands.

C.   Flexors and extensors of the legs and thighs.

D.   Flexors, extensors, supinators and pronators of the lower arm.

E.   Flexors, extensors and rotators of the upper arm.

F.   Extensors of the vertebral column.

G.   Adductors, abductors, elevators and depressors of the shoulder girdle.

H.   Flexors and rotators of the trunk.

POSTURE

1. Correct posture may be defined as maintaining proper anatomical relationships between body parts when the body is in different positions.
   A. The alignment of the body parts should be balanced; there should be minimal tension on all muscles.
   B. Correct body posture exists when the muscular forces required to balance torques produced by the weights of various parts of the body are at a minimum.
2. A correct lying posture in the dorsal recumbent position is the closest possible to good standing posture.
3. A correct lying posture in the prone position is the closest possible to good standing posture with the head turned to the side.
4. A correct lying posture in the lateral position is an approximation of a good sitting posture.
5. The position of function for the hand is similar to that position used in gripping a ball.
6. The position of function for the foot is that position desirable in correct standing posture.
7. The spinal muscles supply the contractions necessary for erect posture. If the reflex mechanisms necessary for this posture are lost, the muscles must be controlled voluntarily. Poor posture and fatigue result.
8. Posture may be related to one's emotional state (e.g., incorrect posture may be associated with depression or excessive tension, while correct posture may be associated with a general sense of well-being).

Physics

1. Force is that which changes or tends to change the linear motion of a body; the motion turns to the same direction as the force.
2. Work is done by a force if the force is allowed to act through a distance.
3. Torque is that force which changes or tends to change the rotary motion of a body.
4. Gravitation is the force of attraction between two objects (e.g., the earth and an object on or near the earth).
   A. The center of gravity of a body is the point where the whole weight of a body may be considered to be concentrated. (The center of gravity in the human body is located at a point approximately 0.57 of the height of the body, considering the total height as 1.0, and measuring up from the base.)
   B. Because of gravitational pull, more force is usually required to lift a heavy object than to push or pull it along a smooth surface.
5. A body is said to be unstable if a slight tipping of the object raises its center of gravity.
   A. A vertical line drawn downward from the center of gravity of a body in stable equilibrium will fall within the base of support. (Increasing the base of support will increase stability.)
   B. In general, a change in the position of the center of gravity upsets equilibrium, and for equilibrium to be regained, changes must be made in forces and/or torques acting on the object (e.g., in standing, when there is a forward shift in

the center of gravity, the muscles of the back must exert more pull to maintain body balance).

6. When a body is in equilibrium:
   A. The sum of all forces acting on the body equals zero; and
   B. The sum of all torques acting at any axis must equal zero.
7. Within the elastic limit, stress is proportional to the strain (Hooke's law):
   A. If the elastic limit of an object is exceeded, the object is either permanently distorted or broken.
   B. Types of stress that may produce characteristic injuries in the body are tension, compression, twisting and bending.
8. A lever is a simple machine comprising a rigid bar which moves about a fulcrum (or fixed axis). Keeping lever arms short decreases the torque produced by a given load.

Pathology

SYMPTOMS AND SIGNS

1. Symptoms and signs of problems involving bones may include:
   A. Abnormalities in contour, alignment, length or continuity of a part or parts.
   B. Absence of, loss of or change in movement of a part.
   C. Feeling or hearing bone break; cracking sounds (crepitus) with movement.
   D. Pain, which may be intense and increase with movement of the body part.
   E. Discoloration of skin due to bleeding from capillaries in injured area.
   F. Localized tissue swelling, possibly hematoma.
2. Symptoms and signs of problems involving voluntary muscles may include:
   A. Muscle weakness, loss of contractility.
   B. Muscle spasms, which may be accompanied by acute cramping pain.
   C. Soreness, tenderness, aching of muscles.
   D. Muscle atrophy.
3. Symptoms and signs of problems involving or associated with the nervous control of muscle function may include:
   A. Spastic or flaccid paralysis.
   B. Involuntary movements, such as convulsions, muscle spasms, tremors.
   C. Changes in strength and/or coordination of muscle contractions.
   D. Loss of equilibrium, difficulty with postural adjustments.
   E. Loss of position sense.
   F. Hypoactive or hyperactive spinal reflexes.
   G. Burning, tingling pain along path of peripheral nerve.
   H. Numbness, coldness of a part.
4. Symptoms and signs of problems involving joints may include:
   A. Change in contour or size of joint.
   B. Limitation of motion in joint, or abnormal motion possible.
   C. Swelling, redness and increased skin temperature around joint.
   D. Local aching or pain that may become severe with movement.
   E. Crackling sounds with movement.
   F. Muscle spasms around joint.

BONE DISORDERS
1. Bone disorders include:
   A. Congenital or acquired deformities.
      [1] Congenital bone defects include absence of bones, shortness of bones, weakness of bones and positional anomalies (e.g., clubbed feet).
      [2] Bone deformities may be acquired through:
          a. Abnormal bone development because of improper nutrition. (See Chapter 3.)
          b. Abnormal bone development due to hormonal imbalance. (See Chapter 8.)
          c. Abnormal pressure exerted against bones, especially during the growth period.
          d. Infections.
          e. Bone tumors, which may be primary or secondary.
          f. Improperly healed fractures.
   B. Conditions in which there is a reduction in the density of bone.
      [1] Osteomalacia is a pathological condition in which the bones become soft and fragile because of deficient mineralization related to nutritional or metabolic faults.
      [2] Osteoporosis is a condition in which there is loss of bone bulk (both matrix and salts). It occurs in relation to muscle disuse and may be seen commonly in the elderly.
   C. Fractures, with or without dislocations.
      [1] Fractures are breaks in the continuity of bone which are usually caused by traumatic injury. If a bone is weakened by disease (e.g., infection or osteomalacia) or by osteoporosis, a very slight injury can cause a fracture.
      [2] Fractures may be classified according to:
          a. The type of injury (e.g., direct or indirect).
          b. The shape of the bone fragments (e.g., transverse, oblique, spiral, or comminuted).
          c. Whether they are open (i.e., there is a connection between the fracture and the outside) or closed. An open fracture is sometimes referred to as a compound fracture.
      [3] Fractures, with or without dislocations, often cause injury to adjacent soft tissues, including muscles, blood vessels and nerves.
   D. Infections.
      [1] Acute osteomyelitis is the infection of bone with pyogenic microorganisms, frequently staphylococcus or streptococcus.
          a. Organisms usually reach the bone through the blood from an infection elsewhere in the body, but they may also be introduced through the wound of an open fracture or in association with bone surgery (including insertion of traction pins).
          b. Because bone is rigid it does not allow swelling. Accumulation of inflammatory exudates may cause severe pain. Periosteal abscesses are formed. The pressure of exudates sometimes interferes with the blood supply, and ischemic bone will separate from living bone as a sequestrum.

[2] Chronic osteomyelitis is almost always preceded by the acute form. There is usually a sinus over the affected bone that drains purulent discharge.
2. Pain associated with bone disorders may be severe.

MUSCLE DISORDERS
1. Muscle disorders include:
   A. Inflammation.
      [1] Myositis is an inflammation of voluntary muscle tissue which is often due to overexercise, prolonged stretching of muscles or a sudden pull. It can also result from chilling (e.g., neck and back muscles). There is muscle tenderness, which may be exquisite, and there may be muscle spasms, which can be extremely painful (e.g., gastrocnemius muscle).
      [2] Trichinosis is a helminth infection. The parasites are ingested and may invade many body organs. When the skeletal muscles are invaded, there is acute muscle pain, especially during muscle contraction.
   B. Those caused by interference with normal innervation of a muscle.
      [1] See the following section for disorders involving nervous control of skeletal muscles.
      [2] Myasthenia gravis is a chronic disease manifested by abnormal fatigue of skeletal muscles. There is interference with the transmission of impulses from nerve to muscle at the myoneural junction.
   C. Those caused by traumatic injury (e.g., associated with fractures, dislocations, crushing injuries, surgery).
   D. Those caused by interference with blood supply. Inadequate arterial blood supply results in:
      [1] Death of muscle fibers.
      [2] Loss of muscle contractility.
      [3] Replacement by fibrous tissue, which may lead to contractures.
   E. Muscular dystrophies, which appear to be inherited. There is progressive weakness and atrophy of various groups of muscles.

NERVOUS SYSTEM DISORDERS
1. Disorders involving the nervous control of skeletal muscles include:
   A. Injuries to the:
      [1] Sensory and/or motor areas of the cerebral cortex.
      [2] Sensory and/or motor pathways in the brain and spinal cord.
      [3] Cerebellum, midbrain or vestibular apparatus.
      [4] Peripheral nerves (spinal nerves, their branches and various nerve plexuses).
   B. Epilepsy.
   C. Degenerative disorders (e.g., multiple sclerosis, Parkinson's disease).
2. Injury to nerve tissue may be due to:
   A. Trauma (e.g., partial or complete severance of a nerve fiber or tract; stretching and tearing of nerve plexus; destruction of nerve cells by a blow, bullet or sharp instrument).
      [1] Spinal cord damage may occur as a result of fractures and/or dislocations of vertebral bodies or processes.

[2] Spinal cord injuries can occur at any level but are most common at the 5th and 6th cervical level and at the 11th and 12th thoracic level. (Injury above the 5th cervical level usually causes death due to respiratory failure.)

B. Inadequate blood supply, which may be caused by pressure exerted on blood vessels by:
   [1] Accumulating fluids (e.g., edema, inflammatory exudates or hemorrhage).
   [2] Abnormal growths.
   [3] Applied bandages, casts, tractions.
   [4] Abnormal positioning of body parts.
C. Inadequate supply of oxygen. (See Chapter 2.)
D. Hypoglycemia. (See Chapter 3.)
E. Vitamin deficiencies. (See Chapter 3.)
F. Infections (e.g., encephalitis, meningitis, poliomyelitis). (See Chapter 20.)

3. Spinal deformities may cause pressure on the spinal cord and spinal nerves that can result in pain and in various sensory and/or motor disturbances.
   A. Spinal deformities may be due to:
      [1] Improper growth of the vertebral column.
      [2] Muscle imbalances.
      [3] Destruction of bones and joints by infections, traumatic injuries or tumors.
   B. Kyphosis denotes excessive posterior curvature of the spinal column.
   C. Scoliosis denotes lateral curvature of the spine. The deformity may be progressive and permanent or only temporary.

4. Symptoms and signs of injury to nervous tissue are determined by the site of the injury (which nerves are involved), the extent of the injury (how much nervous tissue is involved) and the type of injury (the effect of the injury on nerve cells/fibers).

5. Injury to the motor areas of the cerebral cortex, the motor pathways in the brain and spinal cord, the anterior horn cells and/or the peripheral nerves causes some degree of paralysis.
   A. Damage to upper motor neurons impedes passage of motor signals between the cerebral cortex and a particular segment of the spinal cord, causing:
      [1] Spastic paralysis, which initially may be flaccid. (Unless prevented, flexion contractures can develop.)
      [2] Exaggerated spinal cord reflexes. (Muscle spasms, which can be extensive and severe, may be triggered by various physical and/or emotional stimuli.)
   B. Damage to lower motor neurons interferes with passage of motor signals from origin within the spinal cord segment to destination in a peripheral muscle, causing:
      [1] Flaccid paralysis.
      [2] Diminished or lost spinal cord reflexes.
      [3] Muscle wasting, atrophy.
   C. Muscle imbalances lead to deformed posture, abnormal gaits, abnormal movements and can result in fixed deformities.

6. Damage to the motor areas or to motor pathways involving the cerebellum, midbrain or vestibular apparatus causes various types of abnormal motor activity. These include:
   A. Involuntary movements such as convulsions, spasms, tremors. (Convulsions

are caused by abnormal and excessive neuronal activity in the brain. They may be associated with disorders such as epilepsy, brain tumors, cerebral ischemia, metabolic abnormalities, high fever in children and meningitis.)

    B.   Muscle rigidity.

    C.   Muscular incoordination.

    D.   Loss of equilibrium, difficulty with postural adjustments. (Disorders of the vestibular apparatus are included in Chapter 16.)

7. Epilepsy is a chronic disorder characterized by seizures that may involve convulsions.

    A.   The sequence of a grand mal seizure is:

       [1] Loss of consciousness;

       [2] A tonic stage in which the muscles become rigid and the limbs are extended (usually lasts less than 1 minute); then,

       [3] A clonic stage in which muscles contract and relax, moving the head and limbs about violently (rarely last longer than 3 minutes).

    B.   Grand mal seizures probably originate in the reticular activating system and spread to the cortex. They are frequently preceded by an aura, such as a sensation of bright light or a particular odor or sound.

8. Pathology involving the basal ganglia causes excessive motor activity.

    A.   Chorea (or St. Vitus' dance) is a condition in which there are continuous, uncontrolled and random movements of different muscle groups.

    B.   Athetosis involves slow, rhythmic, writhing movements of one or more extremities. These may be increased by strong sensory stimulation or strong emotions. Voluntary movements may be limited or lost.

    C.   Parkinson's disease (paralysis agitans) is a degenerative disorder in which nerve cells in the basal ganglia are destroyed. There is muscle rigidity (localized or generalized), intention tremors, difficulty in initiating movements, with loss of involuntary and associated muscle movements.

9. Cerebral palsy comprises a number of clinical disorders that are characterized by spastic muscular weakness, exaggerated reflexes, muscle imbalances and lack of voluntary control.

    A.   The condition almost always arises in childhood and is associated with brain damage which may occur:

       [1] Prenatally (e.g., due to congenital defect or erythroblastosis that causes damage to the basal ganglia).

       [2] Natally (e.g., birth injuries, cerebral anoxia during birth).

       [3] Postnatally (e.g., due to infection, such as encephalitis).

    B.   The severity varies from person to person.

10. Pathology involving the cerebellum can result in:

    A.   Inability to control how far body parts move (dysmetria).

    B.   Uncoordinated movements (ataxia).

    C.   Jerky movements.

    D.   Loss of equilibrium, especially when movements are rapid.

11. Infections that affect the central nervous system and locomotor activity include:

    A.   Anterior poliomyelitis, an acute febrile disease in which specific causative viruses attack the anterior horn cells.

       [1] The infection can occur at any level of the spinal cord.

[2] The amount and location of paralysis that develops depends upon the amount of nervous tissue affected and the particular segments of the spinal cord involved.

[3] There is flaccid paralysis and painful muscle spasms.

[4] Most of the motor activity that can be regained will be regained within one year. Paralysis of the muscles affected is permanent when nerve cells have been destroyed.

B. Encephalitis (inflammation of the brain), which may be caused by specific neurotropic viruses or may occur as a complication of virus infections such as measles or mumps. There may be disturbances in reflexes, rigidity of the neck and back muscles and paralysis.

C. Meningitis (inflammation of the meninges), which may be caused by a number of different microorganisms, including the *Neisseria meningitidis*. There may be muscle rigidity (especially of the neck), painful muscle spasms and/or convulsions.

D. Rabies (primarily an encephalitis in animals), which can be transmitted to man through the bites of rabid animals. The viruses travel along the peripheral nerves to the central nervous system. There are severe and painful muscle spasms that progress to paralysis. Death ensues.

12. Injury to the sensory areas of the cerebral cortex, to the sensory pathways in the brain and spinal cord or to the peripheral nerves results in loss of sensation from the specific areas of distribution.

A. There may be anesthetic areas, loss of position sense, loss of the vibratory sense and changes in perception of touch, temperature and pain.

B. The loss of sensation due to injury of a peripheral nerve interferes with normal spinal reflexes, including the protective withdrawal reflex.

13. Multiple sclerosis is a progressive degenerative disorder in which there is demyelination of nerves and sclerosing of areas in the brain and spinal cord. There may be disturbances in sensory and/or motor function, as clinical manifestations are determined by the areas affected. Generally there are periods of remission and exacerbation.

14. Over time, injured nerve cells within the central nervous system can regain function. Dead nerve cells do not regenerate.

15. Axons of injured peripheral nerves can regenerate over time, but recovery tends to be poor in older persons, when circulation is impaired or when there is extensive bruising of the nerve.

JOINT DISORDERS

1. Disorders that affect the movements of joints include:

A. Fractures. (See "Bone Disorders," preceding.)

B. Sprains.

[1] Sprains result from traumatic injury. Ligaments are torn, and muscles and tendons are stretched.

[2] Sprains may be accompanied by fractures.

[3] The area of sprain is usually quite painful. Pain increases with joint move-

ment. Edema tends to develop quickly, and there may be ecchymosis.

C. Dislocations.

    [1] A joint is dislocated (or luxated) when its articular surfaces are wholly displaced, one from the other. The joint capsule and ligaments may be torn. When only partly displaced, the joint is referred to as subluxated.

    [2] Dislocations may be congenital, and they may occur spontaneously. However, they are most often caused by traumatic injury.

    [3] Muscle spasms may be severe with dislocations.

D. Inflammatory joint disease.

    [1] Rheumatoid arthritis is an inflammatory condition of joints in which the tissues show inflammatory response (e.g., changes in secretion of synovial fluid, edema, congestion, tissue destruction and fibrosis).

        a. One or more joints may be involved. The knees, ankles, elbows, wrists and proximal joints of the phalanges are most commonly affected.

        b. In the acute stage joints are swollen, red, hot and extremely painful.

        c. Affected joints become enlarged and stiff. Irregularity of the joint surfaces and/or interference with proper lubrication limit function. Unless joints are moved muscles atrophy. Flexion contractures can occur when joints are maintained in flexion.

        d. Entire joints may become spongy and ankylosed.

        e. The cause of rheumatoid arthritis is unknown, but there are some indications that auto-immunity may be an etiologic factor.

    [2] Gout is a chronic inflammatory condition of the joints that is caused by a defect in purine metabolism.

        a. There is an increase in the concentration of uric acid in the blood, and urate crystals are deposited within joints. Usually only a single joint is involved, and the joint is frequently in the foot.

        b. There is pain, redness and swelling of the involved joint.

E. Infections.

F. Degenerative changes; for example, osteoarthritis.

    [1] Osteoarthritis involves hypertrophic changes in joints. The joint becomes enlarged, the articular cartilage becomes thin and there may be calcium deposits within the joint.

    [2] There is joint pain and stiffness, but no inflammation. Motion is limited.

    [3] The condition may follow traumatic injury to a joint or may result from excessive use of a joint, poor posture or excessive weight-bearing.

2. Bursitis is an inflammation of bursae, which may result from traumatic injury, strain or overuse of the muscles and joint around which these structures are found. There is pain with movement.

3. Muscle guarding generally occurs around an injured, painful joint; sustained muscle spasm reduces joint movement.

4. Stress placed on weight-bearing joints (primarily the hips and knees) increases with the amount of weight that must be borne by these joints. Unusual stress increases the likelihood of joint injury and slows the healing process when injury does occur.

Nursing Care

Nursing care should be directed toward assisting the patient to attain, retain or regain the best possible locomotor function.

COLLECTION, EVALUATION AND COMMUNICATION OF DATA

1. Patients should be interviewed, observed and examined to identify symptoms and signs of actual or potential locomotor problems.
   A. Problems may be indicated by:
      [1] Abnormalities in the structure and function of bones, muscles and/or joints.
      [2] Abnormal spinal reflexes.
      [3] Loss of equilibrium or position sense.
      [4] Pain (e.g., aching, tenderness, acute pain) associated with bones, muscles, joints, peripheral nerves.
      [5] Symptoms and signs of impaired peripheral circulation. (See Chapter 1.)
   B. Systematic patient evaluation is of especial importance when the patient:
      [1] Has suffered traumatic injury (e.g., a fall, a car accident).
      [2] Has a disease or injury (e.g., surgery) that involves bones, muscles and joints necessary for normal locomotion.
      [3] Has a disease or injury (e.g., surgery) that involves or may involve the central nervous system and/or peripheral nerves.
      [4] Is partially or completely immobilized.
      [5] Is unconscious.
      [6] Is an infant (especially a newborn), a child or an elderly person.
   C. The structure and function of the neuromusculoskeletal system should be evaluated in relation to:
      [1] Normal size and contour of body parts.
      [2] Normal alignment of body parts.
      [3] Normal range of motions of joints.
      [4] Normal voluntary control of body movements.
      [5] Normal coordination of body movements.
      [6] Normal state of equilibrium and postural adjustments.
      [7] Any diagnosed disorder that involves or might involve the neuromusculoskeletal system.
   D. Data collected should be evaluated not only on the basis of a single deviation from normal (e.g., joint stiffness), but should also be evaluated on the basis of combinations of symptoms and signs that are commonly associated with specific disorders or injuries (e.g., symptoms and signs associated with rheumatoid arthritis).
2. How, when and what data are communicated to the physician and/or other nursing personnel depend upon:
   A. Any potential threat to the patient's well-being (e.g., paralysis or convulsions).
   B. Any particular implications for the physician in relation to:

[1] The patient's progress or lack of progress toward recovery (e.g., change in motor function).

[2] Making a diagnosis (e.g., new objective or subjective data).

[3] The patient's physical and emotional responses to specific diagnostic procedures and therapeutic measures.

C. Any particular implications for nursing (e.g., assisting with activities of daily living).

PROMOTION OF HEALTH AND PREVENTION
OF DISEASE/INJURY

1. Health teaching to promote efficient locomotor function should be concerned with:

A. The importance of:

[1] A balanced program of exercise throughout the life cycle.

[2] Gradual increases in exercise and avoidance of overexercise.

[3] Proper nutrition throughout the life cycle, with adequate protein and calcium intake during growth periods, pregnancy, and lactation; and avoidance of excessive calories.

[4] Properly fitting shoes and hosiery, especially during growth period.

B. Correct posture and correct body mechanics.

C. Effects of shoes (fit, type) and foot problems on posture and body movements.

D. The importance of:

[1] Periodic health evaluations.

[2] Prompt medical evaluation when:

a. There has been traumatic injury such as falls, car accidents.

b. There are early indications of problems involving the neuromusculoskeletal system (e.g., bone pain, loss of motion, deformities, loss of voluntary muscle control).

c. There has been an animal bite.

[3] Immunization against poliomyelitis.

E. Accident prevention.

2. All patients should be protected from injury to the neuromusculoskeletal system. This is of critical importance when the patient:

A. Is dependent upon others for physical care and protection. This includes patients who are:

[1] Unconscious.

[2] Infants, children or elderly people.

[3] Weak or debilitated.

[4] Mentally incompetent (e.g., mentally retarded or having certain psychic disturbances).

[5] Immobilized.

B. Has a condition in which motor function is impaired (e.g., paralysis or involuntary movements).

C. Has a condition in which there is loss of sensory function (e.g., vision, hearing, position sense, pain sense).

   D. Uses special devices for locomotion (e.g., braces, canes, crutches, walkers, artificial limbs).

   E. Has a condition in which loss of consciousness is apt to occur (e.g., postural hypotension associated with circulatory disorder).

3. All patients should be protected from accidents such as falling, slipping or hitting against hard objects.

4. Patients should be positioned in normal anatomical alignment while in any posture, lying, sitting or standing.

   A. All body parts should be adequately supported in functional positions without pressure, drag or strain.

   B. The patient's environment (e.g., lights, tables, special equipment) should be arranged so as to encourage proper alignment of body parts.

5. Patients should have frequent changes of position (at *least* every few hours), within medical orders. When movement is restricted, even slight adjustments in the positioning of body parts are important.

   A. Patients should be moved smoothly, with normal body alignment maintained during the moving process.

   B. Body parts should be handled firmly but gently, always providing support for the head, the limbs and the joints.

6. Unless contraindicated, all major groups of muscles should have active, active-assisted or passive exercise daily.

   A. The freely movable body joints of the trunk and extremities should be moved through their normal and/or anatomically possible ranges of motion at *least* once daily and several times if possible.

   B. Ambulation should be encouraged, within medical orders.

   C. Patients should be encouraged (and assisted as necessary) to assume activities of daily living to the fullest possible extent.

   D. Unless contraindicated, patients with some degree of immobilization should be taught and encouraged to do muscle conditioning exercises frequently during waking hours (e.g., every 1–2 hours). These include muscle-setting and resistive exercises.

7. Patients should be taught and encouraged to use correct body mechanics.

   A. The body should be balanced over a firm base of support in standing, walking, squatting or rising. (Using a wide stance and keeping the body centered over the base of support increases stability of an upright posture.)

   B. When carrying heavy objects, the balance of the body should be shifted from the ankle rather than from the trunk.

   C. Prolonged carrying of objects on one side should be avoided.

   D. The pelvis and lower extremities should provide a firm support for the vertebral column, through use of low-heeled shoes or through standing and walking postures that provide this support.

   E. The least amount of muscular effort necessary to perform a given task should be used.

     [1] Movements should be made smoothly and rhythmically.

     [2] In lifting or carrying heavy objects, the arms should be held close to the body, and the object should be close to the body before lifting is done.

[3] When moving a heavy object, the parts of the body should be placed in such a way as to face in the same direction as the force to be applied.

[4] Objects should be moved or slid along surfaces, if possible, rather than lifted.

[5] Body weight should be utilized whenever possible to push or pull objects.

[6] When performing tasks, the sitting position should be used in preference to standing, whenever possible.

[7] Work levels should be such that muscle strain is minimized.

F. Objects that are too heavy to be moved alone should not be moved without adequate assistance.

G. The muscles best suited to the task to be done should be utilized.

[1] In lifting, pushing or pulling, the muscles of the lower extremities should be used rather than the muscles of the trunk.

[2] In carrying heavy objects, the muscles of the upper extremities should be used rather than the muscles of the trunk.

[3] When reaching upward or working at low levels, the trunk should be maintained in normal alignment, and adjustments should be made by the lower extremities (e.g., rising on toes or squatting).

8. Appropriate methods and precautions should be used in administering intramuscular injections (e.g., site of injection, rate of injection, type and amount of fluid injected).

9. Muscle relaxation may be promoted by:

A. Massage.

B. Positive relaxation exercises.

C. Proper positioning and support of body parts.

D. Warm applications.

E. A quiet, nonstimulating environment.

F. Physical and psychologic comfort.

CARE OF PATIENTS WITH SPECIFIC LOCOMOTION PROBLEMS

1. When fracture of a bone or dislocation of a joint has occurred or is suspected:

A. The affected part should be left in the position assumed until medical assistance is available.

B. If transportation is necessary:

[1] It should be accomplished with the least possible amount of motion of the injured part.

[2] The affected part should be splinted as it lies.

a. Splinting of bones requires immobilization of the joints above and below the injury.

b. If the knee or elbow is injured, the full lengths of the bones on either side of the joint should be splinted in the position that has been assumed.

C. Surgical aseptic technique is indicated when there is an open fracture.

2. Patients who have sustained open fractures or have had bone surgery should be observed closely for clinical manifestations of infection in the involved part, and these should be reported promptly.

3. When a patient has simple muscle spasm (muscle cramp):
   A. The affected muscle may be carefully placed on stretch (e.g., spasm of the gastrocnemius may be relieved by dorsal flexion of the foot).
   B. Gentle massage of the muscle may be helpful. (Note: If there is the possibility of phlebothrombosis, massage should not be used.)
4. When a patient has severe muscle spasms and/or there is spastic paralysis:
   A. The muscles affected should be put at rest in a position of comfort.
   B. Deformities should be prevented by providing normal alignments and functional positions (e.g., by use of pillows, pads, sandbags, rubber balls for hands, footboard, special splints).
   C. Heat should be applied as ordered and as needed for comfort.
   D. Skeletal muscle relaxant drugs should be administered as ordered and promptly as needed.
5. When a patient has flaccid paralysis, the affected part:
   A. Must be supported in proper anatomical alignment at all times.
   B. Must be protected from pressure, stretching, or abnormal motions.
   C. Should have passive range of motion exercises several times daily.
6. When a sprain has been sustained, and periarticular structures of a joint are torn or stretched and inflamed:
   A. The injured joint should be immobilized and protected from further injury.
   B. Cold should be applied immediately to limit congestion. Hot applications may be helpful after 48 hours.
   C. The part should be elevated, if possible, to limit edema.
   D. Prescribed analgesic drugs should be administered as needed to reduce pain.
7. When a patient has rheumatic disease (e.g., rheumatoid arthritis):
   A. All involved body parts should be maintained in functional positions and in alignment as close to normal as possible.
   B. Inflamed joints should be kept at rest and should always be properly supported and handled with great gentleness.
   C. Exercise of involved joints should be done only as ordered, and motion should be carried only to the point of pain.
   D. Splints, when ordered, should be properly shaped and applied to prevent deformities.
   E. Minimally desirable body weight should be encouraged when weight-bearing joints are affected.
   F. Heat should be applied as ordered and as needed for comfort.
   G. Prescribed analgesics should be administered as needed to reduce pain.
8. When a patient has sustained injury to structures concerned with locomotion:
   A. Medical orders relative to positioning, exercise, immobilization and/or traction should be explicit and followed exactly.
   B. Problems in relation to these factors should be reported promptly.
9. When a patient has a cast applied:
   A. The injured part should be supported in proper alignment at all times.
   B. Elevation of an injured extremity, if permitted by medical orders, may be helpful in limiting edema.

  C. Systematic evaluations should be made to identify symptoms and signs of impaired circulation and peripheral nerve damage.

      [1] These include cyanosis, pallor, absence of pulse, swelling, numbness or tingling, persistent pain, inability to move fingers or toes.

      [2] Pain should always be promptly and thoroughly investigated.

      [3] Any indications of impaired circulation or peripheral nerve damage should be reported immediately.

10. When a patient has traction applied and the objective is to immobilize and align a part:

  A. The injured part should be maintained in the exact alignment in which it was placed by the physician.

  B. The traction apparatus should be maintained as it was applied (i.e., weights, alignment of pulleys, amount of countertraction, etc.).

  C. There should be systematic patient evaluation to identify symptoms and signs of impaired circulation or peripheral nerve damage. If an internal fixation device is in place, the site of insertion should be inspected frequently for indications of infection. Any of these findings should be reported promptly.

11. When a patient has a convulsive seizure:

  A. He should be helped to lie down if and when there is a warning signal.

  B. Movements should not be restrained during the convulsion.

  C. Hard objects such as furniture should be moved away or should be padded.

  D. Data about the following should be noted and reported/recorded:

      [1] Presence of an aura.

      [2] Level of consciousness before, during and after convulsion.

      [3] Motor activity—the body parts involved and sequence of involvement.

      [4] Duration of the seizure.

Chapter 12

Bones, Muscles and Body Fluids
that Protect and Support

Certain bones, muscles and body fluids serve to protect and support underlying soft tissues.

Anatomy and Physiology

1. The bones of the skull protect the cranial contents (including the brain, the meninges, blood vessels, the pituitary gland and cerebrospinal fluid.
2. Some of the bones of the skull (frontal, parietal, temporal and occipital) are united in suture lines, which are immovable joints.
   A. At birth, the suture lines are not united, and there are unossified areas between the bones.
      [1] The anterior fontanel lies between the two parietal and frontal bones and normally closes within 1 and 1½ years.
      [2] The posterior fontanel lies between the two parietal and occipital bones and normally closes within 6 months.
   B. The rigidity of the skull allows almost no room for expansion.
      [1] Any increase in mass within the cranium will exert pressure against the soft tissues.
      [2] Downward pressure can compress the medulla oblongata into the foramen magnum, the opening in the occipital bone that provides communication between the cranial cavity and the vertebral canal. (The medulla contains vital nerve centers that function in the control of circulation and respiration. See Chapters 1 and 2.)

212

3. Cerebrospinal fluid is produced constantly in the lateral ventricles of the brain. From there it circulates through the ventricles, the subarachnoid space and the central canal of the spinal cord. The fluid is reabsorbed into the cerebral venous system, primarily in the dural sinuses.
   A. Cerebrospinal fluid is watery, yellowish and somewhat similar to tissue fluid.
   B. In the adult there is about 125 ml. of cerebrospinal fluid.
   C. The fluid has a protective function (among others), in that it serves to cushion the brain and spinal cord.
4. The vertebral column protects the contents of the neural canal.
   A. The vertebrae are connected by anterior and posterior ligaments and intervertebral discs.
   B. The neural canal, containing the spinal cord, meninges and spinal fluid, is formed by the bodies and processes of the vertebrae.
   C. Spinal nerves emerge from the neural canal through the intervertebral foramina, which are posterior to the bodies of the vertebrae and between the bases of successive arches.
   D. The intervertebral discs have an outer layer of fibrous tissue and an inner soft elastic tissue called the nucleus pulposus. The discs act as shock absorbers.
5. The thoracic cage is composed of 12 thoracic vertebrae, which articulate with the 12 pairs of ribs, some of which articulate anteriorly with the sternum and clavicle.
   A. Within the thoracic cage lie the lungs, the heart and the great vessels.
   B. Movement of the ribs by costal muscles plays an important role in breathing.
   C. The diaphragm, which also plays an important role in breathing, originates in part on the ribs and sternum.
6. The pelvic girdle is composed of the hip bones, the sacrum and the coccyx.
   A. The hip bones (or innominate bones) articulate anteriorly at the symphysis pubis. They articulate with the sacrum posteriorly in the sacroiliac joints.
   B. The true pelvis contains the bladder, rectum and (in the female) the nonpregnant uterus and vagina.
7. The muscles of the abdominal wall are flat muscles, which extend from the pelvic girdle or lumbodorsal fascia to the costal cartilages; they help to support and protect the abdominal and pelvic viscera.
   A. The separated rectus abdominis muscles extend from the pubis to the anterior rib cage, and are relatively weak muscles. The umbilicus lies between the separated rectus muscles and transmits the umbilical cord in the unborn child.
   B. The inguinal canal (which transmits the spermatic cord in the male and the round ligament in the female) runs through the lower portion of the abdominal muscles above the inguinal ligament. It has two openings: a superficial one in the external oblique close to the body of the pubis and a deep opening which lies more laterally and opens into the abdominal cavity.
   C. The femoral canal lies in the femoral sheath. Its base is the femoral ring, which lies behind the inguinal ligament. It transmits numerous lymphatic vessels.
8. The muscles of the pelvic floor support part of the weight of the abdominal viscera and pelvic viscera. These muscles include the paired levator ani and coccygeus muscles. (During childbirth the muscles of the pelvic floor are greatly stretched.)
9. The abdominal muscles contract and exert pressure against the abdominal and pelvic viscera during:

A. Forced expiration.
B. Coughing.
C. Vomiting (unless the vomiting is effortless).
D. Micturition, defecation and parturition. (Intra-abdominal and intrapelvic pressures are greatly increased when a person strains to have a bowel movement.)

Pathology

SYMPTOMS AND SIGNS

1. Symptoms and signs of head injury include:
   A. Abnormality in contour, alignment or contiguity of skull bones.
   B. Headache.
   C. Observable bleeding (may be from nose, mouth, ears or in or around eyes).
   D. Drainage of cerebrospinal fluid (e.g., from nose, ears, head wound).
   E. Symptoms and signs of brain injury, which may be due to increased intracranial pressure caused by hemorrhage and/or edema within the rigid skull.
      [1] Changes in cardiovascular function. (See Chapter 1.) At first, there is generally a slowed pulse rate and a rise in systolic blood pressure and pulse pressure. This is followed by a drop in the blood pressure and a rapid, irregular pulse.
      [2] Changes in respiratory function. (See Chapter 2.) Respirations may be deep and noisy at first and then become Cheyne-Stokes in nature.
      [3] Headache.
      [4] Nausea and/or vomiting (often projectile).
      [5] Hyperthermia. (See Chapter 9.)
      [6] Changes in motor function. (See Chapter 11.)
         a. There may be convulsive seizures, muscle rigidity, muscle weakness, paralysis.
         b. There may be incontinence.
         c. There may be hyperactivity.
         d. There may be changes in speech. (See Chapter 18.)
      [7] Changes in sensory function. (See Chapters 11 and 16.)
         a. Loss of visual acuity is an early symptom.
         b. Pupil sizes may vary; reaction to light may be unequal.
         c. Pupils may become dilated and fixed.
      [8] Changes in mental status.
      [9] Progressive loss of consciousness.
2. Symptoms and signs of spinal injury include:
   A. Abnormality in contour, alignment or contiguity of the vertebral column.
   B. Headache, local pain at site of injury or pain along paths of sensory nerves.
   C. Loss of locomotive function involving muscles attached to trunk.
   D. Drainage of cerebrospinal fluid from wound.
   E. Symptoms and signs of spinal cord injury. These depend greatly upon the level of the injury and the extent of the injury and may include:
      [1] Loss of respiratory function.
      [2] Changes in motor function. (See Chapter 11.)

     [3] Loss of bladder and bowel control.

     [4] Loss of sensation and reflexes. (See Chapters 11 and 16.)

3. Symptoms and signs of injury to the bones of the thoracic cage include:
   A. Abnormality in contour, alignment or contiguity of the bones of the thoracic cage.
   B. Sharp pain, especially with respiratory movements.
   C. Changes in respiratory movements. (See Chapter 2.) (Flail chest occurs when ribs that are fractured in parallel fashion move in directions that are opposite to normal respiratory motions. For example, during inspiration the ribs move downward and inward.)
   D. Changes in heart action (which may be caused by direct injury or may be due to a mediastinal shift).

4. Symptoms and signs of injury to the bones of the pelvic girdle include:
   A. Abnormality in contour, alignment or contiguity of the bones of the pelvic girdle.
   B. Loss of locomotive function involving muscles attached to the pelvic girdle. (See Chapter 11.)
   C. Pain, which may radiate down the leg.
   D. Observable bleeding from wound, rectum, urethra, vagina.
   E. Symptoms and signs of internal bleeding. (See Chapter 1.)

5. Symptoms and signs of injury to the abdominal musculature include:
   A. Loss of strength, contractility of abdominal muscles.
   B. Abnormal lumps, especially in groin, scrotum or umbilicus.
   C. Pain, especially with muscle contraction.
   D. Wound separation, possibly with evisceration.

6. Symptoms and signs of injury to the muscles of the pelvic floor include:
   A. Incontinence or retention of urine.
   B. Incontinence or retention of feces.
   C. Feeling of pressure or dragging sensation in pelvic region.
   D. Prolapsed uterus.
   E. Dysmenorrhea.

INJURIES AND DISTURBANCES OF FUNCTION

1. A traumatic head injury can result in:
   A. Loss of consciousness, which may be momentary or prolonged. (A concussion is a temporary disorder caused by injury to the head. There is immediate loss of consciousness. The extent or severity of any other clinical manifestations depends upon the extent and type of injury to the soft tissues within the skull.)
   B. Bone fracture.
        [1] A depressed fracture exerts pressure on the brain and may interfere with the circulation of blood and/or cerebrospinal fluid within the cranium.
        [2] Bone fragments can cause laceration of the soft tissues within the cranium, injuring the brain, meninges, and/or blood vessels. If the meninges are lacerated, cerebrospinal fluid will be lost.
        [3] Injury involving the superior sagittal sinus not only interferes with venous drainage but may prevent proper absorption of cerebrospinal fluid.

C. Inflammatory response with congestion, edema, fibrosis.
D. Hemorrhage.
  [1] Symptoms and signs depend upon the location and size of the hematoma.
  [2] A subdural hematoma develops when veins between the dura and brain are injured. Bleeding is slow, so symptoms and signs may not appear for hours, days or weeks.
  [3] An epidural hematoma develops quite rapidly when meningeal arteries are injured.
E. Loss of cerebrospinal fluid.
2. Hydrocephalus is a condition in which there is excessive cerebrospinal fluid.
A. The condition may be caused by overproduction and/or inadequate absorption.
B. Since the skull bones are not yet fused in the infant, considerable enlargement of the head may develop with this disorder.
3. Disorders of the vertebral column can cause injury to the spinal cord and nerve roots.
A. Injury may be due to:
  [1] Excessive or unusual stress on the vertebral column, which can be caused by tension, compression, twisting or bending movements (e.g., lifting too heavy an object or lifting a heavy object incorrectly).
  [2] Fractures, with or without displacement.
  [3] Bone pathology with subsequent destruction and collapse of vertebrae.
  [4] Abnormal spinal curvatures, such as kyphosis.
  [5] Ruptured or slipped intervertebral discs.
B. Intervertebral discs can become softened, and the nucleus pulposus can become displaced. This stretches the posterior ligament. Sometimes the disc can actually herniate into the neural canal and press on nerve roots.
4. Traumatic injury to the bones of the thoracic cage (may involve splintering, crushing or displacement of bones) can result in damage to the respiratory muscles, pleura, lungs, heart, peripheral nerves and/or great vessels.
5. Traumatic injury to the bones of the pelvic girdle can result in damage to the urinary tract, uterus, lower intestinal tract, spinal nerves and/or large blood vessels.
6. Weakness of the abdominal musculature may be congenital or acquired.
A. A surgical wound that has not healed properly is one way of acquiring weakness.
B. When weakened or injured muscles are placed under tension (e.g., with strenuous exercise, lifting, obesity, pregnancy, abdominal distention, paroxysmal coughing), a hernia may result. If a surgical wound is involved, the wound may open.
C. An abdominal hernia is the protrusion of peritoneum and intestine through a weakened area of the abdominal musculatures.
  [1] An indirect inguinal hernia involves the protrusion of peritoneum and intestine into the inguinal canal and, in the male, on into the scrotum.
  [2] A direct inguinal hernia involves the protrusion of peritoneum and intestine through the posterior inguinal wall.
  [3] A femoral hernia involves the protrusion of peritoneum and intestine into the femoral canal.

[4] An umbilical hernia involves the protrusion of peritoneum and intestine into an umbilical ring that has not closed or is weak.

[5] If the blood supply to protruding tissues is cut off, it is called a strangulated hernia. Tissue necrosis will occur if the blood supply is not restored promptly.

D. If an abdominal incision fails to heal properly, the wound may open, exposing the abdominal viscera. The viscera may actually come to the outside, through the opening.

[1] Circulatory shock often results.

[2] Peritonitis is a possible complication.

7. Weakness of the pelvic floor may be congenital or acquired.

A. Weakness is frequently acquired through childbirth when:

[1] There may be considerable trauma to soft tissues.

[2] There are perineal tears that are either not repaired or are repaired improperly.

[3] Episiotomies fail to heal properly.

B. Uterine displacement may occur, and occasionally, the uterus may actually prolapse through the vagina.

C. Rectoceles and cystoceles may result and interfere with proper elimination from the bladder and rectum.

Nursing Care

Nursing care should be directed toward preventing injury to soft tissues normally protected and supported by bones, muscles and fluid.

COLLECTION, EVALUATION AND COMMUNICATION OF DATA

1. Patients should be interviewed, observed and examined to identify symptoms and signs of problems involving bones, muscles and fluid that protect and support.

A. Problems may be indicated by:

[1] Abnormalities of the vertebral column; symptoms and signs of spinal cord injury.

[2] Abnormalities of the skull; symptoms and signs of brain injury.

[3] Abnormalities of the thoracic cage; symptoms and signs of impaired respiratory and/or cardiovascular function.

[4] Abnormalities of the pelvic girdle; symptoms and signs of injury to structures within the pelvis.

[5] Abnormalities of the abdominal musculature.

[6] Symptoms and signs of inadequate support of the uterus, the urinary bladder and/or rectum.

B. Systematic patient evaluation is of especial importance when the patient:

[1] Has sustained traumatic injury (e.g., due to a fall, an auto accident, a severe blow).

[2] Has a diagnosed disorder or has sustained injury to bones, muscles or fluid that support and protect.

   C. Data collected should be evaluated not only on the basis of a single deviation from normal (e.g., headache) but should also be evaluated on the basis of combinations of symptoms and signs that are commonly associated with specific disorders or injuries (e.g., symptoms and signs associated with increased intracranial pressure).

2. How, when and what data are communicated to the physician and/or other nursing personnel depend upon:
   A. Any immediate threat to the patient's life processes (e.g., symptoms and signs of increasing intracranial pressure).
   B. Any potential threat to the patient's life and well-being (e.g., symptoms and signs of fracture of thoracic spine).
   C. Any particular implications for the physician in relation to:
     [1] The patient's progress or lack of progress toward recovery (e.g., change in level of consciousness).
     [2] Making a diagnosis (e.g., new objective or subjective data).
     [3] The patient's physical and emotional responses to specific diagnostic procedures and therapeutic measures.
   D. Any particular implications for nursing (e.g., in relation to immobilization).

PROMOTION OF HEALTH AND PREVENTION
OF DISEASE/INJURY

1. See Nursing Care in Chapter 11.
2. Infants up to the age of 1½ years should be protected from injury to the fontanels.
3. Proper obstetrical care should be encouraged.
4. When administering external heart massage, fractures of the sternum and/or ribs may be prevented by:
   A. Proper placement of the hands over lower half of sternum, avoiding the xyphoid process.
   B. Proper placement of hands so as to avoid pressure on ribs.
   C. Adjustment of pressure in accordance with the age, size and development of the patient.
5. Abnormal lumps in the groin, scrotum or umbilical area should be medically evaluated when they are first noticed.

CARE OF PATIENTS WITH SPECIFIC PROBLEMS

1. When a patient has sustained a head injury, or this is suspected:
   A. He should be quietly maintained in a horizontal position until a medical evaluation is done.
   B. The head should be supported, immobilized and protected from any further injury.
   C. No object remaining in a head wound should be moved or removed.
   D. Surgical aseptic technique is extremely important in the care of open wounds.
   E. Systematic evaluations should be done to identify symptoms and signs of brain injury or fracture of the cervical spine.
2. When a patient has sustained injury to the spine, or this is suspected:

A. He should be kept quiet in the position he is in until a medical evaluation is done. If it is necessary to transport the patient or change the position:
   [1] Any movement of the head, neck or spine is to be avoided. There should be no bending or twisting of the spine in any direction.
   [2] The head, neck and spine should be evenly supported along the entire length of a firm surface.

B. Medical orders relative to positioning, traction, immobilization and exercise of limbs should be explicit and must be followed exactly.

C. The trunk should be properly supported on a firm surface and in correct alignment at all times. Sudden movement of any body part should be avoided.

D. Systematic evaluations should be made to identify symptoms and signs of spinal cord injury.

E. Appliances such as braces or corsets must be properly fitted and properly applied.

3. When a patient has injury to the thoracic cage, or this is suspected:
   A. He should be kept quiet in the position he is in until a medical evaluation is made.
   B. If it is necessary to transport the patient or change the position, the chest wall should be properly supported and protected from further injury.
   C. Systematic evaluations should be made to identify impaired respiratory and/or cardiovascular function. (See Chapters 1 and 2.)

4. When a patient has sustained traumatic injury to the bones of the pelvic girdle, or this is suspected:
   A. He should be kept quiet and the injured pelvis immobilized in a position of comfort until a medical evaluation is made.
   B. Systematic evaluations should be made to identify symptoms and signs of:
      [1] Internal bleeding.
      [2] Injury to the bladder, rectum and/or uterus.
      [3] Injury to peripheral nerves.

5. When a patient has a weakened area in the abdominal musculature (e.g., an incompletely healed surgical wound):
   A. Strenuous activity involving these muscles should be avoided (e.g., lifting, descending stairs).
   B. Increased intra-abdominal pressure should be avoided.
   C. The weakened area should be properly supported during activities likely to cause strain.
   D. Positioning should minimize tension of affected muscles.
   E. Unhealed abdominal surgical wounds should be inspected closely for separation.
      [1] Wound separation, with or without evisceration, represents a medical emergency.
      [2] Should wound separation occur:
         a. The patient should be kept absolutely quiet and may be placed in low Fowler's position.
         b. A supportive dressing is adequate for an opened wound, but any

exposed organ should be covered immediately with sterile saline compresses and then a supportive dressing.

6. When a patient has weakened muscles of the pelvic floor:
   A. Prolonged standing, and sometimes even sitting, should be avoided.
   B. Increased intra-abdominal and intrapelvic pressures should be avoided.
   C. Indications of possible problems with elimination and/or displacement of the uterus should be reported promptly. (See Chapters 7 and 19.)

Chapter 13

The Skin and Mucous Membranes

Intact healthy skin and mucous membranes serve as the first lines of defense against harmful agents.

Anatomy and Physiology

THE INTEGUMENT

1. The skin is the largest organ of the body. It envelops the entire surface of the body. Its epithelium is continuous with the epithelium of the external orifices of the digestive, respiratory and genitourinary tracts.
2. The healthy intact skin:
   A. Prevents water loss.
   B. Plays a major role in temperature regulation.
   C. Is impermeable to most microorganisms.
   D. Is resistant to many potentially injurious chemical agents.
   E. Is resistant to considerable trauma, cold, heat and to some radiation.
   F. Supplies information about the external environment.
3. The skin is composed of two layers.
   A. The epidermis, or cuticle, is the outer, paper-thin, layer.
      [1] This layer is avascular, nourished by tissue fluid only.
      [2] The cells of the outermost stratum (the stratum corneum) are dead and are constantly being shed, to be replaced by cells moving up from the lower strata.
         a. Cells of the stratum corneum contain keratin, a tough fibrous protein.

b. This horny layer is hygroscopic; that is, it absorbs water readily. Skin that is exposed to moisture over time becomes swollen and wrinkled.

c. The amount of water in the stratum corneum is greatly influenced by the external temperature, relative humidity and air currents. When the atmosphere is very dry, this layer loses water at a faster rate than it can be replaced from below. Chapping results; the skin appears dry and scaly. When the water level falls below a critical level, fissures and cracks expose the underlying epidermis to physical and chemical injury.

[3] The epidermis varies in thickness from about 0.1 mm. on most parts of the body to about 1.0 mm. on the soles of the feet.

a. Infants and children have a soft and delicate epidermis.

b. Rubbing and pressure cause thickening of the epidermis.

c. Corns and calluses are areas of hypertrophied, thickened horny epidermis.

[4] The epidermis acts as a barrier to keep external substances out and prevent water loss from within. Skin without an epidermis is freely permeable.

[5] The epidermal appendages include:

a. Eccrine sweat glands.

b. Apocrine glands.

c. Sebaceous glands.

d. Hair follicles and nails.

[6] The health of the epidermis is dependent upon the health of the body.

B. The dermis, or corium, lies beneath the epidermis.

[1] The dermis, sometimes called the "true skin," is composed of dense connective tissue which contains:

a. Blood and lymph vessels.

b. Sensory nerves that conduct impulses for itching, pain, touch and temperature.

c. Motor nerves for control of glands and blood vessels.

d. Sebaceous glands and sweat glands.

e. Elastic fibers.

[2] The thickness of the dermis varies on different parts of the body; it is exceedingly thin and delicate in the eyelids and male external genitalia, but fairly thick on the hands and soles of the feet.

[3] The dermis is connected to the subcutaneous tissue (or hypodermis) below, which is loose connective tissue that stores fat and acts as a cushion.

a. The subcutaneous tissue is connected with underlying deep fascia, aponeuroses or periosteum.

b. The amount of subcutaneous tissue varies greatly in individuals and in different parts of the body.

c. In old age there is a decrease in the amount of subcutaneous tissue.

4. The skin may be dry, moist, rough or smooth, depending upon the nature and amount of keratinized epidermis and on the amount and nature of the secretions of the cutaneous glands.

A. Sebum is the oily secretion produced by sebaceous glands.

[1] Sebaceous glands are found in most parts of the skin but are especially numerous in the scalp and face; they are very numerous around the nose, mouth, external ear and anus. They are absent in the palms of the hands and soles of the feet.

[2] Sebum prevents water loss from the epidermis.

[3] There is increased production of sebum at the time of puberty.

[4] There is decreased production when the peripheral circulation is impaired (frequently associated with the aging process).

[5] Accumulation of sebum and breakdown products on the skin can cause skin irritation.

B. Eccrine sweat glands are distributed over the entire body; they produce sweat continuously. (See Chapter 4.)

C. Apocrine glands are found primarily in the axilla and in the perianal and genital regions.

[1] These glands begin to secrete very small amounts of a milky white fluid when the secondary sex characteristics appear.

[2] Apocrine secretion increases at times of emotional stress.

[3] Bacteria feeding on apocrine secretions produce chemical substances that have an unpleasant pungent odor.

D. Ceruminous glands are specialized apocrine glands in the external auditory canal. They secrete cerumen (wax), which softens and protects the canal. If allowed to accumulate, the wax hardens and can obstruct the canal.

5. The brown pigment melanin is produced in the lower epidermis as fine granules within the cells.

A. There are great individual variations in the amounts of this pigment contained in the skin.

B. Pigmented skin is more resistant to ultraviolet rays and to chemical and physical trauma.

C. Many individuals are able to produce melanin in response to ultraviolet rays. Persons who are unable to produce melanin sunburn readily.

6. Skin turgor is the normal firmness of the skin and is determined mainly by the amount of interstitial fluid. Normally hydrated skin can be made to rise when pinched but immediately falls when released. Dehydrated skin remains in the pinched position.

7. Individual skins vary in their resistance to injury. Factors which affect this resistance include:

A. The general health of the cells—as determined by adequate circulation, proper nutrition, and so forth.

B. The amount of subcutaneous tissue. (When there is lack of subcutaneous tissue over bony prominences, pressure over these prominences shuts off blood flow very quickly.)

C. The amount of melanin.

D. The degree of dryness.

8. The nails are horny keratin plates that develop continuously from cells in the epidermis.

9. Hairs are found on nearly every part of the body. They vary in length, thickness and color on different parts of the body.
   A. Each hair shaft arises from a hair follicle in the skin. Many hair follicles extend into subcutaneous tissue.
   B. Ducts from one or more sebaceous glands empty into each hair follicle, and the sebum is responsible for the degree of oiliness or dryness of the hair.
   C. Axillary, genital and coarse body hair develop at puberty.
   D. The matrix from which hair grows is one of the most active tissues in the body and is susceptible to systemic stresses that affect the general health.
10. Normal cutaneous vascular response to injury includes:
    A. The white reaction (vasoconstriction).
    B. The red reaction (vasodilatation).
    C. The wheal or hive (localized edema).
    D. The blister (collection of serous fluid between layers of epidermis).
11. Pallor, flushing or uneven pigmentation is normal in many healthy individuals.
12. The temperature of the skin depends largely upon the blood flow through its vessels.
13. Normal physiological response to externally applied heat or cold depends upon:
    A. Normal sensory perception for heat, cold, pain.
    B. Normal vasomotor activity.
14. Prolonged exposure to cold results in marked peripheral vasoconstriction.
    A. Ischemia can cause tissue damage.
    B. Although ischemia of the skin may cause discomfort initially, eventually there will be loss of sensation.
15. Repeated exposures to high temperatures (e.g., hot packs or baths) can result in adaptation of sensory receptors for heat. The skin may be injured if these receptors fail to give warning of the threat of burning.
16. Itching (pruritis) is an unpleasant cutaneous sensation which provokes scratching.
    A. The sensation can occur in the epidermis, in the epithelial layer of transitional epithelium (e.g., in the pharynx) and in mucocutaneous junctions (e.g., anus, femal perineum, auditory canal, nares).
    B. The sensation may be stimulated chemically (e.g., by histamine-like substances), mechanically (e.g., tickling, crawling insects), thermally and electrically.
    C. The sensation may continue long after the original stimulation has ceased.
    D. The sensation can be reawakened by pressure or rubbing.
    E. The nerve endings are made more sensitive by increased heat (e.g., increased blood flow, friction, external heat) and less sensitive by cold and reduced blood flow.
    F. The sensation can occur through stimulation by the higher centers (i.e., by psychogenic factors).
    G. The scratch reflex involves:
       [1] Sensory receptors and sensory pathways in the spinal cord.
       [2] Subcortical centers in the midbrain and thalamus.
       [3] Motor pathways in the spinal cord and peripheral motor nerves.
    H. It is difficult to voluntarily refrain from scratching. Diversion of attention can be helpful if the itching is not too intense.

I. Itching causes scratching, and scratching intensifies itching, which results in even more vigorous scratching.

MUCOUS MEMBRANES

1. The respiratory, gastrointestinal and genitourinary tracts are lined with mucous membranes.
2. Healthy, intact mucous membranes:
    A. Prevent water loss.
    B. Are impermeable to many microorganisms.
    C. Are resistant to many chemical substances, such as the digestive juices.
    D. Have some resistance to trauma.
    E. Contain cells that secrete mucus.
3. Mucus serves to:
    A. Keep the membrane moist.
    B. Act as a lubricant.
    C. Act as a protectant against some chemicals and infectious agents.
4. Irritation of mucous membrane generally causes an increase in mucus production but may cause a reduction.
5. The mucous membrane of the mouth is somewhat similar in structure to the skin.
    A. Except where food is crushed and rubbed (e.g., the hard palate), it is attached to underlying structures by a loose submucosa.
    B. The membrane contains many sensory nerve endings and is very sensitive.
6. The epithelial lining of the vagina is lubricated by mucus made acidic by fermentative action of normal vaginal flora.

Physics

1. Friction is that force which opposes motion between two contacting surfaces.
    A. Friction is caused by surface irregularities.
    B. Friction may be decreased by decreasing the irregularities (e.g., by smoothing surfaces or separating the surfaces with lubricants).
2. Friction produces heat.

Chemistry

1. Surface tension of water may be decreased by soaps and detergents.
    A. Soaps are metallic salts of fatty acids. Some are highly alkaline.
    B. Synthetic detergents can be more efficient than soap in lowering surface tensions.
2. Lowering of surface tension aids in the emulsification of fats.

Pathology

SYMPTOMS AND SIGNS

Symptoms and signs of actual or potential problems involving the skin and/or mucous membranes include:

1. Traumatic breaks in the skin and/or mucous membranes (e.g., scratches, abrasions, lacerations, surgical wounds).

2. Loss of skin (e.g., as with severe burns or desquamation).
3. Abnormal pigmentation.
4. Presence of specific types of lesions.
5. Pruritis (itching).
6. Tenderness or pain.
7. Abnormal skin temperature.
8. Unusual dryness or moistness, possibly with maceration.
9. Loss of normal skin turgor.
10. Alopecia (loss of hair).
11. Abnormal nails (e.g., soft, pitted or grooved).

ABNORMAL PIGMENTATION
1. Abnormal pigmentation of the skin and mucous membranes may be the result of:
   A. An increase in oxyhemoglobin (hyperemia or erythema). This occurs when there is increased blood flow and peripheral vasodilatation due to inflammatory response, elevated body temperature, high skin temperature or as an early response to low skin temperature.
   B. A decrease in hemoglobin (pallor). Pallor occurs when there is decreased blood flow and vasoconstriction, due to injury or cold. It can be observed in scar tissue because of the limited blood supply.
   C. An increase in reduced hemoglobin (cyanosis or mottling). This occurs when there is venous stasis.
   D. A decrease in pigmentation or visible pigmentation. This occurs when there is edema or maceration. It may occur when there is excessive desquamation.
   E. An increase in yellow pigment. This may occur with high intake of carotene in the diet (pigment in yellow vegetables such as carrots) or with jaundice.
   F. An increase in melanin or melanoids. This may occur locally with exposure to ultraviolet rays, with scratching or chafing, with some cancers, with some vitamin deficiencies, in Addison's disease and sometimes with pregnancy.

CLASSIFICATION OF LESIONS
1. A primary lesion is the characteristic, basic lesion that appears early in a disease process. Common primary lesions include:
   A. Macule: a flat, small spot of color change, often red.
   B. Papule: a small spherical mass elevated from the skin, may be colored.
      [1] Nodule: similar to papule, but larger.
      [2] Tumor: similar to nodule, but larger.
   C. Plaque: cluster or merging of papules, nodules or tumors that forms a flat elevated surface.
   D. Vesicle: a small blister containing serous exudate.
   E. Pustule: a small elevated lesion containing purulent exudate.
   F. Bulla: a large blister which may contain serous or purulent exudate.
   G. Wheal or hive: an edematous, hot, raised area, which may vary in size from

very small to very large. It may be white and then redden. It can appear and disappear rapidly. There is usually hyperemia around it. Lesion is characterized by itching.

2. A secondary lesion results from changes in the primary lesion. Secondary lesions include:
   A. Crusts: dried exudate.
   B. Scales: dried flakes of dead epidermis (type of scale may be distinctive).
   C. Erosion: loss of superficial epidermis. There is moist surface but no bleeding.
   D. Excoriation: scraping or abrasion of primary lesion that results in removal of epidermis. (This can occur with scratching.)
   E. Ulcer: necrosis, with loss of epidermis, dermis and, possibly, subcutaneous tissue.
   F. Fissure: linear break in skin or membrane.
   G. Scar: fibrous tissue replacement of injured tissue; does not contain elastic fibers or accessory structures of skin. A keloid is overgrowth of scar tissue.
   H. Lichenification: excessive thickening and toughening of skin from continued irritation, giving a leathery appearance.
3. Other skin lesions include:
   A. Nevus (mole): may be flat or elevated, pigmented or nonpigmented, smooth or irregular and/or hairy or nonhairy.
   B. Verruca (wart): circumscribed, elevated, brownish-colored mass. May appear in crops.
   C. Comedo (blackhead): discolored plug of dried sebum within a hair follicle.
4. The shape (configuration) of a single lesion or patch of lesions has diagnostic significance, as does their distribution on the body parts.

PRURITIS
1. Although pruritis is a very common symptom of skin disorders, it does not occur in all disorders. When skin lesions are present, the absence of itching often has diagnostic significance.
2. Pruritis with resultant scratching is frequently responsible for changes in primary lesions.
3. Pruritis is associated with the following conditions:
   A. Bites and stings of insects, such as spiders and bees.
   B. Bites of animal parasites, such as fleas or lice.
   C. Nervousness, high emotional stress.
   D. Excessive dryness of skin.
   E. Tissue anoxia (e.g., in lower legs when there is venous stasis).
   F. Urticaria (hives).
   G. Some types of dermatitis.
   H. Some infections of skin or mucous membranes (e.g., some vaginal infections can cause intense itching).
   I. Jaundice.
   J. Wound healing.
4. Pruritis is a major symptom of hypersensitivity reactions involving the skin in

which the histamine that is liberated stimulates sensory nerve endings. Itching may precede or follow appearance of skin lesions.

CONDITIONS THAT AFFECT THE SKIN
AND/OR MUCOUS MEMBRANES

1. Disorders of the skin and/or mucous membrane may be caused by:
   A. Inadequate blood supply.
      [1] Decubitus ulcers (pressure sores) are caused by ischemia of the skin with resulting tissue necrosis.
         a. Causative factors include unrelieved pressure over bony prominences; localized pressure areas due to lying or sitting on irregular surfaces; and occlusion of blood vessels due to the sliding of one tissue layer over another.
         b. Factors that contribute to the development of decubitus ulcers include: poor nutritional status, poor circulation, an injured epidermis (e.g., due to friction burns, maceration or chemical irritation).
         c. The earliest sign of a developing pressure sore is skin pallor due to lack of blood in the area. This is followed by erythema, which in turn is followed by edema (with resultant pallor), mottling and cyanosis.
         d. The earliest symptom of a developing pressure sore is pain in the area.
         e. A primary decubitus ulcer involves a superficial erosion only. A secondary decubitus ulcer involves necrosis of the epidermis, dermis and possibly of the subcutaneous tissue. Muscle necrosis may follow.
      [2] Venous stasis in the lower extremities (associated with varicosities) can cause:
         a. Stasis dermatitis, frequently on dorsum of foot and around ankle, characterized by redness, edema, dryness and itching.
         b. Varicose ulcers, in which there is tissue necrosis due to ischemia. Ulcers may develop after the skin has sustained some type of injury.
   B. Improper nutrition (See Chapter 3).
   C. Dehydration or edema.
      [1] Both dehydrated and edematous tissues tend to be prone to traumatic injury.
      [2] The presence of excess tissue fluid interferes with cellular nutrition.
   D. Specific types of injuries. The skin and/or mucous membrane may be injured by:
      [1] Trauma (abrasions, lacerations, pricks, scratches, surgical incisions).
      [2] Burns.
         a. Burns may be caused by chemicals; radiation; electricity; hot gases, solids or liquids; fire and friction.
         b. A first-degree burn involves only the superficial epidermis, causing erythema, slight localized edema and a burning sensation.
         c. A second-degree burn varies in depth but does not involve the full thickness of the skin. The burned area may appear red or white, and

usually there is blister formation. There may be some edema. The burned area is painful and very sensitive to pressure and heat.

d. A third-degree burn involves the full thickness of the skin and may extend to muscles and bones. The burned area may appear blanched or may be charred. Destruction of sensory nerve endings causes anesthesia. The dehydrated dead skin forms a dry, inelastic eschar (slough).

[3] Exposure to irritating chemical agents.

a. Ammoniacal diaper rash involves weeping red papules, which may progress to form tiny ulcers. The skin is irritated by the ammonia produced by breakdown of the urea by bacteria on the skin or clothing.

b. Digestive juices (especially proteolytic enzymes) from a draining stoma cause chemical injury to the skin.

c. Many cosmetics, dental preparations (such as mouthwashes and toothpastes) and vaginal douching preparations contain chemicals that may be injurious.

[4] Too little or too much moisture.

a. Excessive dryness leads to chapping, which may cause cracks in the skin or mucous membrane. These irritated areas cause discomfort, and underlying tissues are exposed to injury.

b. Maceration of the skin is caused by continued wetness. The skin becomes soft and wrinkled, and there is decreased resistance to injury and infection.

2. Specific disease conditions involving skin and/or mucous membrane include:

A. Inflammatory response to endogenous and exogenous irritants (i.e., irritants produced within the body and irritants originating outside the body).

[1] Dermatitis is inflammation of the skin caused by sensitivity to external or internal irritants.

a. The inflammatory response may involve erythema, edema, blister formation, oozing of exudates, crusting, desquamation, lichenification, fissuring and hyperpigmentation. (When this type of inflammatory response occurs in relation to allergens, it is often referred to as eczema).

b. Predisposing causes appear to include such factors as general physical health, susceptibility to allergic reactions, emotional tension, health of the skin and nutritional status.

c. Immediate causes involve specific irritants, such as chemical agents, microorganisms, dusts, radiation.

[2] Contact dermatitis is caused by actual contact with irritants in the external environment. Lesions are limited to the area in contact with the irritating agent.

a. Most contact dermatitis is caused by chemical agents (e.g., in cosmetics, soaps, wool, or plants such as poison ivy).

b. The chemical agents may cause dermatitis immediately or later on, by acting as sensitizers.

[3] Exfoliative dermatitis is frequently the result of allergic response to drugs and may involve massive desquamation.

[4] Atopic eczema or neurodermatitis is an inherited allergic condition in which the lesions tend to be widespread. The distribution is often symmetrical, e.g., both ankles or both wrists. The condition may be precipitated by exposure to specific allergens but is frequently associated with psychogenic factors.

[5] Urticaria is an allergic response that results in hives and, sometimes, generalized edema. Itching is severe.

B. Inflammatory responses to unknown causes.

[1] Psoriasis is a condition in which there are circular patches of dry and scaly eruptions. There are usually exacerbations and remissions.

[2] Pemphigus is a condition characterized by large bullae in the skin and mucous membrane. There is crusting and scarring.

[3] Generalized exfoliative dermatitis involves massive desquamation. The hair and nails may be lost. This condition may arise as a primary condition; may develop secondarily to other chronic skin diseases; or may develop in association with some systemic diseases.

C. Seborrheic dermatoses.

[1] Seborrhea results from overactive sebaceous glands. The skin has a greasy appearance, and there may be scaling with itching. The forehead and scalp are commonly involved.

[2] Seborrheic dermatitis ("cradle cap" in infants) is manifested by a red macular rash over the face, neck and chest. There are dry or greasy scales over the scalp.

[3] Acne vulgaris is a chronic condition that usually occurs in adolescents or young adults. It is often associated with the development of secondary sex characteristics.

a. The ducts of hyperactive sebaceous glands become plugged and then infected.

b. Lesions include pustules, nodules, cysts and scars.

c. The face, chest and back are generally affected.

d. Contributing factors may include an excessively fatty diet and emotional stress.

D. Infections.

[1] Infections caused by bacteria include:

a. Impetigo contagiosa: a superficial infection caused by staphylococcus or streptococcus. It is usually found on the face and hands and can be spread to other parts of the body and transmitted to others. This infection is associated with lack of cleanliness and poor nutritional status.

b. Furuncle (boil): an infection involving a hair follicle and associated sebaceous gland(s), usually caused by staphylococcus. It begins as a subcutaneous swelling and usually becomes a large pustule around the hair shaft. Normally, pimples and boils rupture when the infection is well localized. Purulent drainage is discharged, and healing follows.

c. Carbuncle: a more extensive infection than a furuncle, usually involving several hair follicles. The area is red, swollen and very tender. The infection may not localize but instead become a cellulitis, a diffuse and spreading inflammation of loose connective tissue.

    d. Paronychia: a common infection in the skin at the side of the nail, which may be caused by staphylococcus or streptococcus. The microorganisms enter through a break in the skin (e.g., a hangnail). Unless treated, the infection may progress under the cuticle and then under the nail. The condition can be very painful.

[2] Infections caused by fungi include:

    a. Epidermophytosis (athlete's foot), characterized by superficial vesicles and scaling. Occurs frequently between the toes but may occur in other areas of the body. Itching may be severe.

    b. Tinea (ringworm) of scalp, nails, hands, trunk; characterized by vesicular or pustular lesions, scabs, distorted or lost nails.

    c. Candidiasis (moniliasis), which can cause oral thrush, vaginitis and skin lesions of various kinds. In the mouth and in the vagina there is erythema and white patches. The itching that accompanies the vaginitis may be severe.

[3] Infections caused by viruses include:

    a. Warts, which are benign epithelial tumors which can be spread on the body and may be transmitted to others.

    b. Herpes simplex (cold sore), characterized by a group of small blisters that rupture, crust and heal slowly.

    c. Herpes zoster (shingles), characterized by a chain of blisters that follows the distribution of a nerve or nerves from one or more posterior ganglia; associated with pain and itching.

E. Parasitic infestations.

[1] Pediculosis is caused by lice that may infest the head, the body or the pubic area. Bites cause intense itching.

[2] Scabies is an infestation of the skin caused by a mite.

    a. The mites burrow into the skin and cause itching.

    b. Secondary lesions include vesicles, pustules, excoriations and crusts.

F. Neoplastic disorders.

[1] Benign cysts (sebaceous or mucous) may develop on skin or mucous membrane.

[2] Nevi (moles) are collections of nonfunctioning cells in the upper skin.

    a. If moles are located on a part of the body that is continually being irritated, secondary lesions may develop.

    b. Any change in size or color, the appearance of inflammation, bleeding, crusting or ulceration may indicate the start of a malignancy.

    c. Darkly pigmented moles are sometimes precancerous.

[3] Senile keratosis precedes cutaneous epithelioma and may appear as small reddish or brownish scaling spots, usually on the face.

[4] Cancers of the skin usually grow slowly and remain localized. Development of cancer of the skin is sometimes associated with excessive exposure to the sun.

[5] Any nodule, papule or ulceration that persists (e.g., longer than 3 weeks) may be a beginning malignancy.

3. Various skin manifestations may occur with many of the communicable diseases. Sometimes the causative microorganisms are contained in the lesions.

Nursing Care

Nursing care should be directed toward assisting the patient to retain or regain healthy and intact skin and mucous membrane.

COLLECTION, EVALUATION AND COMMUNICATION OF DATA

1. Patients should be interviewed, observed and examined to identify symptoms and signs of actual or potential problems involving the skin and mucous membrane.
    A. Problems may be indicated by:
        [1] Traumatic breaks in these structures.
        [2] Abnormalities in the color, temperature, texture, turgor and/or moisture of these structures.
        [3] Lesions.
        [4] Symptoms and signs of inflammation. (See Chapter 14.)
        [5] Pruritis, evidence of scratching.
        [6] Pain, tingling, numbness.
        [7] Abnormalities of hair, nails.
        [8] Presence of animal parasites.
    B. Systematic patient evaluation is of especial importance when the patient:
        [1] Has an injury or disorder that involves the skin or mucous membrane.
        [2] Is receiving treatments in which the skin or mucous membrane is involved (e.g., radiation therapy, hot or cold applications, soaks or irrigations, topical medications).
        [3] Has special appliances or equipment in contact with the skin or mucous membrane.
        [4] Is subject to having irritating substances on the skin or mucous membrane (e.g., sweat, urine, feces, gastrointestinal secretions, exudates).
        [5] Depends upon others for physical care or protection (e.g., infants and young children, the weak or debilitated, those who are mentally incompetent, unconscious, paralyzed, immobilized).
        [6] Has impaired circulation.
        [7] Has been living under unhygienic circumstances.
        [8] Has been exposed to a communicable disease in which there are specific types of lesions.
        [9] Is known to have a particularly sensitive or delicate skin.
    C. Data collected should be evaluated not only on the basis of a single deviation from normal (e.g., pruritis) but should also be evaluated on the basis of symptoms and signs that are commonly associated with specific types of problems with the skin or mucous membrane (e.g., symptoms and signs of communicable diseases in which there are skin eruptions).

D. The condition of the skin and/or mucous membrane should be evaluated in relation to such factors as:
  [1] Any diagnosed disease condition that involves or may involve these structures.
  [2] Any injury that has been sustained and the normal healing process.
  [3] Any medications (oral, parenteral or topical) that the patient is or has been using.
  [4] Any history of hypersensitivity.
  [5] The patient's general physical status (e.g., circulation, nutrition, body temperature).
  [6] The patient's emotional status.
  [7] The patient's normal skin coloring.
  [8] The patient's age.

2. How, when and what data are communicated to the physician and/or other nursing personnel depend upon:
  A. Any potential threat to the patient's life and well-being (e.g., skin lesions that persist or change in character).
  B. Any particular implications for the physician in relation to:
    [1] The patient's progress or lack of progress toward recovery (e.g., changes in skin lesions).
    [2] Making a diagnosis (e.g., new objective or subjective data).
    [3] The patient's physical and emotional responses to specific diagnostic procedures and therapeutic measures.
  C. Any particular implications for nursing (e.g., special hygienic measures).

PROMOTION OF HEALTH AND PREVENTION
OF DISEASE/INJURY

1. Health teaching to promote healthy and intact skin and mucous membrane should be concerned with:
  A. Proper nutrition throughout the life cycle.
  B. Proper personal hygiene.
  C. Accident prevention.
  D. Avoidance of excessive exposure to sunlight.
  E. Protection from insect bites and common irritants, such as poison ivy and poison oak.
  F. Environmental hygiene.
  G. The importance of:
    [1] Periodic health evaluations.
    [2] Periodic dental examinations.
    [3] Proper medical attention when:
      a. There is traumatic injury with open wounds.
      b. Skin lesions appear, change in character or persist more than three weeks.
      c. There are symptoms and signs of inflammation or any persistent irritation of the skin and/or mucous membrane.

        [4] Prompt dental consultation when:
            a. Lesions appear in the mouth, change in character or persist.
            b. There is any irritation caused by dentures.

  H. The importance of:
        [1] Promptly discontinuing use of preparations, such as cosmetics, antiperspirants, dentifrices, and douching solutions, if there are indications of irritation.
        [2] Not applying chemical substances on a broken or irritated skin or mucous membrane unless these are medically prescribed.
        [3] Avoiding self-treatment of skin disorders.
        [4] Avoiding continued wetness of skin (e.g., shoes and socks).
        [5] Not squeezing pimples or boils.
        [6] Never plucking hairs in or around the nose.

2. The skin should be protected from injury due to:
  A. Trauma.
        [1] Friction should be avoided by such means as:
            a. Providing and encouraging the use of properly fitted shoes, clothing, supportive devices and dressings.
            b. Moving the patient carefully, avoiding sliding.
            c. Using powders on skin surfaces, especially if surfaces are in contact with each other.
        [2] Special precautions should be taken when sharp objects are used on or around the body (e.g., pins, razor blades, scissors).
        [3] Appliances with sharp edges (e.g., casts) should be carefully padded.
        [4] Skin care should be performed gently with appropriate materials and force. Scratching (e.g., with nails or rings) should be avoided.
        [5] Adhered materials, exudates, secretions or excretions should be removed carefully, gently and by appropriate methods (e.g., with soaking, irrigations, use of special solvents).
        [6] Scratching should be discouraged and prevented as possible.
            a. The cause of itching should be determined and eliminated whenever possible (e.g., lice, irritating fabrics, irritating secretions).
            b. Warmth should be minimized (e.g., by removal of warm clothing or covers or by avoiding exercise).
            c. Cool compresses or soaks may be helpful, unless these are contraindicated.
            d. Cooling lotions may be helpful, unless contraindicated.
            e. Prescribed antipruritic drugs should be administered and/or applied promptly, as ordered and needed.
            f. Mittens, restraints or special coverings for the affected part may be helpful.
            g. Nursing measures to promote rest and sleep should be used.
            h. Nursing measures to divert attention may be helpful.
            i. Itching that cannot be controlled by nursing measures should be reported promptly.

B. An inadequate blood supply.

[1] Continuous pressure against any body part should be avoided; this is of especial importance in relation to pressure over bony prominences.

    a. Special precautions must be taken for patients who are chronically ill, debilitated or weak, immobilized, unconscious, mentally incompetent or paralyzed.

    b. Pressure may be minimized by such means as proper positioning; frequent position changes; padding of natural hollows; use of special pads, mattresses or beds.

[2] Massage, especially of skin over pressure points, should be performed effectively and as frequently as necessary.

[3] Exercise (active or passive) should be provided and encouraged, within medical orders.

[4] Any pain, tingling or numbness in a body part should be investigated promptly.

C. Drying.

[1] Emollients or protectives should be applied as needed.

[2] Excessive washing, use of soaps or other drying agents (such as rubbing alcohol or powder) should be discouraged and avoided. If frequent cleansing is necessary:

    a. The skin should be observed carefully for signs of abnormal dryness.

    b. Appropriate cleaning and nondrying agents should be used with caution.

    c. The skin should be carefully dried.

    d. Emollients and/or protectives should be applied.

[3] Increasing the humidity may be helpful.

[4] Good circulation to the affected part should be promoted (e.g., by positioning, massage, exercise).

D. Excessive moisture.

[1] The skin should be carefully dried whenever it is cleansed.

[2] Clothing or bedding that is wet should be changed promptly.

[3] Moist dressings or pads should be changed as needed, within medical orders.

[4] Drying agents (e.g., powders, antiperspirants, alcohol) or protectives should be applied, unless contraindicated.

[5] When the skin must be moist for prolonged periods (e.g., with frequent or continuous wet compresses or soaks):

    a. Provision should be made for occasional drying.

    b. Normal skin should be protected by appropriate use of a skin protectant.

    c. If the skin shows signs of maceration, this should be reported.

E. Excessive heat or cold.

[1] The temperature of water or solutions used for treatments or baths should be measured or tested. The heat should not exceed that which is safe, comfortable and therapeutically effective.

[2] When local applications of heat or cold are used:

a. The patient should be observed closely for indications of injury to the skin area involved (e.g., burning).

b. Applications should be discontinued if symptoms and signs of injury appear, and this should be reported appropriately.

c. Any heating appliances that are used should be checked frequently and carefully controlled.

F. Radiation.

[1] When treatments involving radiation are used, the time and frequency of the treatment must be followed exactly.

[2] The skin should be observed carefully and frequently for excessive redness or irritation.

G. Chemicals.

[1] Patients should be protected from contact with any known allergens (e.g., drugs, foods, fabrics).

[2] Irritating body secretions, excretions or exudates should be promptly and thoroughly removed from the skin.

[3] Solutions used for treatments must be carefully prepared, in exactly the prescribed strength, and properly applied.

[4] Soap used for cleansing should be thoroughly rinsed off the skin.

H. Bites of insects, animal parasites.

[1] Appropriate means should be used to protect patients from flying or crawling insects.

[2] Clothing and bedding should be maintained clean and free from animal parasites.

[3] The hair should be kept clean and free from animal parasites.

I. Microorganisms.

[1] The skin should be protected from all types of injury. (See A through H above.)

[2] The skin should be kept clean, dry and free from discharges that contain or may contain microorganisms.

[3] Symptoms and signs of injury or inflammation or the appearance of skin lesions should be reported promptly. Appropriate nursing measures should be applied (e.g., use of sterile dressing, medical aseptic techniques).

3. Mucous membranes should be protected from injury due to:

A. Trauma.

[1] Friction should be avoided by:

a. Providing and encouraging the use of properly fitted appliances such as dentures.

b. Using appropriate lubrication when performing treatments involving the nose, moth, esophagus, trachea, pharynx, urethra, vagina, rectum.

[2] Equipment used in treatments involving mucous membranes should be absolutely smooth, padded if necessary and as soft as possible.

[3] No tube or instrument should ever be forced into a body opening. When inserting tubes or instruments, the insertion should be made in the proper direction and for the proper distance to achieve the desired therapeutic effectiveness.

B. Dryness.
    [1] Adequate humidity should be provided (e.g., with use of vaporizers).
    [2] The mucous membranes of the oral cavity should be kept properly moistened; this is particularly important when there is dehydration or mouth-breathing.
    [3] Emollients or protectives may be used at mucous-cutaneous junctions, such as the lips.
C. Excessive moisture. The perineal area should be kept free from secretions, urine, feces or menstrual flow.
D. Heat.
    [1] The temperature of solutions used for treatments should be measured or tested, and the heat should not exceed that which is safe, comfortable and therapeutically effective.
    [2] When local applications of heat are used, careful observations should be made for excessive redness of the involved membrane.
E. Chemicals.
    [1] Only prescribed medications should be applied to mucous membrane.
    [2] Any solutions used in treatments must be carefully prepared, in exactly the strength prescribed, and properly applied.
F. Microorganisms.
    [1] Mucous membrane should be protected from all types of injury. (See A through E above.)
    [2] Mucous membrane should be kept clean and free from possibly infective exudates or excretions.
    [3] Careful observations should be made for indications of irritations, lesions or infections, and these should be reported promptly.

CARE OF PATIENTS WITH SPECIFIC PROBLEMS

1. When a patient has sustained injury to the skin (e.g., cuts, abrasions, burns, infections):
    A. The injured area must be protected from injury due to trauma, excessive moisture, heat, radiation, chemicals or microorganisms.
    B. Tensions around any wound should be avoided.
    C. The injured area should be observed closely for indications of the following, which should be reported promptly:
        [1] Abnormal wound healing.
        [2] Infection (either extension of original infection or presence of secondary infection).
    D. Proper nutrition should be encouraged and provided.
2. When a patient has skin lesions (e.g., pustules, vesicles, desquamation):
    A. The lesions should be protected from injury (especially traumatic injury caused by scratching).
    B. The lesions should not be cleaned nor any preparation applied until medical orders are available.
    C. Medical orders relative to cleansing, application of medications, baths, and so forth should be followed exactly.

   D. Dietary orders must be followed exactly (e.g., limitations of fatty foods or restriction of allergy-causing foods).
   E. Spread of any lesions that are auto-innoculating should be avoided.
   F. Careful observations should be made for any evidence of hypersensitivity and/or possible psychogenic factors, and these should be reported appropriately.
   G. Emotional support should be consistent.
3. When a patient has sustained injury to or has lesions on mucous membranes:
   A. The affected area(s) must be protected from injury due to trauma, dryness, heat, chemicals or microorganisms.
   B. The affected area(s) should be observed carefully for:
       [1] Abnormal healing.
       [2] Infection (either extension of original infection or presence of secondary infection).

Chapter 14

The Inflammatory Response and Immunity

The body produces cellular elements and specific chemical sub-stances to protect itself against injurious agents and assist in tissue repair.

Anatomy and Physiology

PHYSIOLOGICAL DEFENSE MECHANISMS IN GENERAL

1. The body's primary defense mechanisms are those related to natural resistance or innate immunity. These include:
   - A. Healthy, intact skin and mucous membranes.
   - B. The inflammatory response to injury.
   - C. The presence of some nonspecific antibodies in the plasma.
2. The body's secondary defense mechanisms involve the immune process, with the development of specific antibodies. This is "acquired" immunity.
3. The body's ability to resist injury varies among races and individuals.
4. The very young and the aged have less resistance than have individuals in the middle years.

CELLULAR ELEMENTS THAT PROTECT THE BODY

1. The reticuloendothelial system.
   - A. The reticuloendothelial system consists of specialized reticulum cells that are capable of:
     - [1] Phagocytizing bacteria, viruses and other types of foreign matter.

[2] Producing immune bodies.
  B. Reticular cells are sometimes termed "fixed macrophages." They are found:
    [1] In the lining of many blood vessels and lymph channels.
    [2] In bone marrow, the spleen, the liver and lymph nodes.
2. Histiocytes.
  A. Histiocytes are found in all body tissues and have functions similar to those of the reticular cells of the reticuloendothelial system.
  B. Histiocytes can become mobile, and when they do they are called macrophages.
3. White blood cells (leukocytes)
  A. Leukocytes are mobile protective cells which are transported by the circulating blood.
  B. Granulocytes are formed (and, to some extent, stored) in bone marrow, while the monocytes and lymphocytes are formed mostly in the lymph nodes.
  C. Plasma cells, formed in bone marrow and lymph nodes, are the primary source of circulating immune globulins.
  D. White blood cells are capable of ameboid movement and are able to emigrate through the walls of blood vessels.
  E. Normally, there are 5,000 to 10,000 mature leukocytes per cubic ml. of blood.
    [1] Polymorphonuclear neutrophils represent 62.0 percent of that number. These cells are sometimes called microphages. They phagocytize and digest foreign matter and liberate enzymes that dissolve both foreign matter and themselves.
    [2] Polymorphonuclear eosinophils represent 2.3 percent of mature leukocytes. The function of these cells is unknown, but they are found in the blood in large numbers following the injection of foreign protein, during hypersensitivity reactions and with parasitic infections.
    [3] Polymorphonuclear basophils represent 0.4 percent. The function of these cells is also unknown. Their structure is similar to the mast cells in connective tissue, which liberate histamine when damaged.
    [4] Monocytes represent 5.3 percent. These cells are capable of becoming powerful macrophages.
    [5] Lymphocytes represent 30 percent. Although not all the functions of these cells are known, they do play an important role in cellular immunity and appear to function in tissue repair.

LYMPHOID TISSUE
1. Lymphoid tissue is present in small amounts in bone marrow and the spleen and is scattered through the mucous membranes of the alimentary canal and respiratory passages. It forms lymph nodes.
2. Lymphoid tissue produces lymphocytes and serves to filter out and destroy foreign matter such as microorganisms.
3. There is a circular band of lymphoid tissue that guards the respiratory and digestive tracts. The anterior part of the ring is formed by the lingual tonsil, the posterior by the pharyngeal tonsil (adenoids). The palatine tonsils lie on either side of the pharynx between the palatoglossal and palatopharyngeal arches.
4. Lymph nodes are small bodies located along the courses of lymphatic vessels. They consist of lymphocytes (free cells) and reticular cells (fixed macrophages).

A. All lymph passes through one or more lymph nodes before entering the general circulation.

B. The major groups of lymph nodes that may be palpated easily when enlarged include:

[1] Those of the head (e.g., occipital and around the ears).

[2] Those of the neck (e.g., submaxillary and cervical).

[3] Those in the axilla.

[4] Those in the groin (inguinal nodes).

THE INFLAMMATORY RESPONSE

1. Almost all the tissues of the body respond to injury by the process of inflammation.

2. The two basic purposes of the inflammatory response are:

A. Destruction, neutralization or limitation of the effects of injurious agents.

B. Assistance with tissue repair.

3. Essentially, the inflammatory response involves localized vascular changes; the formation of inflammatory exudate; and specialized functions of white blood cells, histiocytes and reticular cells.

A. Injured cells release histamine, which brings about the body's immediate response to injury. Later, chemical substances in the blood, called kinins, serve to extend the response.

B. Following a momentary vasoconstriction, vasodilatation increases blood flow to the injured tissues.

C. Capillaries in the area of injury become increasingly permeable, allowing plasma containing fibrinogen to leak into the tissues.

[1] The leakage causes a local extracellular edema.

[2] In most instances the tissue fluid clots, due to the fibrinogen and tissue exudates. Fibrin helps to wall off the injured area and delay spread of the invading agent.

D. Neutrophils circulating in the blood and histiocytes in the tissues are attracted to the area of damaged tissue and begin phagocytosis of injurious agents and cellular debris.

E. Many inflammations, especially those initiated by bacteria, cause the release of a leukocyte-promoting factor that stimulates the bone marrow to:

[1] Release large numbers of granulocytes, especially neutrophils. The total white blood cell count may increase up to 20,000 to 30,000 per cubic ml. of blood.

[2] Increase production of these leukocytes as long as they are needed.

4. Lymphatic drainage from an inflamed area may increase 7 to 8 times.

5. Healing of injured tissues generally does not begin until the acute inflammatory process has subsided to a nearly inactive state.

6. See also "Inflammation" in the Pathology section of this chapter.

TISSUE REPAIR

1. Healing may occur by:

A. Recuperation of the injured cells.

B. Regeneration, which involves cellular reproduction and organization.

[1] Regeneration depends upon such factors as:

a. The type of cell involved.

   b. The severity of the injury (e.g., approximation of wound edges).
   c. The presence of infection.
   d. Blood supply.
   e. Nutritional status.
   f. The age of the individual (healing is more rapid in the young).
[2] Nerve tissue, muscle tissue and elastic tissue have practically no ability to regenerate, although squamous cells are easily regenerated.
C. Fibrous tissue substitution, which involves the formation of granulation tissue and fibrosis:
   [1] Granulation tissue is composed of connective tissue, blood vessels and lymphatics. It is soft and grayish-red, and it bleeds easily.
   [2] As collagen fibers and hyaline substances increase in amount, contraction occurs, the blood vessels are closed off and the scar becomes nearly avascular.
   [3] Scarring helps by establishing continuity, reinforcing the area, and walling off infective agents.
   [4] Scarring can result in contractures when it occurs around joints.
   [5] Contractures around hollow organs are called strictures and may interfere with normal flow of substances through the organ(s) involved.
   [6] In areas where scars are subjected to repeated stress, the inelasticity may result in stretching and weakening of the part.
       a. A weakness in the abdominal musculature may result in a hernia.
       b. A weakness in the heart muscle may result in a rupture.
2. Wounds may heal by first or second intention.
   A. Healing by first intention involves:
      [1] The formation of a blood clot, which closes the wound, protects underlying tissues from injury and provides a framework for new growth.
      [2] The growth of epithelial tissue across the wound.
      [3] The development of granulation tissue and subsequent fibrous tissue substitution; generally the wound is covered and granulation tissue formed by the 7th or 8th day after injury.
   B. Healing by second intention involves the extensive development of granulation tissue because epithelial tissue cannot cover the wound. This may occur with a particularly large wound or because of wound infection. Healing requires a much longer time, and scarring is extensive.

THE IMMUNE PROCESS

1. The body has the ability to develop immunity against specific invading agents, such as bacteria, viruses, toxins and foreign tissues.
2. Humoral immunity involves the body's production of a specific antibody in response to exposure to a specific agent. The antibody modifies the effects of the antigen.
   A. Antigens are usually large protein molecules, large polysaccharides or a combination of these.
      [1] Haptenes are chemicals with smaller molecular weights that can act as antigens when combined with a macromolecule antigenic substance. The

antibody produced will then react against either the antigen or the haptene.

[2] Haptenes may be drugs, chemicals found in dust or used in industry, or parts of animal skin or hair.

B. Antigen may be introduced into the body by ingestion, inhalation, injection or contact with skin or mucous membrane.

C. Antibody is produced from portions of gamma globulin; each antibody has a specific chemical structure.

D. Antibody reacts with antigen in some specific way that prevents harmful effects of the antigen and facilitates the work of phagocytic cells.

E. Once the body has made a specific antibody, it can usually produce that antibody again rather quickly when it is needed.

[1] When the body is initially exposed to an antigen, a small amount of antibody is produced in a few days and then disappears from body fluids.

[2] Following the second exposure (optimal time is one month), the antibody response is greatly increased, and antibody remains in the body fluids over a longer period.

[3] This accelerated response provides the basis for protective immunization.
    a. Although the response usually persists for life, the extent of the response decreases over time.
    b. Small "booster" immunizations reinforce the accelerated response.

F. Active immunity may be acquired (artificially) against the following diseases:

[1] Routinely: diphtheria, pertussis, tetanus, smallpox, measles, poliomyelitis, rubella.

[2] Under special circumstances: cholera, typhoid, paratyphoid, influenza, mumps, tuberculosis, typhus, plague, rabies, yellow fever.

G. Antibodies that pass from the mother to the baby through the placenta (and to some extent through the mother's milk) can provide immunity for the baby for approximately 6 months after birth.

3. Cellular or lymphocyte immunity involves the sensitization of lymphocytes that are then capable of reacting with and destroying the foreign agent.

A. Cellular immunity protects against foreign protein not taken care of by the inflammatory reaction or by immunoglobin antibodies.

B. This type of immune response appears in some chronic infections (e.g., tuberculosis) and may play a role in some types of contact dermatitis.

Pathology

SYMPTOMS AND SIGNS

1. Symptoms and signs of the body's inflammatory response to injury include:

A. Local symptoms and signs.

[1] The cardinal symptoms and signs of inflammation are:
    a. Redness.
    b. Heat.
    c. Swelling.
    d. Pain.
    e. Loss of function.

       [2] Enlargement and tenderness of lymph nodes.
       [3] Red, inflamed lymphatic vessels (seen as red lines in skin).
       [4] Presence of exudates.
       [5] Lesions of skin or mucous membranes. (See Chapter 13.)
   B.   Systemic symptoms and signs:
       [1] Fever, with associated symptoms and signs. (See Chapter 9.)
       [2] Leukocytosis.
   C.   Progressive tissue repair, wound healing.

2. Systemic symptoms and signs that are frequently associated with the inflammatory process include:
   A.   Lassitude, malaise, weakness.
   B.   Anorexia, nausea, vomiting.
   C.   Headache.

3. Symptoms and signs of inadequate inflammatory response include:
   A.   Infections of mouth, throat or colon (possibly with ulcerations).
   B.   Susceptibility to bacterial infections.
   C.   Delayed tissue repair, wound healing.

4. Symptoms and signs of hypersensitivity reactions may include:
   A.   Those related to immediate hypersensitivity.
       [1] In systemic anaphylactoid reactions:
          a. Itching of scalp, tongue.
          b. Flushing of skin.
          c. Wheezing and dyspnea.
          d. Symptoms and signs of circulatory shock. (See Chapter 1.)
       [2] In localized reactions:
          a. Sneezing, excessive production of watery mucus, nasal congestion.
          b. Wheezing, dyspnea.
          c. Skin lesions (e.g., hives, rash).
   B.   Those related to delayed hypersensitivity.
       [1] Symptoms and signs of inflammatory response.
       [2] Skin lesions such as those associated with eczema. (See Chapter 13.)
   C.   Those related to agglutination and/or hemolysis of red blood cells. (See Chapter 1.)

INFLAMMATION

1. Tissue injuries that evoke the inflammatory response may be caused by:
   A.   Physical mechanisms (e.g., foreign bodies, trauma, radiation, heat or cold).
   B.   Chemicals such as strong acids, strong bases or poisons.
   C.   Hypersensitivity reactions.
   D.   Microorganisms.

2. The cardinal symptoms and signs of local inflammation are caused by specific physiologic changes in the area of injury.
   A.   The redness and heat are due to increased blood supply to the area.
   B.   The swelling is due to leakage of plasma into the injured tissues.
   C.   The pain is due to swelling of the tissues with resultant pressure on nerve endings and to the liberation of irritating chemicals within injured tissues.

[1] The more dense the tissue the more intense the pain.

[2] Throbbing pain is caused by additional blood being forced into the area with each heart beat.

D. The loss of function is due to cellular damage and cellular death, caused by both the injury and the inflammatory response. Affected tissues are disrupted, and function is impaired.

3. Inflammatory responses vary in duration.

A. Acute inflammations have a rapid onset and are of short duration, rarely lasting longer than two weeks.

B. Chronic inflammations are low-grade and prolonged, lasting from months to years.

[1] The inflammatory destruction of tissue may be progressive.

[2] Granulomas are specialized forms of chronic inflammation that involve the proliferation of cells at the site of injury.

a. Lymphocytes and epitheloid cells serve to wall off invading microorganisms.

b. Granulomas are formed in tuberculosis, syphilis and with some fungus infections.

4. Inflammatory responses vary in the type of exudate produced.

A. Purulent exudate (pus) contains dead or dying polymorphonuclear neutrophils, tissue debris, products of proteolytic digestion and microorganisms that may be dead or alive. This type of exudate is commonly associated with staphylococcal infections.

[1] The local accumulation of pus in any tissue is called an abscess.

[2] Drainage of the exudate may be spontaneous or may need to be brought about by surgical incision.

a. If all the exudate is drained, healing can progress. If not, the infection persists.

b. Superficial abscesses generally erode to the skin.

c. A tract from an abscess to the skin is called a sinus.

d. A tract from an abscess to the skin and to a second area (e.g., the intestinal tract) is called a fistula.

e. Sinuses and fistulae rarely heal by themselves.

[3] Deep abscesses may erode into areas where the infection can spread, or the erosion may cause critical tissue damage, such as erosion of a major blood vessel.

[4] Sometimes pus is absorbed and the area heals, leaving only some scar tissue.

B. Serous exudate resembles blood serum, containing little fibrin or blood cells. This type of exudate is frequently caused by streptococcal infections. Serous cavities are frequent sites for the collection of serous exudate.

C. Fibrinous exudate contains large amounts of fibrin. It is commonly produced in inflammation of serous membranes (visceral and parietal pleura, pericardium and peritoneum). As fibrin forms, the serous surface becomes rough and causes friction. If the inflammation progresses, the fibrin may be replaced by fibrous tissue, and this forms an adhesion.

    D.   Mucous or catarrhal exudate is produced when mucous membrane is inflamed. Initially there is a serous exudate, and this is followed by the mucous. When pyogenic microorganisms are involved, the exudate becomes mucopurulent.

5. When microorganisms capable of causing disease gain entrance into the superficial skin or mucous membrane, there is normally a localizing process with the formation of pimples, furuncles or superficial abscesses.

    A.   Polymorphonuclear leukocytes, fibrin and edema fluid containing nonspecific antibodies surround the microorganisms. Lymphocytes surround these, then macrophages, which cause some granulation.

    B.   Phagocytosis and proteolytic action result in the formation of a purulent exudate.

    C.   The inflammatory exudate may be absorbed or drained from a body opening (spontaneously or through surgical intervention).

    D.   The more intense the inflammatory response, the more likely the successful localization.

    E.   Localization is impeded by any injury to or movement involving the inflamed area.

6. When the localizing process fails, the microorganisms:

    A.   May cause a spreading cellulitis.

        [1] Cellulitis occurs most frequently in loose tissue such as subcutaneous tissue.

        [2] Some highly invasive microorganisms are able to spread very quickly through the ground substance (e.g., erysipelas is a rapidly spreading subcutaneous infection caused by *Beta hemolytic streptococcus*).

    B.   May be drained with tissue fluid into the lymphatic vessels, where they may cause an inflammation (lymphangitis).

    C.   May reach the lymph nodes and other lymphoid tissues, where they may:

        [1] Be destroyed by the action of mobile and fixed phagocytic cells.

        [2] Cause a local inflammation (e.g., lymphadenitis, cervical adenitis, tonsillitis).

7. When microorganisms capable of producing disease enter the circulating blood, either directly or indirectly through lymph drainage:

    A.   The fixed macrophages in the liver, spleen and bone marrow attempt to destroy the microorganisms and may be successful.

    B.   The liver, spleen and bone marrow may themselves become sites of inflammation.

    C.   A state of septicemia exists, and all the body tissues are subject to infection.

    D.   When microorganisms reach the lymphatic vessels that drain the face, they can be carried to the venous sinuses of the brain, where they can cause a meningitis and, possibly, a venous sinus thrombosis.

8. The release of almost any incompletely broken-down protein substance into the blood stream can cause a toxic reaction, resulting in malaise, anorexia, headache, fever.

9. The inflammatory response is impaired whenever blood flow to an injured body part is impaired.

10. Large amounts of cortisol or any other glucocortocoid block all stages of the inflammatory process.

11. The inflammatory response is impaired whenever there is a decrease in the normal numbers of mature white blood cells.
    A. When the white blood count falls below 5,000 per cubic ml. of blood, the condition is known as leukopenia. Possible causes include:
       [1] Viral infections.
       [2] A massive bacterial infection.
       [3] Disorders involving leukocyte-producing tissues.
    B. In agranulocytosis there is a marked reduction in the production of granulocytes. Depression of bone marrow function may be due to injury caused by large doses of radiation or by certain drugs and poisons. Early manifestations of this problem are ulcerations of the mucous membranes of the mouth, throat and the colon. There is increased susceptibility to infection.
    C. In leukemia (a neoplasm that may originate in the bone marrow or lymphoid tissue), there is an uncontrolled production of white blood cells. In some types of leukemia the cells are mostly immature forms that cannot function properly. Infections can be severe and may prove fatal.
    D. When the white blood count falls below 1,000 per cubic ml. of blood, any infection is potentially life-threatening.

IMMUNOPATHOLOGY
1. Inappropriate immune responses include:
   A. Production of too little antibody, which allows microorganisms to cause infectious diseases.
   B. Exaggerated response or overreactions, which cause undesirable physiological responses.
   C. Reactions against the self: one's own tissues and/or tissue products.
2. Hypogammaglobulinemia is a condition in which there is a deficiency in immune globulin.
   A. This condition may be inherited or acquired.
   B. Disorders that can lead to the development of hypogammaglobulinemia include those that affect the production of lymphocytes and/or plasma cells and those in which plasma proteins are lost (e.g., in nephrosis or with extensive burns).
3. Hypersensitivity represents an inflammatory condition caused by exaggerated antigen-antibody reactions. This is frequently termed an allergic response.
   A. Undesirable physiological responses may involve:
      [1] Blood vessels, resulting in congestion, swelling and edema.
      [2] Smooth muscle, causing spasms.
      [3] Exocrine glands, causing increased secretions.
   B. Immediate hypersensitivity generally occurs within minutes after the antigen has been introduced. Antibody is circulating in the serum.
      [1] Previous sensitization must have occurred at least 10 days previously.
      [2] Anaphylaxis is the most severe type of hypersensitivity and may be caused by:
         a. Protein substances, such as horse serum, insulin, dextran, allergen extracts and trypsin.

      b. Drugs, such as penicillins, salicylates, local anesthetics, mercurial diuretics.

[3] A generalized anaphylactoid response involves generalized vasodilatation and edema that results in acute hypotension. There may also be bronchial spasms.

[4] Examples of more localized anaphylactoid responses include:

      a. Bronchial asthma. Sensitivity is to foreign protein, such as pollen, house dust, animal hair, bacteria or virus. The primary response is contraction of the smooth muscle of the small bronchi. (See Chapter 2.)

      b. Hay fever. Hypersensitivity is to pollens or molds, and the target organ is nasal mucosa. There is seasonal edema, excessive sneezing and hypersecretion of the nasal mucosa.

      c. Allergic rhinitis. Hypersensitivity may be to many types of inhalants, foods, physical agents or bacteria. Symptoms are similar to hay fever.

      d. Urticaria, swelling of the tongue and laryngeal edema. Hypersensitivity may be to various inhalants, foods, drugs, insect bites. Capillaries in the inflamed area become greatly dilated and are highly permeable to leakage of plasma.

[5] Cytolytic or cytotoxic reactions are also examples of immediate hypersensitivity. Included are transfusion reactions and hemolytic disease of the newborn. (See Chapter 1.)

4. Auto-immune diseases are conditions believed to be the result of inappropriate immune response to one's own tissues or tissue products.

    A. It is possible that normal tissues or tissue products are not properly identified as of the self or that normal body components have been altered in some way that causes them to act as antigens.

    B. Disorders that may involve auto-immune response include rheumatoid arthritis, rheumatic fever and lupus erythematosus.

Nursing Care

Nursing care should be directed toward assisting the patient to attain, retain, or regain proper inflammatory and immune processes.

COLLECTION, EVALUATION AND COMMUNICATION OF DATA

1. Patients should be interviewed, observed and examined to identify symptoms and signs of actual or potential problems involving the inflammatory and immune processes.

    A. Problems may be indicated by:

      [1] Poor inflammatory response to injury, including poor wound-healing.

      [2] Symptoms and signs of hypersensitivity reactions.

    B. Systematic patient evaluation is of especial importance when the patient:

      [1] Has sustained an injury, most particularly if circulation is impaired.

      [2] Is known to have an infection.

      [3] Has leukopenia.

[4] Has a condition in which there is hypersecretion of glucocorticoids or is receiving steroid therapy.

[5] Has been exposed to a communicable disease.

[6] Has a protein deficiency due to improper diet or abnormal loss of body protein.

[7] Has a history of hypersensitivity.

[8] Has been or is receiving drugs that are frequently associated with hypersensitivity reactions.

[9] Is receiving treatments which may depress bone marrow function.

C. Data collected should be evaluated not only on the basis of a single deviation from normal (e.g., itching) but also on the basis of symptoms and signs that tend to occur when there are specific problems involving the inflammatory and/or immune processes (e.g., symptoms and signs of anaphylactoid shock).

D. The inflammatory response of individual patients should be evaluated on the basis of the body's normal inflammatory response to injury.

2. How, when and what data are communicated to the physician and/or other nursing personnel depend upon:

A. Any immediate threat to the patient's life processes (e.g., symptoms and signs of anaphylactoid shock or laryngeal edema).

B. Any potential threat to the patient's life and well-being (e.g., indications of a spreading infection).

C. Any particular implications for the physician in relation to:

[1] The patient's progress or lack of progress toward recovery (e.g., progress of wound-healing).

[2] Making a diagnosis (e.g., new objective or subjective data).

[3] The patient's physical and emotional responses to specific diagnostic procedures and therapeutic measures.

D. Any particular implications for nursing (e.g., in relation to need for special precautions to prevent infections).

PROMOTION OF HEALTH AND PREVENTION
OF DISEASE/INJURY

1. Health teaching to promote proper inflammatory and immune processes should be concerned with:

A. Proper nutrition.

B. A balanced program of exercise throughout the life cycle.

C. Adequate sleep and rest.

D. The importance of appropriate and prompt medical care when injuries are sustained and/or there are indications of infections.

E. Proper care of superficial skin injuries, infections.

F. The importance of:

[1] Protection against infections by routine immunizations and special immunizations when indicated.

[2] Avoiding any known allergens and instituting prompt treatment if exposure occurs.

[3] Protection against dangerous amounts of irradiation.

[4] Avoiding self-medication.

2. Localization of an infection may be hastened by:
   A. Warm, moist applications that increase blood flow to the part.
   B. Restricting motion of the inflamed part.
3. Venous return and lymphatic drainage from an inflamed area may be increased by elevation of the part above the level of the heart. This can serve to reduce swelling (and pain) and improve blood flow within the part.
4. When exudate is draining from an inflamed part, positioning should promote the drainage.
5. Healing wounds should be protected from any type of injury (traumatic, physical or chemical), from infections and from stresses such as pulling and stretching.
6. Patients with protein-wasting conditions should be provided special protection against infections. (See Chapter 20.)
7. Known hypersensitivities should be ascertained, and patients should be protected against exposure to these antigenic substances.
8. When pharmaceutical preparations likely to cause hypersensitivity reactions are administered (e.g., desensitizing drugs, antitoxins):
   A. The patient should be observed closely for indications of local or systemic reactions for at least 15 minutes after administration.
   B. Epinephrine and equipment for administration should be ready for immediate administration.

CARE OF PATIENTS WITH SPECIFIC PROBLEMS
1. When a patient has impaired inflammatory response (e.g., due to agranulocytosis, acute leukemia, steroid therapy), special precautions should be taken to protect him from *any* type of tissue injury. In some instances reverse isolation may be indicated to protect patients from infections.
2. When a patient has a superficial infection (e.g., a pimple, furuncle):
   A. The affected area should be protected from trauma (e.g., squeezing). This is of special importance when the infection is around the nose and mouth.
   B. Warm, moist packs may be applied to assist in localization.
   C. The inflamed area should be observed for signs of spreading of infection, and these should be reported promptly.
   D. The inflamed area should be observed for progress of tissue repair, and this should be reported/recorded appropriately.
3. When a patient has sustained injury requiring extensive tissue repair, a nutritious diet high in protein is indicated.
4. When a patient develops symptoms and signs of a hypersensitivity reaction:
   A. This should be reported promptly.
   B. Any possible antigenic substance should be promptly removed from the environment.
   C. Drugs that may be antigenic should be withheld pending prompt notification of the physician.
   D. Appropriate nursing actions should be taken in accordance with the undesirable physiological response(s) evoked.
   E. Prescribed antihistamine preparations should be administered promptly.

Chapter 15

Pain

The sensation of pain gives warning that body tissues are being damaged.

Anatomy and Physiology

1. Pain receptors are free nerve endings. They are widespread in the superficial skin layers and in some internal tissues, such as the arterial walls, periosteum, joint surfaces and the tentorium within the skull. They are diffusely distributed in other deeper tissues.
   A. Some regions of the body have sensory receptors that are primarily, if not exclusively, for pain. These include viscera of the chest, abdomen and pelvis; the teeth; the tympanic membrane; and the cornea.
   B. Localization of pain is difficult when an area is supplied almost entirely by pain fibers, because localization is largely dependent upon stimulation of the tactile receptors along with the pain receptors.
   C. Muscles and tendons possess exquisite pain sensitivity.
   D. Although very localized injuries do not cause severe pain in regions that have only a diffuse distribution of pain receptors, generalized stimulation of the receptors can result in severe pain.
   E. Brain tissue itself has no pain receptors.
2. Fast pain fibers (small type A fibers) transmit pricking-type pain sensations to the spinal cord and up the spinothalamic tracts to the thalamus. From the thalamus signals are conducted to the somatesthetic area of the cortex.
   A. Type A fibers are also found in the sensory portion of cranial nerves.
   B. Pricking-type pain sensations quickly alert a person to the presence of a painful stimulus and cause immediate reflex actions to remove the stimulus.

251

3. Slow pain fibers (type C fibers) transmit burning- and aching-type pain sensations to the spinal cord and up the spinothalamic tracts to the thalamus. These signals tend to spread through the reticular areas of the medulla, pons and midbrain before entering the thalamus.
   A. Type C fibers may be carried directly to the brain via the sensory portion of cranial nerves.
   B. Burning and aching pain sensations follow the initial pricking pain sensation and tend to become increasingly painful over time.
4. Pain is consciously but indiscriminately perceived at the level of the thalamus. The cerebral cortex functions to localize the pain, discern the quality of pain and give meaning to the pain.
   A. Conditioning impulses from higher centers probably modify the strength of the transmission of pain signals.
   B. If the axon or the dorsal root of a pain fiber is stimulated, pain is perceived as coming from the terminal end.
5. It is postulated that damaged cells release proteolytic enzymes that split bradykinin and similar chemicals from globulins in the interstitial fluid and that it is these compounds that stimulate the pain receptors.
   A. The histamine that is released from damaged cells probably acts as an irritant, also.
   B. It is possible that the lactic acid that accumulates in the tissues during anaerobic metabolism also acts as a painful stimulus.
6. When the blood flow to a part is blocked, the ischemic tissue becomes very painful.
   A. The higher the metabolic rate of the involved part, the more quickly the pain appears.
   B. Ischemia of muscle tissue (cardiac, skeletal and smooth) causes severe pain.
7. Pain may be designated as being superficial or cutaneous; deep (from muscles, tendons, joints, bone, fascia) or visceral.
   A. Cutaneous pain may be caused by burning or by traumatic injuries such as abrasions, lacerations or pricks.
   B. Deep pain may be due to tissue damage caused by traumatic injuries, the inflammatory process, pressure from abnormal growths or ischemia.
   C. Visceral pain may be caused by:
      [1] Blocking of the blood supply to a fairly large area.
      [2] Traumatic or chemical damage to visceral surfaces.
      [3] Smooth muscle spasm or stretching of smooth muscle fibers.
      [4] Stretching of supporting ligaments.
8. Visceral pain may be referred pain.
   A. Referred pain is pain felt in the body surface although originating in the viscera. The pain is not felt directly over the organ but in the dermatome of the segment from which the visceral organ was originally derived in the embryo.
   B. Branches of the visceral pain fibers synapse in the spinal cord with neurons that receive pain fibers from the skin. Signals being transmitted from the viscera (especially if intense) spread to neurons that conduct pain sensation from the skin.
   C. Heart pain may be felt in the upper thorax and in the shoulders, possibly radiating down the left arm.

D. Gallbladder pain may be felt in the right shoulder.

E. Pain from an inflamed appendix may be felt around the umbilicus.

9. Visceral pain may be localized in two surface areas when there are two pathways for the transmission of pain—i.e., visceral pain fibers and parietal pain fibers.

    A. While the visceral pain is referred to a surface area not directly over the involved organ, stimulation of pain fibers in the irritated parietal peritoneum, pleura or pericardium causes pain directly over the irritated area.

    B. The pain associated with an inflamed appendix is referred to the umbilical region but may also be experienced in the right lower quadrant of the abdomen.

10. There are both physical and emotional responses to pain.

    A. Severe superficial pain generally excites physiological defense mechanisms associated with the alarm pattern. Stimulation of the sympathetic nervous system causes:

        [1] Peripheral vasoconstriction, with a rise in blood pressure.

        [2] A stronger and more rapid heart beat.

        [3] An increase in the respiratory rate.

        [4] A decrease in the motility of the gastrointestinal tract.

        [5] Increased muscle tension.

        [6] General mental alertness.

        [7] Sweating.

    B. With severe deep or visceral pain there may be a failure of defense mechanisms, with resultant hypotension, weakness, bradycardia and nausea and vomiting.

11. Although thresholds for pain do not appear to vary significantly among individuals, personal reactions to pain vary greatly.

12. Individuals may respond to the experience of pain by:

    A. Vocal expressions, such as crying out, whimpering, gasping.

    B. Changes in facial expression (e.g., grimaces, frowns, general tenseness).

    C. Crying.

    D. Certain kinds of body movements.

        [1] Holding very still in rigid posture, possibly clenched fists.

        [2] Moving about aimlessly, restlessly.

        [3] Protective postures such as knees drawn up to abdomen or holding onto the painful part.

        [4] Rocking motions.

        [5] Rubbing of painful part.

    E. Withdrawal into self, with limited responsiveness to external environment.

    F. Irritability.

    G. Use of various psychologic defense mechanisms.

13. The pain that an individual experiences depends upon:

    A. Physiological variables such as:

        [1] The type, duration and intensity of the painful stimulus.

        [2] The level of consciousness.

        [3] The integrity of the sensory mechanism.

        [4] The degree of fatigue. (Fatigue lowers tolerance to pain.)

    B. Psychologic variables such as:

        [1] Past experiences with pain.

[2] Degree of threat to the life situation.

[3] Degree of understanding of the origin and significance of the pain.

[4] Basic personality type in relation to reaction to stimuli (i.e., whether one tends to minimize, maximize or moderate personal reactions).

[5] Learned attitudes, values and reaction patterns (may be related to particular sociocultural groups or to one's sexual role).

[6] Presence of other stressful stimuli. (Emotional tension increases reaction to pain.)

[7] The amount of attention given to the pain.

14. Pain involves and affects the whole person. Dealing with pain requires energy.

Pathology

SYMPTOMS AND SIGNS

1. Symptoms and signs of pain may include:
   A. Crying, moaning, yelling.
   B. Unusual quietness, withdrawal, depression.
   C. Generalized local muscle rigidity; fists may be clenched.
   D. Tense facial expressions.
   E. Unusual body movements or postures (e.g., knees drawn up to abdomen).
   F. Pulse and blood pressure changes.
      [1] With superficial pain pulse may become rapid, and there may be a rise in the arterial blood pressure.
      [2] With deep pain there may be a decrease in the heart rate and a fall in the arterial blood pressure.
   G. Respiratory changes (e.g., rate may be increased, decreased or irregular).
   H. Changes in skin color and temperature. (Skin may be flushed and hot or pale and cold.)
   I. Nausea, vomiting, anorexia.
   J. Sweating.
   K. Rubbing of body part.
   L. Restlessness, agitation, irritability, insommnia.

2. Significant information about experienced pain includes:
   A. The type of pain (e.g., aching, burning, cramping, constrictive, dull, sharp, stabbing, stinging).
   B. Severity of the pain.
   C. The location of the pain.
   D. Any change(s) in the type, severity and/or location.
   E. The duration of the pain.
      [1] Pain is usually not constant for long periods of time.
      [2] Pain indicates that tissue damage is occurring. When injury is severe, the pain receptors and fibers may be damaged so that pain signals are no longer received from the injured tissue.
   F. Recurrence of the pain.

DISORDERS RELATED SPECIFICALLY TO THE
SENSATION OF PAIN
1. Hyperalgesia exists when pain fibers are extremely sensitive to painful stimuli.
   A. The pain receptors may be hypersensitive due to some type of injury (e.g., a sunburned skin is more sensitive to painful stimuli than is a normal skin).
   B. Transmission of pain signals may be increased by the presence of lesions within the brain (e.g., a lesion within the thalamus may cause pain sensations to be intensified).
2. Central pain (sometimes called phantom pain) is felt as peripheral pain but does not originate in the periphery. Instead, the pain results from injury to nerve trunks, pain tracts or areas of the brain that are concerned with the perception of pain. Injury may be due to trauma (e.g., surgery), abnormal growths or an inflammatory process.
3. Trauma or neural disease involving peripheral nerves, pain tracts in the spinal cord or brain or sensory areas in the brain may interfere with transmission of pain signals and pain perception. There is loss of pain sensation. (Transection of the spinal cord is an example of an injury in which the sensation of pain is lost in regions no longer connected with the central nervous system.)
4. Neuritis is an inflammation of one or more peripheral nerves. If sensory nerves are involved there is pain as long as the nerves are still able to function.
   A. The nerves may be injured by trauma (e.g., overstretching, blows), by the pressure of abnormal growths, by irritating chemicals injected into them or near them or by infections.
   B. Polyneuritis, involving numerous nerves, especially those of the arms and legs, may be caused by a deficiency of B vitamins. (See Chapter 3.)
   C. Trigeminal neuralgia, sometimes called *tic douloureux*, is characterized by stabbing paroxysms of pain in one or more branches of the trigeminal nerve (ophthalmic, maxillary, mandibular).
      [1] This condition tends to develop in later life. The cause is unknown.
      [2] The pain, which is experienced superficially, may be started by stimulation of the nerve endings of the affected branch(es).

HEADACHES
1. Headaches resulting from intracranial disturbances may be caused by:
   A. Traction on the venous sinuses.
   B. Injury to the tentorium cerebelli (the transverse shelf of dura mater separating the cerebellum from the occipital lobe of the cerebrum).
      [1] When the upper surface of the tentorium is affected, pain is experienced in the upper part of the head anterior to the ear.
      [2] When the under surface of the tenorium is affected, pain is experienced in the occipital region.
   C. Stretching of the dura at the base of the brain or trauma to or stretching of dural blood vessels.
      [1] In meningitis, the irritation of the dura and increased sensitivity of areas around the venous sinuses cause severe headaches.
      [2] Headaches associated with brain tumors may be generalized or localized. They are usually intermittent.

[3] Severe headaches may occur in association with arterial hypertension.
2. Migraine headaches are thought to be related to vascular changes within the dura and/or the scalp. These recurrent headaches are usually severe and may last for hours or days.
   A. Classic migraine headaches often begin with prodromal sensations such as visual auras, loss of vision, transient paresthesia or nausea.
   B. This type of headache tends to occur in families. Personality factors appear to contribute.
   C. The headaches are often accompanied by excessive irritability, photophobia, nausea and vomiting, chills and sweating.
3. Extracranial headaches include:
   A. Muscle contraction (tension) headaches.
       [1] These headaches usually involve the neck, shoulders and occipital region.
       [2] They are often associated with emotional tension.
       [3] There are sustained contractions of the neck and head muscles.
   B. Eyestrain headaches are caused by eye problems, such as refraction errors or overuse of the eyes in inadequate lighting.
       [1] There are sustained contractions of the extraocular muscles.
       [2] Muscle spasms may cause pain in the frontal, temporal or even the occipital regions.
   C. Sinus headaches are associated with inflammation of the paranasal sinuses.
       [1] Pressure changes occur within the sinuses when the mucous lining is congested and drainage is blocked.
       [2] The location of the pain depends upon the sinus(es) involved.
4. Vascular and tension headaches frequently occur under specific circumstances or conditions.
   A. Specific factors such as alcohol, emotional stress, fatigue or menstruation may trigger a headache; sometimes it may be a combination of such factors.
   B. Sometimes an attack appears to follow a series of certain kinds of experiences or situations.

Nursing Care

Nursing care should be directed toward preventing pain whenever possible, alleviating pain and protecting the patient who is insensitive to pain.

COLLECTION, EVALUATION AND COMMUNICATION OF DATA
1. Patients should be encouraged to report the presence of pain.
2. Any pain reported by a patient should be promptly and thoroughly investigated.
3. Patients should be interviewed, observed and examined to identify and evaluate pain.
   A. Observations should be made for behaviors commonly associated with the pain experience. These include:
       [1] Crying and other vocal expressions indicative of pain.
       [2] Tense, anxious facial expressions.

      [3] Unusual body positions and/or movements.

      [4] Sweating.

      [5] Changes in vital signs.

      [6] Unusual emotional behavior.

  B. Systematic patient evaluation is of especial importance when the patient:

      [1] Complains of having pain.

      [2] Has a diagnosed disorder in which pain is usually experienced.

      [3] Is likely to experience pain as a consequence of a particular diagnostic or therapeutic procedure.

      [4] Might develop a particular complication (related to a diagnosed disorder or to a diagnostic or therapeutic procedure) which would be indicated by pain.

      [5] Is not fully conscious.

      [6] Is very young or elderly.

      [7] Tends to minimize discomfort experienced.

  C. A patient's reported pain experience should be evaluated in relation to:

      [1] The location of the pain, the type of pain and common causes of this type of discomfort in this particular location.

      [2] The patient's diagnosis and pain commonly associated with the particular pathophysiology involved or with common complications of this disorder.

      [3] Any recent diagnostic or therapeutic procedures and pain commonly associated with these or with possible complications of these procedures.

      [4] The severity and duration of the pain.

      [5] The patient's age.

      [6] The patient's anxiety level.

      [7] The patient's fatigue level.

      [8] Possible stress-producing factors in the environment.

4. Factors that are helpful in assessing the severity of the pain experienced by a patient include:

  A. Age, sex, sociocultural background.

  B. Facial expressions.

  C. Posture assumed.

  D. The amount and type of physical activity.

  E. The presence or absence of muscle rigidity.

  F. Changes in the pulse rate, respiratory rate and/or blood pressure.

  G. Presence or absence of sweating.

  H. Presence of anxiety.

  I. Presence of fatigue.

  J. Manner in which patient talks about the pain.

  K. Distractability from the pain.

5. How, when and what data about a patient's experienced pain are communicated to the physician and/or other nursing personnel depend upon:

  A. Any immediate threat to the patient's life processes (e.g., pain associated with vital organs, such as the heart).

  B. Any potential threat to the patient's life and well-being (e.g., any severe pain).

C. Any particular implications for the physician in relation to:
[1] The patient's progress or lack of progress toward recovery (e.g., change in pain experienced).
[2] Making a diagnosis that can result in initiation of specific therapeutic measures (e.g., new objective or subjective data).
[3] The patient's physical and emotional responses to specific pain-relieving measures.
D. Any particular implications for nursing (e.g., in relation to nursing measures to prevent or alleviate pain).

PROMOTION OF HEALTH AND PREVENTION
OF DISEASE/INJURY
1. Health teaching should be concerned with:
    A. The function of pain in terms of providing warning of injury to the body.
    B. The importance of prompt medical evaluation when pain is severe, persistent or recurring.
2. All patients should be protected from injury to body tissues. (See Nursing Care in each chapter).

CARE OF PATIENTS WHO HAVE OR MAY HAVE PAIN
1. The amount of pain experienced by a patient during or immediately following a painful procedure may be reduced by:
    A. Explaining, appropriately, what is to be done.
    B. Informing the patient about what sensations can be expected.
    C. Remaining with the patient and responding appropriately to the patient's anxiety.
    D. Encouraging as much muscle relaxation as possible.
2. Nursing actions to alleviate pain should be in accordance with the determined or probable source of the pain, for example:
    A. Distention of hollow organs may be relieved by providing for elimination of gases, fluids and/or solids causing the distention.
    B. External pressure exerted against body tissues may be relieved by:
        [1] Changes in position.
        [2] Proper support of body parts.
        [3] Use of light-weight covers or no covers directly over painful body parts.
        [4] Loosening of constricting bandages or binders (unless this is contraindicated).
    C. Joint strain or muscle strain may be relieved by:
        [1] Proper alignment and support of body parts.
        [2] Changes in position.
    D. Muscle spasms may be relieved by:
        [1] Warm applications.
        [2] Massage, placing muscle on stretch.
        [3] Administration of muscle relaxants.
    E. Pain in an injured body part (e.g., a joint) may be reduced by immobilization of the part.

    F.   Hyperactivity of the gastrointestinal tract may be reduced by the administration of prescribed antispasmodic drugs.

    G.   Local congestion and edema may be reduced by:

        [1] Warm and/or cold applications.

        [2] Elevation of the affected body part above the level of the heart.

        [3] Active or passive exercises.

    H.   Chemical irritation of the gastric or duodenal mucosa may be reduced by the administration of prescribed antacids.

    I.   Painful exposed dermis may be covered with a light dressing.

    J.   Infiltration of I.V. fluids should be promptly stopped.

    K.   See also Nursing Care in other chapters throughout Part II.

3. Nursing actions to alleviate pain should include those which serve to alter other stimuli the patient is receiving, for example:

    A.   Reducing disturbing environmental stimuli, such as bright lights, loud noises, upsetting visitors or nearby patients may help to reduce acute pain.

    B.   Firm massage or pressure against the area around or over the painful spot may reduce the pain sensation.

    C.   The amount of pain that is perceived may be reduced by distraction from the sensation through some type of interesting, different experiences that require attention. These might include watching television, reading, writing, talking with visitors or handcrafts of various types.

4. Pain may be reduced by relieving muscular tension (e.g., by massage, warmth or positive relaxation exercises).

5. Nursing actions to alleviate pain should include those that serve to decrease the patient's anxiety and promote adaptation to the existing situation. (See Part III.)

6. When a patient's anxiety appears to be increasing with the amount of pain experienced, a prescribed sedative or tranquilizing drug may be helpful in alleviating pain.

7. Analgesic preparations should be administered as prescribed and as needed by the patient experiencing pain.

    A.   New pain, not yet evaluated by a physician, should not be masked by drugs.

    B.   Analgesic preparations should be administered in time to prevent severe pain.

8. Pain should be alleviated to the greatest possible extent in order to provide adequate sleep and rest and to prevent fatigue.

9. When a patient has an injured skin (e.g., first- or second-degree burns), the involved area should be carefully protected from heat, pressure or friction.

10. When a patient has a condition (e.g., trigeminal neuralgia) in which the pain sensation may be triggered by certain stimuli (e.g., cold or pressure), great care should be taken to prevent stimulation of the trigger region.

11. When a patient experiences a headache:

    A.   A quiet, nonstimulating environment should be provided.

    B.   Physical rest should be encouraged and provided as possible.

    C.   Emotional support should be consistent.

    D.   Coughing or straining should be avoided. (This is especially important in vascular headaches.)

    E.   Gentle massage of the neck and shoulder muscles may be helpful.

    F. Exercise of neck and shoulder muscles may be helpful (e.g., in tension head-
        aches).
    G. The eyes should be rested (particularly in eyestrain headaches).
    H. Drainage from congested sinuses should be promoted (sinus headaches).
    I. Analgesic drugs should be administered as prescribed and needed.
    J. Prescribed medications specifically for migraine headaches (e.g., vasocon-
        strictors) should be administered promptly as needed.
12. When a patient is insensitive to painful stimuli (e.g., is comatose):
    A. Systematic evaluations should be made to identify indications of injury and/or
        inflammation.
    B. Special precautions should be used to protect the patient from any type of
        injury (e.g., careful positioning, frequent position changes, provision for
        proper elimination, protection from burns).

Chapter 16

The Sensory Processes Other than Pain

Vision, hearing, tactile and thermal sensations, smell and taste provide the body with information about the external environment.

Anatomy and Physiology

VISION

1. The eye, the organ of vision, is a spherical body that is suspended within a bony orbit by means of muscles, ligaments, blood vessels, nerves and a fat cushion.
2. The wall of the eyeball consists of three concentric layers.
   A. The external layer consists of:
      [1] The sclera: the white fibrous covering of the sides and posterior portion of the eye. The sclera contains numerous blood vessels and nerves.
      [2] The cornea: the transparent tissue over the pupil. The cornea is supplied by a rich plexus of pain fibers but has very few blood vessels.
   B. The vascular middle layer consists of:
      [1] The choroid, which contains many blood vessels.
      [2] The ciliary body, which has both secretory and muscular functions.
      [3] The iris: the muscular diaphragm that has a circular aperture, called the pupil.
   C. The innermost layer, the retina, lines the posterior part and sides of the eyeball and contains the sensory receptors for light.
      [1] Each retina contains millions of nerve cells able to react to light and millions more that coordinate and transmit visual signals to the optic nerve.

[2] There are two types of visual cells.
   a. The cones are used in daylight vision. They detect specific colors.
   b. The rods are very sensitive and used for vision in dim light. They detect light of any color except red.

3. The cavity of the eye contains:
   A. The aqueous fluid that fills the anterior and posterior chambers.
       [1] The anterior chamber lies behind the cornea and in front of the iris and central part of the lens. The posterior chamber is a narrow slit behind the peripheral part of the iris and in front of the suspensory ligament of the lens and the ciliary process.
       [2] The aqueous fluid is produced continuously by the ciliary body which encircles the eye, starting just behind the iris.
       [3] The fluid contains nutrients that nourish the lens.
       [4] The fluid circulates anteriorly through the pupil and out of the eye through a meshwork called the trabecular spaces. The fluid empties through the Canal of Schlemm into tiny scleral veins.
   B. The vitreous humor that fills the cavity posterior to the lens.
       [1] This viscous fluid is formed during growth of the eye and remains essentially the same throughout life.
       [2] "Floaters," perceived as tiny floating objects, are shadows cast upon the retina by minute particles contained in the vitreous gel. These may occur normally due to:
       a. Remnants of embryonic blood vessels.
       b. Changes in the gel that tend to occur with aging.
   C. The crystalline lens, the transparent, biconvex, circular structure which lies suspended behind the center of the pupil.
       [1] The lens is composed of a strong elastic capsule filled with gelatinous protein fibers.
       [2] The lens is suspended behind the pupil by tiny ligaments (zonular fibers) that are attached to the ciliary body.
       a. Tension of the zonular fibers is controlled by the contraction or relaxation of the ciliary muscle.
       b. Changes in the shape of the lens are effected by changes in the tension of the zonular fibers.
       c. Ciliary muscle contraction is under parasympathetic nervous control.
       [3] In the aging process the lens structure tends to lose some of its elastic nature and may lose varying degrees of its transparency. Both interfere with visual acuity.

4. The intraocular fluid pressure is determined by the rate of aqueous humor production and the resistance to outflow.
   A. Normally the pressure is between 12 and 22 mm. of Hg.
   B. Because intraocular pressure reflects changes in the choroidal capillary and venous blood pressures, both physical and emotional factors can cause a rise in the intraocular pressure.

5. The exposed part of the eyeball is covered by the conjunctiva, a delicate epithelial tissue, which continues onto the inner surfaces of the eyelids.

   A.   The eyelids are covered with skin on the outer surface; eyelashes develop from the free edges.

   B.   The meibomian glands (tarsal glands) are located on the inner surfaces of the eyelids.

       [1]   There are approximately 30 of these modified sebaceous glands on each lid.

       [2]   Oily secretions from these glands help to prevent tears from overflowing onto the surrounding skin.

6. The conjunctival surfaces are kept moist and clean by a film of tears, the slightly hypertonic, clear, watery fluid that secreted by the lacrimal glands.

   A.   Tears are delivered through several fine ducts into the superior conjunctival fornix.

   B.   Reflex movements of the eyelids (blinking) keep the exposed cornea moist with tears. Corneal ulcers develop rapidly (within hours) if the cornea is dry.

   C.   Tears drain through the lacrimal duct into the nose. The outflow is dependent upon both blinking and gravity.

   D.   Tear secretion is induced reflexly by stimulation of the cornea or conjunctiva.

   E.   Fluids having a salt concentration greater than 1.5 percent or less than 0.16 percent tend to be irritating to the eyes of most people. Plain water does not injure the eyeball.

7. Blinking is a reflex or a voluntary act.

   A.   Blinking helps to protect the eye from the entrance of foreign particles.

   B.   Closure of the eyes is accomplished by contraction of muscles around the eye that are under the control of branches of the facial nerve.

   C.   Opening of the eyes is accomplished by contraction of muscles of the eyelid under the control of the oculomotor nerve.

   D.   Normally, stimulation of the cornea or conjunctiva causes blinking.

8. The extrinsic eye muscles move the eyeball in its orbit.

   A.   There are three separate pairs of muscles, which are controlled by the third, fourth and sixth cranial nerves.

   B.   Normally, movements of the eyeballs are very well coordinated, so that both eyes are aimed at the same point. Lack of coordination results in double vision.

   C.   At birth eyes are not well coordinated with each other; but by the third month, a common visual direction is usually attained.

   D.   Eye as well as head movements are closely associated with the vestibular apparatus and the maintenance of equilibrium. Visual disturbances may cause vertigo and nausea.

9. The optic nerve, formed by hundreds of thousands of nerve fibers from the retina, leaves the eyeball at a point called the optic disc.

10. The 2 optic nerves pass backwards to the optic chiasm, where some fibers cross to the opposite side. From the chiasm the 2 optic tracts continue posteriorly through the midbrain, to the visual cortex in the occipital lobe of the cerebrum.

   A.   Visual images are perceived in the primary visual cortex.

   B.   Visual information is further processed in adjacent visual association areas.

   C.   Interpretation of visual sensations is accomplished largely in the posterior temporal lobe and angular gyrus of the cerebral cortex.

11. Light rays enter the eye through the pupil, and the refraction of the rays (primarily through the cornea and crystalline lens), normally causes them to focus on the retina.
    A. The iris serves as an opaque screen which adjusts the amount of light allowed to enter the eye.
       [1] Parasympathetic stimulation of circular muscles in the iris causes constriction of the pupil (miosis).
       [2] Sympathetic stimulation of radial muscles in the iris causes dilation of the pupil (mydriasis).
       [3] In bright illumination the pupil is constricted; in dim light, the pupil is dilated.
           a. The pupil of the human eye can vary from 0.8 mm. to 1.8 mm. in diameter. The amount of light that is allowed to enter the eye can vary as much as 30 times.
           b. Contraction of the pupil when light is shone into the eye is called the pupillary light reflex.
    B. The adjustment of the eye, by which it focuses the image of both near and far objects on the retina, is called accommodation.
       [1] Accommodation is accomplished by changes in the convexity of the crystalline lens.
       [2] Convergence of the eyes and constriction of the pupils occur when there is accommodation for near objects.
       [3] Generally, the mechanisms of accommodation are not well developed until after the second or third month of life.
       [4] The ability to accommodate generally decreases after the age of 40.
       [5] Eyestrain, leading to eye fatigue, occurs when the ciliary muscles become tired due to prolonged contraction (e.g., when eyes are used for fine work for long periods).
12. The retina is stimulated most effectively by light, but crude visual sensations can be evoked by pressure.
13. Very bright illumination near an object being observed causes glare.
    A. When there is glare, visual acuity is decreased, and eyestrain occurs.
    B. Squinting helps to reduce glare.
14. Clarity and efficiency of vision are reduced by inadequate lighting.
    A. How much illumination is desirable for best vision and avoidance of eye fatigue depends largely upon the amount of visual acuity demanded for the job and the contrast between light and dark in what is being observed.
    B. A general overall illumination of a room with increased illumination on the working surface produces a minimum of glare and helps to prevent eye fatigue.
15. Binocular vision is important for depth perception and for the largest possible visual field.
16. Visual acuity is expressed by a mathematical fraction denoting the ratio of one's visual acuity to that of the normal person. Thus, 20/20 vision (normal) means that a person placed 20 feet from a test chart can see letters of a certain size that he normally should be able to see at that distance; 20/30 vision denotes that a person sees at 20 feet what a normal person can see at 30 feet; and so forth.

HEARING

1. The ear contains the sensory receptors for sound and the sensory organ that detects sensations concerned with equilibrium.
    A. The external ear is composed of the pinna (or auricle) and the auditory canal.
        [1] The pinna contains elastic cartilage and is covered with skin.
        [2] The ear canal in the adult is a slightly S–shaped channel, approximately 1 to 1¼ inches in length. It ends blindly at the flexible tympanic membrane (ear drum).
            a. The ear canal in the child is relatively straight.
            b. The outer half of the canal is lined with skin containing wax-secreting and sweat glands and is attached to cartilage.
            c. The inner half of the canal is lined with a thin epithelium that is attached closely to the underlying bone.
            d. The tympanic membrane is normally a pearly gray color. It is a fairly tough membrane.
    B. The middle ear is a tiny chamber situated in the temporal bone; it contains three articulating miniature bones (ossicles).
        [1] The malleus articulates with the tympanic membrane; the incus is in the center; and the stapes articulates with the oval window in the posterior wall.
        [2] The middle ear is filled with air that is maintained at atmospheric pressure by means of an air passageway through the eustachian tube.
        [3] The middle ear is lined with mucous membrane, which is continuous with that of the eustachian tube, the nasopharynx and the mastoid antrum (cavity in the mastoid process).
        [4] The posterior wall of the middle ear has an opening into the mastoid antrum.
            a. The mastoid process is the posterior portion of the temporal bone, located behind the ear.
            b. The mastoid contains a deep groove for the lateral sinus of the brain.
            c. The mastoid cells are separated from the brain by only a thin plate of bone.
            d. The mastoid cells are spaces containing air. There is a direct connection between the mastoid cells and the middle ear.
        [5] A branch of the facial nerve lies very close to the middle ear.
    C. The internal, or inner, ear contains a bony labyrinth and a membranous labyrinth. The sensory receptors lie within the membranous labyrinth.
        [1] The bony labyrinth is a series of communicating cavities within the temporal bone. It consists of the vestibule, the semicircular canals (concerned with equilibrium) and the cochlea (concerned with hearing).
            a. The vestibule is in the central portion; its lateral wall contains the oval window.
            b. There are three bony semicircular canals which open into the vestibule. They are unequal in length and lie in different directions.
            c. The cochlea is a conical structure, with spirals that form a canal.
        [2] The membranous labyrinth is a series of communicating sacs and ducts

that lie within the osseous labyrinth. It consists of the utricle and the saccule within the vestibule; the semicircular ducts within the semicircular canals; and the cochlear duct within the cochlea.

[3] In the space between the membranous labyrinth and the bony labyrinth is a clear fluid, perilymph, which acts as a cushion.

[4] The membranous labyrinth is a closed system and contains the fluid endolymph.

[5] Hair cells in the utricle, saccule and semicircular ducts act as rotary and gravity receptors. Nervous impulses are carried to the brain by way of the vestibular nerves. (See Chapter 11 in regard to equilibrium.)

[6] Within the cochlear duct, on the surface of the basilar membrane lies the organ of Corti, which contains the receptive end-organs for hearing (thousands of hair cells). The hair cells are stimulated by vibratory stimuli. Auditory signals are carried to the brain by way of the cochlea nerve, a division of the auditory nerve.

2. Hearing is a mechanoreceptor sense. Sound waves cause the tympanic membrane to vibrate. The vibratory motions are transmitted through the ossicles in the middle ear and through the oval window in the vestibule. The perilymph in the inner ear is set in motion, and this in turn causes the motion of the endolymph. The vibrations of the basilar membrane in the cochlea excite the receptor hair cells of the organ of Corti. Vibratory stimuli are then converted into nervous impulses.

A. The tiny ossicles in the middle ear concentrate the vibrations received from the tympanic membrane. Pressure exerted on the cochlear fluid is about 20 times greater than the pressure that is exerted by sound waves on the tympanic membrane.

B. Each frequency of sound causes a different pattern of vibration, and these are interpreted as variations in pitch.

C. The loudness of sound that is perceived depends on the rate at which the hair cells are stimulated and on the number of cells stimulated.

D. Awareness of the direction from which a sound comes appears to depend on the differing speeds with which sound waves hit each ear drum.

E. The delicate ear structures can be damaged by very loud sounds.

3. Centers for auditory reflexes (e.g., jumping at loud noises) are located in the midbrain.

4. Sound is perceived and interpreted in the auditory cortex, which is located in the superior temporal gyrus of the cerebral cortex.

5. Continued and/or excessive stimulation of the auditory nerves gives rise to general fatigue and nervous irritability. Individuals vary in their tolerance to noise.

6. Hearing is generally the last sense to be lost when there is loss of consciousness.

7. When heated or cooled quickly, the fluid in the semicircular canals causes sensations of position change that may result in vertigo and nausea.

THE TACTILE SENSES

1. The tactile senses include the senses for touch, pressure and vibration.

A. All of these sensations are detected by the same types of mechanoreceptors.

B. Touch sensation results from stimulation of tactile receptors in the skin or directly under the skin.

   C. Pressure sensation results from stimulation of receptors in the deeper tissues, when these tissues are "deformed."

   D. Vibration sensation results from very rapid stimulation of these receptors.

 2. There are a number of types of tactile receptors.

   A. Some free nerve endings are found everywhere in the skin and in many other tissues.

   B. Meissner's corpuscles, which are very sensitive, are especially numerous on the fingertips and lips. They adapt quickly. (See "Sensory Adaptation," following.)

   C. Expanded-tip tactile receptors are found in areas where there are Meissner's corpuscles. These receptors do not adapt so quickly.

   D. A hair end-organ is found at the base of every hair on the body. These can detect even the slightest movement of the hair.

   E. Ruffini's end-organs are found in the dermis and in deeper tissues. They do not adapt readily.

   F. Pacinian corpuscles are also found in the dermis and deeper tissues. They are stimulated by very rapid stimuli and adapt within a fraction of a second.

 3. Tactile sensations are transmitted via sensory nerve fibers that enter the spinal cord through the posterior roots. Upon entering the cord, the fibers separate into medial and lateral divisions.

   A. The medial fibers enter the dorsal columns of the cord and ascend the full length of the cord.

   B. The lateral fibers synapse with other neurons which form the spinothalamic tracts that ascend the spinal cord in the ventral and lateral columns. The spino-thalamic tracts transmit crude touch and pressure sensations and tickle and itch sensations.

 4. The sensory nerve fibers from the separate body parts are maintained in a definite spatial relationship from where they originate in the dorsal columns to the cerebral cortex.

   A. Second-order neurons originating in the medulla cross to the opposite side before passing upward to the thalamus.

   B. Third-order neurons originating in both sides of the thalamus project almost entirely to the postcentral gyrus of the cerebral cortex. This area is termed Somatic Sensory Area I.

 5. Somatic Sensory Area I enables the conscious individual to:

   A. Localize sensations.

   B. Distinguish degrees of pressure exerted against body parts.

   C. Judge the shapes, forms and textures of objects (without visual sense).

THERMAL SENSATION

 1. Sensory receptors for warmth and cold are found peripherally, especially in the skin.

 2. Thermal receptors respond to:

   A. Steady states of temperature.

   B. Changes in temperature.

 3. Gradations of temperature are difficult to discern unless a fairly large surface area

is stimulated. The larger the area stimulated, the smaller the differences that can be detected.
4. When the temperature is very cold or very hot, the pain fibers are stimulated.
5. Thermal receptors adapt to a great extent.
6. Thermal signals are transmitted very quickly. The thermal fibers travel in the spino-thalamic tract.
7. Thermal sensations are perceived in the somesthetic cortex.

TASTE
1. Tastebuds, located mainly on the anterior and lateral surfaces of the tongue, are stimulated by chemical substances in solution.
2. Although many taste variations can be experienced, there appear to be four primary taste sensations: sour, salty, sweet and bitter.
3. A bitter taste usually causes the individual to reject the substance (a protective mechanism).
4. Most taste receptors respond to more than one type of taste stimulus.
5. Taste signals are transmitted by cranial nerves (fifth, seventh and tenth) to the brain stem, then via the thalamus to the somesthetic cortex, where the taste is perceived.
6. Taste reflexes help to control secretion of the salivary glands during eating.

SMELL
1. There are millions of receptor cells for smell within the olfactory epithelium, which lies in the superior portion of each nostril.
2. Only a very minute amount of stimulus is needed to stimulate the smell receptors, whose main function is to detect the presence or absence of odors.
3. To stimulate the smell receptors the substance must be volatile, soluble in lipids and at least partially soluble in water.
4. Smell signals are sent to the olfactory bulb and through the olfactory tract to two major olfactory areas, located medially and laterally in the brain.
   A. Secondary tracts pass into the thalamus, hypothalamus and brain stem. These areas control the automatic body responses to the olfactory sensations, e.g., salivation and emotional responses.
   B. Secondary tracts also pass into the temporal cortex and prefrontal cortex, where the smell sensations are perceived and interpreted.

SENSORY ADAPTATION
1. All sensory receptors adapt either partially or totally to their various stimuli over a period of time.
   A. When stimuli are applied continuously, receptors respond at a very rapid impulse rate at first, then more and more slowly. Some fail to respond at all after a certain period of time.
   B. Pain receptors, sound receptors and receptors in the vestibular apparatus adapt at a very slow rate.
2. Adaptation to smell and taste sensations occurs rapidly and is thought to be related more to psychological factors than to receptor adaptation.

Physics

1. Light is a form of electromagnetic radiation (gamma rays, x-rays, ultraviolet rays, visible light rays and infrared rays).
2. Illumination varies with 3 factors:
   A. The power of the source of light.
   B. The distance from the source of light.
   C. The angle of incidence at which the light strikes a surface and is reflected.
3. Refraction is the bending of a ray of light as it passes from one medium to another medium of different density.
4. A converging lens causes, through refraction, the convergence of parallel light rays on the opposite side of the lens at a point called the principal focus.
5. Sound originates in vibrations, and the waves, which are set up in some medium (solid, liquid or gas), travel outward from the source of sound.
6. Pitch indicates the brain's interpretation of the frequency of sound waves.
7. The intensity of sound is heard as loudness.
8. Pressure is the force exerted on a unit area.
9. Pressure exerted on a confined liquid is transmitted undiminished to all parts of that liquid.
10. Heat is a form of energy; and temperature is the measure of the intensity of heat.

Pathology

VISION DISORDERS
1. Symptoms and signs of disorders that involve or may involve vision include:
   A. Visual abnormalities, including:
      [1] Loss of vision.
      [2] Loss of visual acuity, blurred vision.
      [3] Diplopia (double vision).
      [4] Sudden appearance of many floaters.
      [5] Flashes of light.
   B. Redness of the eye.
   C. Pain in or around the eye.
   D. Foreign body sensation.
   E. Headache (frontal, temporal or occipital).
   F. Photophobia (unusual intolerance of light).
   G. Abnormal pupils. (Pupil irregularities or constriction or dilatation of one or both pupils that is inappropriate to lighting may indicate serious neurological disease.)
   H. Burning, irritation of eyes and/or eyelids.
   I. Itching of eyes, eyelids; edema of lids.
   J. Tearing.
   K. Presence of inflammatory exudate.
   L. Lesions of eyeball or eyelid.
   M. Bleeding in or around eyeball.
   N. Eye fatigue.

O. Abnormal positions or movements of eyeballs.

P. Difficulties in postural adjustments, determination of distances.

Q. Vertigo and nausea.

2. Refraction errors result in reduced visual acuity and discomfort from using the eyes.

A. Most refraction problems are inherited and involve the curvature of the cornea, the power of the lens or the length of the eye. In some cases problems may result from disease or injury.

B. Myopia is nearsightedness, i.e., light rays are focused in front of the retina.

[1] Objects must be at a close range to be seen clearly.

[2] Myopia exists when the cornea or lens refracts too much or when the eyeball is unusually long.

C. Hyperopia is farsightedness, i.e., light rays are focused in back of the retina.

[1] Objects must be at a distance to be seen clearly.

[2] Hyperopia exists when the cornea or lens does not refract enough or the eyeball is unusually short.

D. In presbyopia, accommodation cannot occur normally, due to loss of lens elasticity. This condition tends to develop after the age of 40.

E. In astigmatism vision is blurred, due to uneven curvature of the cornea.

4. The eyeball may be damaged by:

A. Traumatic injuries (e.g., penetrating injuries or contusions).

B. Chemical burns.

C. Ultraviolet burns.

D. Burns from excessive heat.

E. Presence of foreign bodies (especially if these are rubbed against the surface of the eye).

5. Inflammations of the eye or eyelid include:

A. Minor superficial infections (frequently caused by staphylococci).

[1] A sty (hordeolum) is an infection of an eyelash follicle and the associated gland. A tiny abscess is formed.

[2] A chalazion is a small hard cyst of the meibomian glands. The cyst can irritate the eyeball.

[3] Blepharitis is inflammation of the eyelids, generally caused by infection. There is edema, redness of the lid, exudate production and small ulcerations along the lid.

B. Conjunctivities.

[1] Acute inflammation of the conjunctiva results in redness, tearing, pain, exudate production and photophobia.

[2] The inflammation may be caused by a large variety of microorganisms or other irritants.

[3] Conjunctivitis in the newborn is most frequently caused by gonococcus coming in contact with the baby's eyes during the birth process. These organisms invade and destroy the cornea.

C. Keratitis is inflammation of the cornea, which may result from traumatic injury, hypersensitivity reactions or infection. Corneal infections occur easily after injury. If the inflammatory process is severe, there is ulceration and scarring, and blindness results.

   D. Uveitis is inflammation of all or part of the uveal tract (iris, choroid and ciliary body). There may or may not be granuloma formation, depending upon the etiologic agent.

   [1] Iritis, the most common inflammation, causes pain, redness around the cornea, blurring of vision, a constricted pupil and photophobia.

   [2] If the inflammation is anterior, the condition may contribute to the development of glaucoma. Adhesions can prevent proper drainage of aqueous fluid.

   [3] If the inflammation is posterior, the lens may not receive proper nourishment from the aqueous fluid, and cataract may result.

6. Glaucoma comprises several pathologic conditions that are caused by an abnormal increase in intraocular pressure.

   A. Glaucoma is the most common preventable cause of blindness.

   B. The condition generally occurs in persons over 40 years of age and is due to faulty drainage of aqueous fluid.

   C. Chronic simple glaucoma is the most common form.

   [1] The tendency to develop this type of glaucoma appears to be inherited.

   [2] Symptoms develop very gradually and include:

      a. Eye fatigue.

      b. Gradual loss of peripheral vision first, then of central vision.

      c. Seeing halos around lights.

   D. In acute glaucoma there is severe eye pain and blurred vision. If untreated, eye structures are damaged by the increased pressure within the eyeball. Blindness results.

   E. Some forms of glaucoma appear to be associated with vasomotor disorders, emotional disturbances and/or endocrine imbalance.

   F. Secondary glaucoma may develop following traumatic eye injury or iritis or may be caused by the pressure of an abnormal growth.

7. Cataract is an opacity (cloudiness) of the lens, caused by both chemical and physical changes within it.

   A. Although most cataracts are caused by slow degenerative changes associated with the aging process, they also may be caused by some types of damage to the lens.

   B. It is possible that the tendency to develop cataracts is inherited.

   C. Cataracts may develop in one eye or in both eyes, and the consequence is gradual loss of vision.

8. When the retina becomes separated from the choroid or when the layers of the retina become separated, the condition is called "detached retina."

   A. The separation may occur as a result of a head injury, tumor growth, inflammation of the choroid or retinal hemorrhages.

   B. Symptoms include:

   [1] Sudden appearance of many floaters, caused by bleeding.

   [2] Sudden flashes of light, resulting from stimulation of the retina.

   [3] Partial or complete loss of vision in the involved eye.

   C. If the detachment is partial, degeneration of the retina usually does not begin for several days.

9. Vision may be impaired by injuries or disease conditions that affect the optic nerves, the optic tracts, the midbrain or the occipital lobe of the cerebral cortex (e.g., cerebrovascular accidents, tumors, increased intracranial pressure).

10. Retrolental fibroplasia is a condition in which there is overgrowth of fibrous tissue posterior to the lens. There is a proliferation of blood vessels in the retina and vasodilatation with edema and hemorrhaging. There may be retinal separation.
   A. The condition develops in premature infants when they are exposed to high concentrations of oxygen (over 40 percent) for prolonged periods.
   B. The condition can progress quite rapidly, leading to blindness.

11. Strabismus (crossing of the eyes) occurs when eye movements are not coordinated and both eyes cannot be used simultaneously to see an object.
   A. In paralytic strabismus there is inability to use one or more of the extraocular muscles to move the eyeball.
       [1] The condition may be caused by nerve damage or by a disorder affecting one or more of the muscles. The damage or disorder may be the result of traumatic injury, tumor growth, infections or brain injury.
       [2] Double vision occurs.
   B. In nonparalytic strabismus there is a defect in the positions of the two eyeballs in relation to each other. The person cannot fix on an object with both eyes simultaneously.
       [1] This is an inherited abnormality.
       [2] In monocular strabismus the individual uses one eye constantly for vision.
       [3] In alternating strabismus either eye may be used for vision.

12. Deficiency of Vitamin A can cause night blindness and keratinization of the cornea, with resultant loss of corneal transparency.

HEARING DISORDERS

1. Symptoms and signs of problems concerned with hearing include:
   A. Auditory disturbances:
       [1] Loss of hearing.
       [2] Tinnitus (buzzing, roaring, ringing, pounding sounds).
       [3] Auditory hallucinations.
   B. Indications of hearing impairment, such as:
       [1] Asking to have things repeated.
       [2] Inattentiveness, unresponsiveness.
       [3] Strained or intense facial expressions.
       [4] Tendency to withdraw from social activities.
       [5] Delayed speech and language development.
       [6] Behavior suggestive of delayed emotional development.
   C. Pain in or around the ear, may vary from dull ache to excruciatingly acute pain. Moving ear lobes may increase pain.
   D. Feeling of fullness in the ears.
   E. Discharge from the auditory canals (e.g., blood, exudates).
   F. Lesions of the auditory canal, redness, edema, itching.

2. Symptoms and signs of facial paralysis, indicate disturbance of a facial nerve and thus possible auditory pathology. They may include:

    A.   Inability to close eye on the affected side.

    B.   Inability to use facial expressions on the affected side (e.g., smile).

    C.   Mouth drawn over to the unaffected side.

3. Symptoms and signs of inflammation of the mastoid cells include redness, heat, swelling and pain (can become severe) in the mastoid region.

4. The auditory canal may be injured by:

    A.   Trauma (e.g., foreign bodies or sharp objects inserted into the canal).

    B.   Allergic manifestations (e.g., eczema).

    C.   Microorganisms (e.g., fungus infections, furuncles).

5. The tympanic membrane may be perforated by:

    A.   Severe blow to the side of the head.

    B.   The insertion of sharp or pointed objects through it (e.g., hairpins or matchsticks).

    C.   Pressure exerted against the membrane by accumulating exudate in the middle ear.

    D.   Pressure exerted against the membrane by fluids injected forcibly into the auditory canal.

    E.   Excessive pressure of air against the membrane when the eustachian tubes are closed or plugged.

6. Otitis media, inflammation of the middle ear, may be acute, chronic, purulent or sterile. The inflammation may be caused by:

    A.   Abnormal pressures in the middle ear (e.g., during high-altitude flying or when eustachian tubes become plugged).

    B.   Microorganisms (e.g., these may gain entrance to the middle ear through the eustachian tubes or through a perforated ear drum).

    C.   Symptoms vary with the severity of the infection.

        [1] Pain in or about the ear is an early symptom. The pain may become severe, as pressure exerted by accumulating exudate within the middle ear increases.

        [2] There may be loss of hearing and unusual noises in the affected ear.

        [3] If the tympanic membrane perforates spontaneously, the pain is greatly relieved.

    D.   A middle ear infection can spread to the mastoid cells.

        [1] If the inflammatory exudate cannot drain out of the mastoid cells through the middle ear, the pressure within the bone causes severe pain.

        [2] Infection in the mastoid cells can spread to the meninges, the lateral venous sinuses or the brain itself.

7. Otosclerosis is a condition in which the bony capsule of the labyrinth becomes spongy and the stapes becomes ankylosed in the oval window. The other ossicles may also become fixed. The tendency to develop this disorder seems to be inherited. There is a very gradual loss of hearing.

8. Loss of hearing may be caused by:

    A.   Impairment of the middle ear mechanism for transmitting sound to the cochlea. This is termed conductive hearing loss.

    B.   Impairment of inner ear mechanisms for the reception of sound and/or of the central nervous system pathways for the transmission of auditory signals. This is termed sensorineural loss of hearing.

9. Sensorineural loss of hearing may be caused by:
   A. Infections (usually viral).
   B. Tumor growth.
   C. Head injuries.
   D. Some drugs that are toxic to the inner ear.
10. A baby may be born deaf, due to damage to the inner ear, if its mother had German measles (Rubella) during the first trimester of pregnancy.
11. Some loss of hearing generally occurs in the aging process.
12. Hearing loss is sometimes associated with psychogenic factors, in which case no pathophysiology can be identified.
13. Labyrinthitis is an inflammation of the inner ear, usually caused by an infection. Vertigo is severe.
14. Meniere's disease is a condition that affects the inner ear. The cause is not known, but the dysfunction has been associated with increased pressure within the endolymph channels and vasospasms in the inner ear. Symptoms are vertigo (severe and occurring with great suddenness), unilateral hearing loss and tinnitus.
15. Tinnitus, sometimes referred to as a ringing in the ears, is produced in a number of different conditions. The character of the sound heard varies. Tinnitus may occur when there are problems involving:
   A. The external ear (e.g., a plug of wax).
   B. The middle ear (e.g., perforation of the ear drum, otosclerosis, plugged eustachian tubes).
   C. The inner ear (e.g., labyrinthitis, salicylate toxicity).

TACTILE AND THERMAL SENSE DISORDERS

1. Symptoms and signs of abnormalities involving the tactile and/or thermal senses include:
   A. Anesthesia (loss of sensation).
   B. Hyperesthesia (unusual sensitiveness to sensory stimuli).
   C. Paraesthesias (abnormal sensations that occur without observable stimuli).
   D. Astereognosis (inability to recognize objects or forms by touch).
2. Disorders involving the tactile and thermal senses may be caused by:
   A. Dysfunction of the sensory receptors, which may be due to disorders of the skin or mucous membrane.
   B. Dysfunction of peripheral nerves, which may be the result of traumatic injury, inflammation, inadequate circulation or Vitamin B deficiency.
   C. Injury to posterior nerve roots, which may be due to spinal injuries, to lesions caused by the spirochete of syphilis or to the pressure of abnormal growths.
   D. Interference with normal functioning of the sensory pathways in the spinal cord and brain, or the somesthetic areas of the cerebral cortex, which may result from:
      [1] Degenerative disorders, such as multiple sclerosis.
      [2] Traumatic injuries.
      [3] Increased intracranial pressure.
      [4] Neoplasms.
      [5] Impaired circulation, anoxia, hypoglycemia.

DISORDERS OF TASTE AND SMELL

1. Inflammatory disorders of the tongue impair taste sensation.
2. Lesions affecting the fifth, seventh and/or tenth cranial nerves; the thalamus; and/or the inferior portion of the postcentral gyrus may result in impairment of the sense of taste or in taste hallucinations.
3. Inflammation of the nasal mucosa impairs smell sensation.
4. Lesions affecting the olfactory tract, olfactory areas or the temporal cortex may result in impairment of the sense of smell or in olfactory hallucinations.
5. Very strong or unpleasant tastes or smells may give rise to nausea and result in vomiting.

Nursing Care

Nursing care should be directed toward assisting the patient to attain, retain or regain the best possible sensory function.

COLLECTION, EVALUATION AND COMMUNICATION OF DATA

Vision

1. Patients should be interviewed, observed and examined to identify symptoms and signs of actual or potential problems involving vision.
   - A. Problems may be indicated by:
     - [1] Visual abnormalities.
     - [2] Discomforts of the eye and/or eyelid.
     - [3] Symptoms and signs of inflammation of the eye and/or eyelid.
     - [4] Abnormalities in eye or eyelid movements or in positions of eyeball(s).
     - [5] Pupil abnormalities.
     - [6] Lesions of the eye or eyelid.
     - [7] Bleeding in or around the eye.
     - [8] Difficulties in postural adjustments, judgment of distances.
     - [9] Headaches.
   - B. Systematic evaluation is of especial importance when the patient:
     - [1] Has an injury or a diagnosed condition that involves or may involve:
       - a. The structures of the eyeball.
       - b. The eyelid and its movement.
       - c. The extrinsic eye muscles, the movement of eye muscles.
       - d. Nervous tissue concerned with vision (e.g., the optic nerves, optic tracts, specialized nuclei in the brain, the visual cortex).
     - [2] Has loss of consciousness.
     - [3] Is an infant or a young child.
     - [4] Has only one good eye for vision.
   - C. A patient's vision should be evaluated in relation to:
     - [1] Normal vision.
     - [2] The patient's usual vision.
     - [3] Any diagnosed disorder that involves vision.
     - [4] Any diagnostic procedures or therapeutic measures that may have an affect on vision.

D. Data collected should be evaluated not only on the basis of a single deviation from normal (e.g., eye fatigue) but also on the basis of combinations of symptoms and signs that are commonly associated with specific problems involving vision (e.g., symptoms and signs associated with inflammation of the internal eye structures).

2. How, when and what data are communicated to the physician and/or other nursing personnel depend upon:
   A. Any potential threat to the patient's life and well-being (e.g., persistent, severe eye pain).
   B. Any particular implications for the physician in relation to:
      [1] The patient's progress or lack of progress toward recovery (e.g., change in visual acuity or field of vision).
      [2] Making a diagnosis (e.g., new objective or subjective data).
      [3] The patient's physical and emotional responses to specific diagnostic or therapeutic procedures.
   C. Any particular implications for nursing (e.g., in relation to special safety precautions).

Hearing

1. Patients should be interviewed, observed and examined to identify symptoms and signs of actual or potential problems involving hearing.
   A. Problems may be indicated by:
      [1] Hearing abnormalities.
      [2] Discomforts in or around the ear.
      [3] Symptoms and signs of inflammations of ear or mastoid.
      [4] Symptoms and signs of facial paralysis.
      [5] Bleeding from the ear.
   B. Systematic evaluation is of especial importance when the patient:
      [1] Has an injury or a diagnosed disorder that involves or may involve:
         a. The structures of the ear.
         b. The nasopharynx or eustachian tubes.
         c. Nervous tissue concerned with hearing.
      [2] Is young or elderly.
   C. A patient's hearing should be evaluated in relation to:
      [1] Normal ranges of hearing ability.
      [2] The patient's usual hearing.
      [3] Any diagnosed disorder that involves or may involve hearing.
      [4] Any diagnostic procedure or therapeutic measure that may have an effect on hearing.
   D. Data collected should be evaluated not only on the basis of a single deviation from normal (e.g., tinnitus) but also on the basis of combinations of symptoms and signs that are commonly associated with specific problems involving hearing (e.g., symptoms and signs associated with inflammation of the middle or inner ear).

2. How, when and what data are communicated to the physician and/or other nursing personnel depend upon:

   A. Any potential threat to the patient's life and well-being (e.g., symptoms of acute otitis media).

   B. Any particular implications for the physician in relation to:

      [1] The patient's progress or lack of progress toward recovery (e.g., change in hearing).

      [2] Making a diagnosis (e.g., new objective or subjective data).

      [3] The patient's physical and emotional responses to specific therapeutic measures.

   C. Any particular implications for nursing (e.g., in relation to special safety precautions).

Tactile and Thermal Senses, Taste and Smell

1. Patients should be interviewed, observed and examined to identify symptoms and signs of problems that involve the tactile sense, the thermal sense, taste and/or smell.

2. Systematic evaluation is of especial importance when the patient:

   A. Has or may have interference with peripheral circulation.

   B. Has or may have disorders involving the peripheral nerves, the spinal cord and/or the brain.

   C. Has or may have disorders involving sensory nerve pathways and sensory areas in the brain concerned with taste or smell.

3. How, when and what data are communicated to the physician and/or other nursing personnel depend upon:

   A. Any potential threat to the patient's life and well-being (e.g., numbness or tingling in a peripheral body part).

   B. Any particular implications for the physician in relation to:

      [1] The patient's progress or lack of progress toward recovery (e.g., change in sensations experienced).

      [2] Making a diagnosis (e.g., new objective or subjective data).

      [3] The patient's physical and emotional responses to specific therapeutic measures.

   C. Any particular implications for nursing (e.g., in relation to special safety precautions).

PROMOTION OF HEALTH AND PREVENTION
OF DISEASE/INJURY
Vision

1. Health teaching to promote proper vision should be concerned with:

   A. Accident prevention, especially in relation to children and occupational hazards.

   B. Proper first aid care of common eye injuries.

   C. The importance of not rubbing eyes.

   D. The avoidance of unprescribed eye drops, washes or ointments.

   E. The prevention of injuries or infections in relation to:

      [1] Use of eye cosmetics.

      [2] Use of hair sprays.

        [3] Use of contact lenses.

        [4] Use of sun lamps or exposure to the sun.

  F. Proper nutrition.

  G. The importance of periodic health evaluations throughout the life cycle.

  H. The importance of:

        [1] Obtaining appropriate medical evaluation when visual changes occur (e.g., loss of visual acuity).

        [2] Using corrective lenses when these are needed and prescribed.

  I. The importance of periodic eye examinations by an ophthalmologist:

        [1] After the age of 40 years.

        [2] When corrective lenses are prescribed and used.

        [3] When there is a known eye disorder.

  J. Danger signals for which a qualified physician should be consulted.

2. Patients should be protected from eye injuries.

  A. Protection is of particular importance when the patient:

        [1] Already has an eye disorder.

        [2] Is an infant, a small child or elderly.

        [3] Is irresponsible (e.g., mentally incompetent).

        [4] Has loss of consciousness.

        [5] Is unable to close eye(s).

        [6] Has an anesthetized eye.

  B. Cleanliness should be maintained in all eye care, and surgical aseptic technique should be used whenever indicated by a patient's particular eye disorder.

  C. Eyes should be protected from trauma.

        [1] When there is faulty eye closure, the eyes should be carefully protected and adequately lubricated.

        [2] Eyes should not be rubbed.

        [3] Great caution should be used in the manipulation of any equipment near the eyes; this is of particular importance when the patient is irresponsible or lacks control.

        [4] Only very soft materials should be used to touch the conjunctiva.

        [5] When eye irrigations are performed, the force should be minimal.

  D. Eyes should be protected from excessive heat (e.g., the temperature of the solution used for warm eye compresses should be tested and must be safe for application).

  E. Dilated eyes should be protected from bright light.

  F. Prophylaxis of a newborn's eyes should be performed properly.

3. Proper first aid measures should prevent further eye damage. (See "Vision" under Care of Patients with Specific Problems.)

4. Extreme caution must be used in the administration of all prescribed eye medications.

5. When a premature infant is receiving prescribed oxygen therapy, the oxygen concentration should not exceed 40 percent over any extended period of time.

Hearing

1. Health teaching should be concerned with:

  A. Accident prevention through:

        [1] Safe cleaning of ears.

  [2] Protecting small children from damaging ears by inserting objects into the ear canal.

  [3] Proper protection of ears from high-intensity sounds (e.g., in industry, military service).

 B. Proper nose-blowing.

 C. The importance of periodic health evaluations.

 D. The importance of obtaining prompt medical attention when:

  [1] There is any noticeable change in hearing ability.

  [2] There is impacted cerumen in the auditory canal.

  [3] There is a foreign object impacted in the ear.

  [4] There are frequent upper respiratory infections, with sore throats and ear-aches.

  [5] There is ear pain, discharge from the ear or ear sounds.

 E. Noise control.

2. Patients should be protected from ear injuries and infections.

 A. Great caution should be used in performing any treatments involving the ear. This is of particular importance when the patient is a child or lacks control.

 B. Cleanliness should be maintained in all ear care, and surgical aseptic technique should be used whenever indicated by the patient's particular ear disorder.

3. Drainage of exudate or blood from the auditory canal should be promoted, not prevented (e.g., by positioning).

4. When a patient tends to develop ear infections, the auditory canal should be kept dry and protected from water during swimming or bathing. Diving may be contraindicated.

CARE OF PATIENTS WITH SPECIFIC PROBLEMS
Vision Problems

1. When a patient's eyes are burned by chemicals:

 A. The eyes should not be rubbed.

 B. The eyes should be washed immediately and continuously with copious amounts of water for at least 15 minutes.

 C. Appropriate medical consultation should be obtained promptly.

2. When a patient's eyes have been burned by ultraviolet rays:

 A. Cold compresses may be applied to the lids.

 B. The eyes should be protected from light.

 C. Appropriate medical consultation should be obtained promptly.

3. When there is bleeding from the eye or eyelid:

 A. Appropriate medical evaluation should be obtained promptly.

 B. No action should be taken to stop the bleeding.

4. When there is a penetrating wound of the eyeball:

 A. This is a medical emergency.

 B. The eye should not be touched, and it should be carefully protected from any pressure.

 C. Physical exertion should be avoided.

5. When there is a foreign particle on the conjunctiva:

 A. The eye should not be rubbed.

    B. Strict cleanliness of the hands or any equipment must be maintained.

    C. The inner lids should be checked for the particle.

    D. The eyeball or lid can be gently irrigated with physiologic saline solution, or with plain water if necessary.

    E. If the particle is not embedded in the conjunctiva or on the clear cornea, a soft swab or piece of soft material may be used to gently remove the particle. *The cornea must not be touched.*

6. When there is a foreign particle or scratch on the clear cornea (may be seen or may be indicated by pain and excessive tearing):

    A. The eye should be protected from any pressure.

    B. The patient should be treated by an ophthalmologist immediately.

7. When an eye has been bruised sufficiently to cause a "black eye":

    A. Cold applications may help to limit edema, bleeding and pain.

    B. Appropriate medical evaluation should be obtained.

8. When a patient has symptoms and signs of a detached retina:

    A. The patient should be placed in a horizontal position, with the retina of the affected eye maintained in a dependent position.

    B. Head movements should be avoided.

    C. Physical exertion should be avoided.

    D. The eyes may be lightly covered to minimize eye movements.

    E. Appropriate medical consultation should be obtained promptly.

9. When a patient has photophobia, the eyes should be protected from light.

10. When a patient has eye fatigue:

    A. The eyes should be rested.

    B. The application of cold compresses may be helpful.

    C. Appropriate medical consultation should be obtained if fatigue is persistent or recurs frequently.

11. When a patient has a traumatic injury (e.g., surgery) or a disorder that involves the internal structure of the eyeball:

    A. Medical orders concerning the following factors should be explicit and must be followed exactly:

        [1] The use of protective covering over the affected eye(s).

        [2] The amount and type of lighting allowed.

        [3] The amount and type of physical activity permitted.

        [4] Positioning.

    B. The eye(s) should be protected from any external pressure.

    C. The head should be kept still. There should be no rapid or jerky movement and no jarring.

    D. Physical and emotional factors that tend to raise the intraocular pressure should be avoided. These include:

        [1] Sneezing, coughing, straining with defecation.

        [2] Physical exertion, such as lifting of heavy objects, raising arms over the head.

        [3] Bending over, stooping.

        [4] Emotional upsets.

    E. In general, lighting should be reduced.

F. Infections should be prevented.

G. Close observations should be made for restlessness, unusual eye pain (or increase in pain) and abnormal drainage from eye or nose. These should be reported promptly.

12. When a patient has glaucoma, it is important that he be helped to understand the need for continued medical supervision and strict adherance to the prescribed therapeutic regimen.

13. When a patient has an external eye inflammation:
    A. Special precautions should be made to:
       [1] Prevent infection in the injured eye.
       [2] Prevent any further infection in an already-infected eye.
       [3] Prevent spread of infection from one eye to the other.
    B. Lighting should be as dim as necessary to prevent discomfort.

14. When a patient has partial or total loss of vision:
    A. Special precautions should be taken to prevent accidents.
    B. The patient should be given adequate information about his environment to provide for physical safety and psychologic comfort at all times.
    C. The patient should be assisted with the activities of daily living as necessary and helped to learn how to take care of his own needs to the greatest possible extent.
    D. The immediate environment should be arranged in such a way as to allow the patient to meet his needs safely and satisfactorily.
    E. Psychologic support should be consistent.
    F. The patient should be encouraged to develop increased use of his remaining senses, especially hearing and touch, to obtain information about the external environment.

Hearing Problems

1. When a patient has a disorder or has had surgery that involves the middle or inner ear:
    A. Medical orders relative to the following factors should be explicit and must be followed exactly:
       [1] The use, changing or reinforcing of any dressings.
       [2] Positioning.
       [3] The extent and type of physical activity permitted.
    B. The head should be kept quiet; this is of particular importance when the inner ear is involved. There should be no jarring and no quick or jerky movements, and position changes should be made slowly, at the patient's own rate.
    C. Nose-blowing should be discouraged. Sneezing, coughing should be prevented as possible.
    D. Close observations should be made for indications of vertigo, facial paralysis, mastoid involvement. These should be reported promptly.

2. Any prescribed ear drops instilled into the ear should be at room or body temperature, never cold or hot.

3. When a patient has an inner ear disorder that affects his sense of balance:
    A. Head movements should be minimal.

    B.   Appropriate means of accident prevention should be utilized.

    C.   The patient should be maintained in a horizontal position while dizziness exists; keeping the eyes closed is usually helpful.

    D.   The patient should be encouraged to move only at his own rate.

    E.   Psychologic support should be consistent.

4. When a patient has loss of hearing:

    A.   Appropriate methods of accident prevention should be used.

    B.   Psychologic support should be consistent.

    C.   The efficiency of oral communications should be maintained or reestablished as possible, by such means as:

        [1] Providing assistance in learning to "read" speech.

        [2] Providing assistance in learning how to listen more effectively.

        [3] Facilitating lip-reading.

           a. The patient's attention should be obtained in some nonstartling manner.

           b. The light should be on the speaker's face.

           c. The speaker should look directly at the patient.

           d. Speech should be slow and distinct.

           e. The speaker should move closer as necessary and speak toward the better ear.

           f. Important messages should be repeated as necessary.

           g. Enough time should be allowed for interpretation.

        [4] Encouraging the use of hearing aids when they can improve hearing.

        [5] Speech-training.

    D.   Written communications can be used as necessary.

Problems of Tactile and Thermal Senses, Taste and Smell

1. When a patient has anesthesia of a body part, special precautions should be taken to prevent injury to that part.

2. When a patient has hyperesthesia of a body part, special precautions should be taken to minimize stimulation of the part.

Chapter 17

Intellectual Processes

Intellectual processes are functions of the cerebral cortex.

Anatomy and Physiology

1. The cerebral cortex, the outer gray matter of the cerebrum, contains approximately 75 percent of all the nerve cell bodies in the entire nervous system.
2. Analysis and interpretation of sensory signals are functions of the sensory areas of the cerebral cortex.
   A. Sensory signals received in the cortex are analyzed and interpreted on the basis of past experience. Vast amounts of information are stored in the cortex.
   B. Analysis and interpretation of sensory experiences (visual, auditory and somatic) occur primarily in the temporal lobe and in the angular gyrus, where the parietal, temporal and occipital lobes come together.
   C. A thought probably involves simultaneous stimulation of several parts of the brain.
      [1] Stimulated areas in the thalamus and reticular formation appear to be responsible for the crude nature of thought (e.g., general and unrefined awareness of somatic sensations).
      [2] Stimulated areas in the sensory areas of the cerebral cortex appear to be responsible for discrete qualities of thought.
   D. Complex thought associations appear to be made in the temporal lobe and angular gyrus.
3. Cognition involves the dynamic organization of thoughts so that what is perceived is given meaning.

4. Abstract thought processes probably occur in the prefrontal lobe and in large areas of the temporal and parietal lobes.
5. Memory, the ability to recall information, is a function of the cerebral cortex.
   A. Memory is classified as "temporary" when information can be recalled only for minutes or hours after it has been received.
   B. "Fixed" memory may be short-term or long-term.
      [1] With short-term memory, information can be recalled for days.
      [2] With long-term memory, information can be recalled for months and years.
   C. Different areas of the cortex are probably able to store memories for differing periods of time. Memory storage in temporal lobe areas seems to be short-term and temporary.
6. Communication is a function of the cerebral cortex.
   A. Communication involves visual abilities, auditory abilities, verbal abilities, graphic ability, vocalization and body language.
   B. Understanding the spoken word is a function of the auditory sensory areas.
   C. Understanding the written word is a function of the visual sensory areas.
   D. Understanding the meaning of words when used to express thoughts is probably a function of the temporal lobe or angular gyrus.
   E. Selection and sequencing of words for the expression of thoughts probably occurs in the lower somesthetic areas.
   F. Broca's area, in the motor cortex of the dominant hemisphere, controls vocalization. (See Chapter 18.)
7. Usually intellectual processes are highly developed in only one cerebral hemisphere, known as the dominant hemisphere.
   A. Although the hemispheres have equal capacity for development, the left hemisphere is dominant in about 9 out of every 10 persons.
   B. Both hemispheres receive sensory signals; the dominant hemisphere also receives sensory information from the nondominant side.
   C. If the temporal lobe or angular gyrus of the dominant lobe is not able to function properly after the age of 6 years, intellectual processes can be developed only very slightly in the nondominant side. Prior to that age, the opposite side can be developed.
8. The prefrontal areas, which lie anterior to the motor cortex, function in:
   A. Maintaining attention and motivation.
   B. Abstract thought processes, such as planning, prediction and complex problem-solving.
   C. Behavior control.
9. Learning implies changes in behavior based on changes in the central nervous system.
10. Intellectual functions develop in systematic patterns during the normal growth and development of individuals. The rate and extent of development depend upon both internal and environmental factors.
    A. Internal factors include both neurologic and psychologic variables.
    B. Environmental factors include overall life experiences and specific maturational opportunities.

Pathology

1. Symptoms and signs of impairment of intellectual processes include:
   A. Faulty sensory perceptions.
   B. Confusion, disorientation.
   C. Disorganized thought processes, unusual distractibility, irrationality.
   D. Learning difficulties.
   E. Loss of memory (recent or remote).
   F. Various forms of aphasia.
2. Injury to the nerve cells, projection fibers and/or association fibers of the cerebral cortex may be caused by:
   A. Traumatic injuries of the brain (e.g., birth injuries, head injuries due to accidents, brain surgery).
   B. Increased intracranial pressure (e.g., due to bleeding, edema, tumors).
   C. Inadequate blood supply.
   D. Anoxia.
   E. Hypoglycemia.
   F. Hyperthermia.
   G. Toxemias (e.g., resulting from accumulation of certain metabolites or caused by bacterial toxins or certain poisons).
   H. Encephalitis.
   I. Abnormal growths, such as cysts or tumors.
   J. Degenerative disorders.
3. Mental retardation may be associated with microcephaly, mongolism and hypothyroidism.
4. Mongolism (Down's syndrome) appears to be caused by abnormalities in embryologic development. The condition can often be recognized at birth by some typical physical characteristics, including the structure of the face and head, lack of muscle tone and a protruding tongue. Both physical and mental development are slow, and the intellectual level rarely progresses beyond the age of 7 years.
5. Impairment of intellectual processes may be associated with emotional disorders. (See Part III.)
6. Loss of consciousness involves loss of ability to perceive and react to one's environment.
   A. There may be only mental confusion, disorientation and hyperirritability to external stimuli.
   B. There may be drowsiness, with very slow responses to stimuli and incoherent speech.
   C. There may be stupor, with only reflexive muscle responses to painful stimuli.
   D. When deep coma occurs there is total lack of response to stimuli. The sense of hearing is the last sense to be lost.
7. Aphasia is the inability to express oneself properly through speech and/or understand words.
   A. Motor aphasia is caused by disorders involving Broca's area. The individual

knows what he wants to say but is unable to speak his thoughts. (See Chapter 18.)
  B. Sensory aphasias include:
    [1] Auditory aphasia, in which there is inability to understand the spoken word. A disorder of the auditory cortex of the temporal lobe is involved.
    [2] Visual aphasia, in which there is inability to understand the written word. A disorder of the visual cortex in the occipital lobe is involved.
  C. Disorders that affect the temporal lobe and angular gyrus region can result in inability to formulate intelligible thoughts.
  D. Disorders involving the lower portion of the somesthetic area can result in inability to put words together in proper sequence to express formulated thoughts.

Nursing Care

Nursing care should be directed toward assisting patients to attain, retain or regain the best possible intellectual functioning.

COLLECTION, EVALUATION AND COMMUNICATION OF DATA
  1. Patients should be interviewed, observed and examined to identify symptoms and signs of impaired intellectual processes.
    A. Problems may be indicated by:
      [1] Faulty sensory perceptions.
      [2] Confusion, disorientation, irrationality.
      [3] Disorganized thought processes, unusual distractibility.
      [4] Learning difficulties.
      [5] Loss of memory.
      [6] Various forms of aphasia.
      [7] Speech difficulties.
    B. Systematic evaluation is of especial importance when the patient:
      [1] Has an injury or diagnosed disorder that involves or may involve the cerebral cortex.
      [2] Is an infant, a child or elderly.
      [3] Is emotionally disturbed.
    C. Data should be evaluated on the basis of:
      [1] Intellectual processes expected in different stages of normal growth and development.
      [2] The patient's usual intellectual functioning.
      [3] Any diagnosed physical or psychic disorder.
  2. How, when and what data are communicated to the physician and/or other nursing personnel depend upon:
    A. Any potential threat to the patient's life and well-being (e.g., irrational behavior).
    B. Any particular implications for the physician in relation to:
      [1] The patient's progress or lack of progress toward recovery (e.g., a change in reasoning ability).

[2] Making a diagnosis (e.g., new objective or subjective data).

[3] The patient's physical and emotional responses to specific diagnostic procedures and therapeutic measures.

C. Any particular implications for nursing (e.g., in relation to special safety precautions or assistance with activities of daily living).

PROMOTION OF HEALTH AND PREVENTION
OF DISEASE/INJURY

1. Health teaching should be concerned with:
   A. Normal development of intellectual processes.
   B. The importance of periodic health evaluations throughout the life cycle.
   C. The importance of seeking prompt professional consultation when abnormalities in intellectual processes occur.
   D. Avoidance of drugs that affect the intellectual processes (e.g., hallucinogenic drugs, narcotics, excessive alcohol).
2. Patients should be protected from injury to the brain caused by:
   A. Traumatic injuries. (See Chapter 12.)
   B. Inadequate blood supply. (See Chapter 1.)
   C. Anoxia. (See Chapter 2.)
   D. Hypoglycemia. (See Chapter 3.)
   E. Fluid, electrolyte and/or acid-base imbalances. (See Chapters 4, 5 and 6.)
   F. Hyperthermia. (See Chapter 9.)

CARE OF PATIENTS WITH IMPAIRED
INTELLECTUAL FUNCTIONING

1. When a patient has impaired intellectual functioning:
   A. He should be protected from causing harm to himself or others.
   B. He should be helped as much as necessary to meet his basic physiological needs.
   C. Psychologic support should be consistent.
   D. Specialized education and training may be indicated.
2. See also Part III.

Chapter 18

Speech

Speech provides an important means of communication.

Anatomy and Physiology

1. Communication through language involves both sensory and motor elements in the use and understanding of symbols for the expression of ideas.
   A. Sensory elements include the abilities to understand both the written and spoken word.
   B. Motor elements include the abilities to write and speak words.
2. Broca's area, in the motor cortex of the dominant hemisphere, controls the patterns of muscle movements needed for vocalization. The muscles involved include those of the larynx, pharynx, tongue, soft palate, lips and jaw and the respiratory muscles.
3. The larynx produces vocal sounds, but the actual articulation of words is accomplished by the shape given to the mouth, pharynx and soft palate and the movement and positions of the lips and tongue.
   A. Vocal sounds are produced by the vibration of the vocal folds in the larynx, caused by the controlled passage of air through the larynx.
   B. Changes in the position and tension of the vocal folds (causing changes in voice pitch) are brought about largely by muscles that move the cartilages of the larynx.
   C. The recurrent laryngeal nerves, branches of the vagus nerves, innervate all but one of the laryngeal muscles.
4. Speech is learned.
   A. A child hears sounds and copies them. Word-sounds are associated with objects in the external environment, and the information is stored as memories. Eventually, the sounds of words are associated with visual symbols of language

(the written word). Through association of auditory and visual experiences and through the development of motor skills, the child learns to write.

B. Response to vocal sounds occurs within a few months after birth; imitation of word-sounds usually begins before the end of the first year of life.

C. A child usually begins to comprehend speech and is able to formulate intelligible words between the ages of 1 and 2 years.

D. Proper articulation of words requires practice, as complex patterns of muscle movements must be learned. Precise articulation of vowel and consonant sounds and combinations of these is usually achieved by the time a child is 7 to 8 years of age.

E. Writing and understanding the written word can be learned after the 4th or 5th year, sometimes earlier.

F. Deafness prevents learning speech through usual means.

Pathology

1. Symptoms and signs of disorders related to speech include:
    A. Loss of voice.
    B. Production of unclear, slurred, garbled or meaningless noises.
    C. Hoarseness.
2. The larynx may be injured by trauma, inflammatory processes (e.g., due to infections or overuse of vocal cords) and tumor growth. Hoarseness is an early and primary symptom.
3. Predisposing factors in the development of cancer of the larynx include excessive smoking, excessive use of alcohol and chronic laryngitis.
4. The laryngeal muscles may be paralyzed due to injury to the motor nerves (e.g., injury may be trauma or pressure from tumor growths or aneurysms).
5. Injury to Broca's area may result from traumatic injury, tumor growth, thrombosis or hemorrhage. There may be inability to speak, or there may be unclear and garbled speech or production of meaningless noises.
6. Voice loss may occur in some psychic disorders.

Nursing Care

Nursing care should be directed toward assisting the patient to attain, retain or regain the function of speech.

COLLECTION, EVALUATION AND COMMUNICATION OF DATA

1. Patients should be interviewed, observed and examined to identify symptoms and signs of problems involving speech.
    A. Problems may be indicated by:
        [1] Loss of voice.
        [2] Hoarseness.
        [3] Unclear, slurred or garbled words or meaningless noises.
        [4] Poor articulation, stuttering, unusual voice quality.
    B. Systematic evaluation is of especial importance when the patient has a disorder that involves or may involve:
        [1] The larynx.

    [2] The motor nerves that innervate laryngeal muscles.

    [3] The motor cortex concerned with speech.

2. How, when and what data are communicated to the physician and/or other nursing personnel depend upon:

  A. Any potential threat to the patient's life and well-being (e.g., persistent hoarseness).

  B. Any particular implications for the physician in relation to:

    [1] The patient's progress or lack of progress toward recovery (e.g., a change in speech).

    [2] Making a diagnosis (e.g., new objective or subjective data).

    [3] The patient's physical and emotional responses to specific diagnostic procedures and therapeutic measures.

  C. Any particular implications for nursing (e.g., in relation to assistance with communication).

PROMOTION OF HEALTH AND PREVENTION
OF DISEASE/INJURY

1. Health teaching should be concerned with:

  A. The importance of periodic health evaluations throughout the life cycle.

  B. The importance of obtaining prompt medical consultation when hoarseness persists longer than 2 weeks.

  C. The importance of stimulating and encouraging young children to learn speech.

  D. The importance of obtaining medical consultation when a child's speech does not develop normally.

  E. Avoidance of misuse of the voice (e.g., excessive singing or shouting, especially when out of normal voice range).

  F. Avoidance of excessive use of tobacco or alcohol.

2. See also Chapter 2, concerning the respiratory system.

CARE OF PATIENTS WITH SPEECH DISORDERS

1. When a patient is hoarse:

  A. The vocal cords should not be used; other means of communication should be initiated.

  B. Steam inhalations may be helpful in reducing irritation and congestion.

2. When a patient is unable to use speech effectively for communication:

  A. Writing may be used or some other means of communication may need to be developed.

  B. Close observations should be made for indications of the patient's needs.

  C. Psychologic support should be consistent.

  D. The patient should be assisted in obtaining specialized training to learn the following, as indicated and as possible:

    [1] Proper articulation and/or speech rhythms.

    [2] The use of artificial speech methods (e.g., esophogeal or pharyngeal speech).

    [3] Other means of communication (e.g., hand language).

Chapter 19

Reproduction

Human sexuality provides for reproduction of the human species.

Anatomy and Physiology

FEMALE

1. The female organs of reproduction include:
   A. The external genitalia (the structures of the vulva), which include:
      [1] The mons pubis.
      [2] The labia majora and the labia minora.
      [3] The clitoris.
      [4] The vestibule, which has four openings:
         a. The urinary meatus.
         b. The vaginal orifice.
         c. Ducts of Bartholin's glands, located on either side of the vagina.
         d. Ducts of Skene's glands, which lie on either side of the urethra.
   B. The internal organs.
      [1] The ovaries are two nodular bodies located on either side of the uterus and attached to the back of the broad ligament of the uterus.
         a. At birth each ovary contains thousands of germ cells (the primordial ova).
         b. The ovaries function in the development and expulsion of the ova and in the secretion of estrogen and progesterone.
      [2] The two uterine tubes (fallopian tubes) extend from either side of the uterus outward toward each ovary.
         a. The tubes are composed of smooth muscle; they are lined with mucous

      membrane that is continuous with that in the uterus, and they are covered with peritoneum.

b. The outer ends of the uterine tubes are fimbriated and open to the abdominal cavity. One fimbria of each tube is attached to the ovary on that side.

c. The uterine tubes provide a means for the ova to reach the uterine cavity and a means for the spermatozoa to reach an ova. Fertilization generally occurs in a tube.

[3] The uterus is a hollow and thick-walled muscular organ which lies (in the nonpregnant state) between the bladder and the rectum.

a. The smooth muscle fibers of the uterine wall are arranged in all directions, allowing the uterus to expand and to compress downwards (during contractions) in all directions. During pregnancy there is considerable hypertrophy of the muscle fibers.

b. Blood vessels, nerves and lymphatics lie between the muscle layers.

c. There is a large blood supply to the uterus, and this supply increases during pregnancy.

d. Sympathetic nerves cause muscle contractions and vasoconstriction; parasympathetic nerves inhibit contractions and allow vasodilation.

e. Mild contractions of the uterus occur fairly frequently and without sensation, but strong contractions cause cramping discomfort, which can become severe. Dilation of the cervical canal causes contractions felt as cramping discomfort.

f. The cervix is the lower constricted cylindrical portion of the uterus which projects into the vagina. It becomes effaced and dilated during labor.

g. The uterus is lined with mucous membrane, which is called endometrium.

h. The uterus is suspended and freely movable. It is supported by three sets of ligaments (broad, round and uterosacral) and by the pelvic floor. The lower anterior wall of the uterus is connected to the bladder by a layer of connective tissue.

i. The position of the uterus is normally slightly antiflexed, but its position is influenced by the position of the individual and the sizes of the bladder and the rectum.

[4] Through hormonal effects, the endometrium of the uterus is periodically prepared for the implantation of a fertilized ovum. When a fertilized ovum implants in the endometrium, the uterus normally retains it, provides for its nourishment, enlarges as the products of conception grow and expels the infant and placenta at term.

[5] The vagina is a dilatable muscular tube (3 to 5 inches long in the adult), which extends from the vestibule to the cervix.

a. The vaginal walls are arranged in thick folds and are lined with mucous membrane. Changes in the vaginal epithelium at puberty cause it to become more resistant to trauma and infection.

     b. The vagina ends in a blind vault, into which the cervix projects. The recesses around the cervix are called fornices.

     c. The hymen is a thin fold of mucous membrane which lies across the vaginal orifice. It is sometimes imperforate, sometimes partly torn and sometimes absent.

2. The secondary sex characteristics appear at puberty (between the ages of 11 and 15 years). They include:

    A. Development of the female body form, with breast enlargement.

    B. Growth of axillary and pubic hair.

    C. Onset of menses.

    D. Increased sexual awareness and the appearance of the sexual drive.

3. At puberty gonadotropins produced by the adenohypophysis exert effects upon the ovaries which bring about sexual maturity.

    A. The follicle-stimulating hormone (FSH) causes the periodic development of follicles (and ova) and the secretion of estrogens. (See #4, below.)

    B. The interstitial cell-stimulating hormone (ICSH), also called luteinizing hormone [LH], is necessary for:

      [1] Final growth of follicles and ovulation.

      [2] Development of the corpus luteum and subsequent secretion of estrogen and progesterone.

    C. The luteotropic hormone (LTH) (prolactin) probably maintains secretion of estrogen and progesterone by the corpus luteum. It also stimulates milk production following parturition.

4. Ovulation involves the periodic development of a follicle and the ovum it contains and the release of the ovum into the fimbriated end of the uterine tube.

    A. Following ovulation, a yellow body (the corpus luteum) develops in the ruptured follicle.

    B. More than 20 follicles may develop at approximately the same time, but usually only one ruptures, so that only a single ovum is released.

5. Estrogens, produced by the ovaries, are responsible for the development and maintenance of female sexuality.

    A. Two forms of estrogen have major physiological effects. These are beta-estradiol and estrone.

    B. At puberty the estrogens promote:

      [1] Growth of the uterus, fallopian tubes and vagina.

      [2] Development of the external genitalia.

      [3] Development of the breasts.

    C. Estrogens initiate periodic endometrial development, in preparation for implantation of a fertilized ovum.

6. Progesterone, produced by the corpus luteum, increases the growth of the endometrium and promotes glandular activity within it.

    A. Mucous glands in the endometrium secret mucin that is high in glycogen content.

    B. Progesterone also promotes development of the breasts in preparation for milk secretion.

7. If the mature ovum is not fertilized within about 36 hours of its release from the ovary, the production of estrogen and progesterone gradually decreases, and this hormomonal change brings about the breakdown of the proliferated endometrium. The blood, mucus and epithelial cells from the endometrium escape from the uterine cavity through the cervix and vagina. This is termed menstruation.

8. The periodic preparation of the uterus for implantation of a fertilized ovum is called the menstrual cycle.

   A. The menstrual cycles begin at puberty (normally between the ages of 11 and 15 years, with the average being 12 years). Climate, race and general physical health may affect the time of onset of menstruation.

   B. Menstrual cycles continue from puberty until menopause (except during pregnancy).

   C. The menstrual cycle averages 28 days, but it may vary with different individuals and, to some extent, from month to month. Ovulation generally occurs about midway through the cycle but may occur at various times during the cycle.

   D. The onset of menstruation indicates the end of a menstrual cycle.

      [1] The amount of menstrual flow differs between individuals, sometimes from month to month and usually decreases in amount as menopause approaches.

      [2] The menstrual flow may vary normally from about 60 to 180 ml. and last from 4 to 6 days.

      [3] A few days prior to menstruation and at the onset of menstruation, there may be some pelvic discomfort (feelings of pressure or fullness, a mild backache). There may be varying degrees of breast tenderness and varying degrees of emotional instability (e.g., mild depression). There may be a slight degree of water retention, which can be noted in some ankle edema and a feeling of abdominal fullness; there may be a tendency toward constipation.

   E. The menstrual cycles may be temporarily interrupted or delayed by such factors as changes in environment (e.g., moving to an area in a different climate), marked changes in daily activities (e.g., a new job) and strong emotional upsets.

9. Normally, there may be a slight amount of mucoid vaginal discharge. This discharge may increase in amount or appear just before menarche and just before a menstrual period begins. Occasionally, in some individuals there may be a very slight brownish discharge at the time of ovulation.

10. Menopause indicates the cessation of ovarian activity and the end of the female reproductive period.

    A. Menopause may occur as early as age 40 or as late as the middle 50s. It usually begins between 45 and 50 years of age.

    B. Menstrual periods become scanty, irregular, then cease altogether.

    C. Loss of estrogens accounts for:

       [1] Some of the vasomotor symptoms that may be associated with menopause (e.g., hot flashes).

       [2] Atrophic changes in the sexual organs, for example:

      a. The vaginal epithelium becomes thin and is easily damaged.

      b. The breasts atrophy and lose support.

      c. The pubic hair becomes thinner.

  D. Menopause is sometimes accompanied by psychic changes, associated with a woman's personal reactions to the aging process and the cessation of her reproductive capacity.

MALE

1. The male reproductive organs include:
   A. The gonads, which form the sex cells.
   B. A series of tubes, which carry the sex cells to the exterior.
   C. Accessory structures, which produce secretions in which the sex cells are transported and can survive outside the body.

2. The testes are two glandular structures which form the male sex cells (spermatozoa) and secrete the male sex hormone, testosterone.
   A. The testes are in the abdominal cavity in early fetal life, but normally they descend along the inguinal canal into the scrotum before birth.
   B. The testes are suspended in the scrotum by the two spermatic cords. These cords extend from the abdominal inguinal ring to the back part of each testis. The cords are composed of arteries, veins, lymphatics, nerves and the excretory ducts of the testes (the ductus deferens).
   C. Mammalian spermatozoa cannot adjust to the high environmental temperature inside the body.
   D. Each testis consists of many lobules. Each lobule consists of minute convoluted tubules (the seminiferous tubules).
      [1] Specialized cells within the seminiferous tubules are transformed into spermatozoa (the male sex cells).
      [2] The tubules are supported by loose connective tissue, which contains groups of "interstitial cells."
   E. The tunica vaginalis is the serous covering of the testes. It is derived from the peritoneum when the testes descend from the abdominal cavity.
   F. The cremaster is a thin layer of muscle located in the inguinal canal, which extends in loops around the spermatic cord as far as the testes. When the cremaster muscles contract, the testes are drawn upward toward the subcutaneous inguinal ring.

3. The seminiferous tubules merge into progressively larger convoluted ducts that become one long tortuous channel—the epididymis—which lies on the side of the testis.

4. The ductus (or vas) deferens is a continuation of the canal of the epididymis. It passes in the spermatic cord up through the inguinal canal and the abdominal inguinal ring, and then it enters the pelvic cavity, where it crosses in front of the ureter, and then downward toward the seminal vesicles.

5. The seminal vesicles are two membranous pouches located between the fundus of the bladder and the rectum. They secrete a fluid which is added to the spermatozoa. The lower part of each seminal vesicle joins each ductus deferens to form the two ejaculatory ducts.

6. The ejaculatory ducts run downward between the lobes of the prostate gland and open into the prostatic portion of the urethra. The urethra then continues to the outside (acting as a passageway for both semen and urine).

7. The prostate gland consists of glandular and smooth muscle tissue. The glandular tissue produces a secretion which is part of the semen. The gland is located just below the bladder (around the urethra) and in front of the rectum.

8. The bulbourethral glands (Cowper's glands) are tiny bodies located behind the membranous portion of the urethra. Their excretory ducts open into the cavernous urethra. They secrete a viscid fluid which becomes part of the semen.

9. The penis contains the greatest part of the urethra. The penis is composed of three cylindrical sections of cavernous tissue (tissue that contains spaces) bound together by fibrous tissue and a strong outer capsule.
   A. The medial cavernous body (the corpus cavernosum urethrae) contains the urethra.
   B. The penis is covered with skin; at the end of the penis the skin leaves the surface and folds over on itself to form the prepuce (or foreskin).
   C. The covering of the glans penis is continuous with the urethral mucous membrane and the internal layer of the prepuce.
   D. The glans penis is the anterior end of the corpus cavernosum urethrae, expanded into a cone shape.
   E. Under cerebral or spinal stimuli, the arterial blood supply to the blood sinuses of the cavernous tissue is increased. The increased blood causes compression of the veins, preventing venous return. The engorgement of the cavernous tissues with blood is responsible for the erection of the penis.

10. The erect penis and the contractions of smooth muscle along the male reproductive tract make possible the introduction of semen into the female reproductive tract.
    A. Semen is composed of spermatozoa and fluid produced in the seminal vesicles, the prostate gland and Cowper's glands.
    B. Normally, 3 ml. of semen contain approximately 400,000,000 sperm.
    C. Sperm can live for many weeks in the male ducts but can survive only 1 to 3 days after being ejaculated (at body temperature).

11. At puberty the adenohypophysis produces:
    A. Follicle-stimulating hormone (FSH), which stimulates the formation of spermatozoa in the seminiferous tubules.
    B. Interstitial cell-stimulating hormone (ICSH), or luteinizing hormone [LH], stimulates the interstitial cells in the testes to secrete testosterone, the male sex hormone.

12. Before birth, testosterone is partly responsible for the development of male characteristics of the male baby and is necessary for proper descent of the testes into the scrotum before birth.

13. At puberty (approximately 12 years of age) testosterone causes development of secondary sex characteristics. These include:
    A. Development of the male body form, with enlargement of the penis, scrotum and testes.
    B. Growth of facial and body hair.
    C. Changes in the larynx that result in a lowering of voice pitch.

D. Increased sexual awareness and the appearance of the sexual drive.
14. Testosterone is necessary for final maturation of the spermatozoa.
15. There is a gradual decrease in the secretion of testosterone after the age of 40.
16. The adrenal cortex secretes androgens, which contribute to male sex characteristics.

Pathology

FEMALE REPRODUCTIVE DISORDERS

1. Symptoms and signs of problems related to the female reproductive organs or reproductive functions include:
    A. Absence of secondary sex characteristics after the age of puberty.
    B. Menstrual disorders.
    [1] Amenorrhea (except as related to pregnancy).
    [2] Severe and/or persistent dysmenorrhea.
    [3] Menorrhagia (prolonged, excessive menstrual flow).
    C. Metrorrhagia (uterine bleeding between regular menstrual periods or at irregular intervals).
    D. Gross bleeding from the vagina, possibly containing clots and/or tissue fragments.
    E. Abnormal vaginal discharge.
    F. Symptoms and signs of inflammation of the external genitalia, vagina and/or groin.
    G. Lesions of the external genitalia.
    H. Lower backache, sensation of heaviness in pelvic region, urinary incontinence.
    I. Urine or feces draining from the vagina.
    J. Painful or difficult coitus.
    K. Infertility or habitual abortions (miscarriages).
    L. Symptoms and signs of abortion (miscarriage).
    [1] Vaginal bleeding.
    [2] Uterine cramping.
    [3] Loss of products of conception.
2. The normal development of secondary sex characteristics in the female may be delayed or prevented by:
    A. Hypogonadism, which may be due to:
    [1] The absence of ovaries or improperly formed ovaries.
    [2] Insufficient secretion of gonadotropins.
    [3] Acquired ovarian disorders.
    B. Hypothyroidism. (See Chapter 8.)
3. Menstruation may be accompanied by symptoms and signs caused by both physiologic and psychic factors.
    A. Symptoms and signs sometimes associated with menstruation include:
    [1] Dysmenorrhea, which may precede the onset of menses and extend through the first day or so of the menstrual period, or it may be experienced just at the beginning of the period.
    [2] Water retention, possibly some dependent edema or abdominal "bloating" prior to the onset of menses.

[3] Nausea and vomiting.

[4] Changes in emotional behavior prior to or during menstruation (e.g., depression).

B. Dysmenorrhea may be caused by:

[1] Increased intrapelvic pressure, due to congestion of blood in the pelvic vessels, constipation or tumor growth.

[2] Hormonal imbalances.

[3] Hypersensitivity of the uterus to painful stimuli.

[4] Strictures of cervical canal.

4. Amenorrhea, when not due to pregnancy, may be caused by:

A. Factors listed in #2 above.

B. An imperforate hymen.

C. Severe physiological or emotional stress.

5. Infertility may be due to:

A. Ovarian disorders.

B. Uterine disorders (e.g., infantile uterus, tumor growth, inflamed uterus, displaced uterus).

C. Strictures of fallopian tube(s).

6. Uterine displacements may involve antiflexion, retroversion and retroflexion and prolapse.

A. Displacements may be caused by:

[1] Congenitally weak ligaments or an acquired weakness of ligaments due to strain related to pregnancies.

[2] Injury to muscles of pelvic floor (e.g., with childbirth). (See Chapter 12.)

[3] Formation of adhesions following surgery or infections.

B. Backward displacement generally causes lower backache and a dragging sensation in the pelvis.

C. A prolapsed uterus causes symptoms similar to those experienced with backward displacement, and because the urinary bladder is pulled downward, there are symptoms of urinary disorders.

[1] Urinary incontinence is common; there may be retention.

[2] A severely prolapsed uterus may protrude from the vagina.

7. Menorrhagia may be caused by:

A. A bleeding tendency. (See Chapter 1.)

B. Hormonal imbalances.

C. Tumors of the reproductive tract.

8. Metrorrhagia is most frequently caused by uterine tumors.

9. Vaginitis may be caused by many types of microorganisms (bacteria, fungi, protozoa).

A. Infections are more likely to occur when there is trauma to the tissues, a poor blood supply, atrophic changes in the epithelium or a poor nutritional status.

B. Infections usually cause local discomfort (e.g., itching, burning) and exudate production. The exudate may be irritating to the tissues. The type of exudate varies with the causative organisms (e.g., it may be purulent, watery, cheesy, white, yellow, bloody, foul-smelling).

10. Fistulas may occur between the bladder and vagina, between a ureter and the

vagina or between the rectum and the vagina. They may be caused by traumatic injury, infections or radiation burns.

11. Disorders of the cervix may be caused by infections, trauma (which may occur with childbirth) and tumor growth. Erosions due to unknown causes sometimes appear on the cervix.

   A. Cervical inflammations generally result in profuse leukorrhea. There may be some bleeding from injured cervical tissue.

   B. Malignancies of the cervix usually spread very rapidly throughout the surrounding tissues and the pelvis. The earliest symptom is usually an abnormal vaginal discharge. Cervical erosions and chronic cervical infections appear to predispose to the development of cervical cancer.

12. Disorders involving the body of the uterus include:

   A. Infections. (These may result from improper techniques used during childbirth or retained placental tissue following childbirth, or infections may ascend from the cervix.)

   B. Tumor growths, which may be benign or malignant.

   [1] Fibroids are benign fibroid tumors within the uterus. They may be a cause of sterility. They are a frequent cause of uterine bleeding (e.g., menorrhagia or metrorrhagia).

   [2] A hydatidiform mole is a benign neoplasm in the uterus caused by degeneration of placental tissue. The growth consists of clusters of many vesicles. There is uterine enlargement and uterine bleeding.

13. Ovarian disorders include cyst development and tumor growth. Cysts may become quite large. Sometimes endometrial cysts develop on the ovary. They fill with blood during the menstrual cycle and then rupture, spilling their contents into the pelvic cavity.

14. Disorders of the fallopian tubes include infections and strictures, which may be congenital or caused by inflammation.

15. Endometriosis is a condition in which pieces of endometrium-like tissue grow outside of the uterus. Tissue may be attached to the ovary, the uterosacral ligaments, the peritoneum and/or other structures located within the pelvic cavity. The tissue responds to hormonal influences, causing periodic "menstrual bleeding" into the pelvic or abdominal cavity. The irritation and the resulting inflammatory process (which includes adhesion formation) cause abdominal and/or pelvic discomfort. Other symptoms vary, depending on the location and extent of adhesions that are formed.

16. Pelvic inflammatory disease is an inflammation of the pelvis that may involve the fallopian tubes, the ovaries and other pelvic structures, such as the peritoneum, blood vessels and connective tissue.

   A. The inflammation is usually caused by microorganisms that gain entrance to the reproductive tract through the vagina. Causative organisms include the gonococcus, streptococcus and staphylococcus. Occasionally the infection may be caused by tubercle bacilli that are transported by the blood and/or lymph.

   B. The inflammatory process usually localizes in abscesses. Adhesions form.

   C. There may be foul-smelling and possibly purulent vaginal discharge.

D. The condition may be acute or become chronic. In addition to local symptoms of inflammation, there generally are systemic effects, such as malaise, fever, nausea and vomiting.

E. Pelvic inflammatory disease is a cause of menstrual disorders, sterility and ectopic pregnancies.

17. Ectopic pregnancies are those that occur outside the uterine cavity, most frequently in a fallopian tube. The tubal wall usually ruptures within several weeks following conception. There is sudden, severe pain. There are symptoms and signs of internal hemorrhage. Circulatory shock develops rapidly. (See Chapter 1.)

18. An abortion is the termination of a pregnancy before the fetus has reached the stage of viability.

A. A spontaneous abortion is threatened when, in early pregnancy, there is vaginal spotting and possibly some mild uterine cramping.

B. An incomplete or partial abortion is one in which only part of the product of conception is passed. Bleeding (which may be profuse) persists until remaining tissues are lost or surgically removed.

C. A complete abortion is one in which the products of conception are lost, accompanied by bleeding and usually some cramping. The cramping and bleeding then subside.

D. Spontaneous or habitual abortion (miscarriage) may occur because of:
[1] Some defect in the product of conception.
[2] Abnormalities of the reproductive tract (e.g., an infantile uterus).
[3] Hormonal imbalance.

MALE REPRODUCTIVE DISORDERS

1. Symptoms and signs of problems related to the male reproductive organs or reproductive functions include:

A. Absence of testes in the scrotal sac.
B. Absence of secondary sex characteristics after the age of puberty.
C. Urinary retention.
D. Urgency, frequency, burning in relation to urination.
E. Abnormal discharge from urethra (e.g., purulent, bloody).
F. Lesions of the external genitalia or groin.
G. Inability to retract or reduce the foreskin.
H. Symptoms and signs of inflammation of the scrotum and/or groin.
I. Enlargement of one or both testes (may be painless).
J. Sterility.
K. Impotence.

2. Development of secondary sex characteristics may be delayed or prevented by hypogonadism, which may be due to:

A. Congenital absence of testes.
B. Cryptorchidism (undescended testes).
C. Insufficient secretion of gonadotropic hormones.

3. Sterility of the male may be caused by:

A. Disorders of the testes that affect production and/or maturation of spermatozoa.

    B.   Strictures of the genital ducts, which may be congenital or acquired. Acquired strictures are usually the result of inflammation.

4. Impotence may be caused by both neurologic and psychic factors.

5. Cryptorchidism is a condition in which one or both testes have failed to descend into the scrotum.

    A.   This condition is found most frequently when birth was premature.

    B.   Failure of descent may occur because of:

        [1] Anatomic defects.

        [2] Deficiency of testosterone secretion in the developing fetus.

    C.   The warmth of the abdominal cavity prevents proper development of spermatozoa within the seminiferous tubules. Eventually the testes atrophy.

6. Disorders of the penis include carcinoma, skin lesions and phimosis.

    A.   Ulcerations may be associated with infections which may be venereal.

    B.   Phimosis is a disorder in which the foreskin cannot be retracted behind the glans penis. It may be a congenital disorder or acquired as a result of an inflammatory process.

    C.   Paraphimosis is a disorder in which the foreskin cannot be reduced after retraction. Stricture of the urethra may result. Paraphimosis is usually caused by an inflammatory edema resulting from infection or traumatic injury.

7. Urethritis, inflammation of the urethra, is generally caused by invasion of the urethra by microorganisms that gain entrance from the outside.

    A.   Infection is frequently caused by the gonococcus.

    B.   The inflammation causes urgency, frequency and burning related to urination. There is often exudate production.

    C.   Infections can ascend along the reproductive tract, thus affecting the accessory glands, the genital ducts and the testes.

8. The prostate gland is a frequent site of benign or malignant tumors.

    A.   Prostatic tumors tend to develop after the age of 50.

    B.   Enlargement of the prostate nearly always causes some degree of urinary obstruction. (See Chapter 7.)

9. Disorders of the testes include inflammations, hydrocele and carcinoma.

    A.   Orchitis (inflammation of the testes) may be caused by traumatic injury but is most often caused by infections.

        [1] Mumps, a communicable virus disease that causes inflammation of the salivary glands, frequently causes orchitis.

        [2] There are local symptoms and signs of inflammation, and there may be systemic manifestations.

    B.   A hydrocele is a collection of serous fluid within the membrane covering of a testis. The production of fluid is usually asociated with an inflammatory process which occurs in response to infection or traumatic injury.

        [1] There is enlargement of the testis involved.

        [2] Sometimes the fluid is gradually reabsorbed.

    C.   Carcinoma of the testes usually develops in young men during their most sexually active years. The involved testis becomes progressively larger, and usually the enlargement occurs without pain. Metastasis occurs in the immediate area, and cancer cells may be carried to other parts of the body via blood and lymph.

10. A variocele involves the enlargement of veins within the spermatic cord. The swelling causes discomfort in the groin.

VENEREAL DISEASES

1. Venereal diseases are those infections that are usually spread by direct contact during sexual activity. They include syphilis, gonorrhea, chancroid and lymphogranuloma venereum.
2. Syphilis is an acute and chronic venereal disease.
   A. The causative spirochete enters the body at the contact site and usually causes the development of a primary lesion. The primary lesion is a papule followed by erosion and ulceration. Sometimes the ulcer takes the form of a hardened chancre.
   B. Within 4 to 6 weeks the secondary stage begins. There is involvement of the skin and mucous membrane, with development of a rash that may be macular or papular in nature. There may be alopecia and patches of erosive lesions in the mouth or on the external genitalia. The lesions may disappear in weeks or months.
   C. The third stage may begin within weeks, months or years. There are periods of latency and relapse. The spirochetes may invade and cause destruction of practically every part of the body, including bone, skin, eyes, heart, blood vessels and the central nervous system.
3. Gonorrhea (gonococcal urethritis) is an infection caused by the gonococcus.
   A. In males the infection results in acute inflammation of the urethra, with production of a thick, purulent, yellow exudate. The infection may ascend the genitourinary tract to involve the epididymis and the prostate gland. The infection can become chronic. The organisms may enter the blood stream and infect other body structures.
   B. In the female the infection has 3 stages.
      [1] Following exposure, there may be a mild urethritis or cervicitis, or there may be no symptoms.
      [2] In the second stage, the infection ascends to cause acute pelvic inflammatory disease.
      [3] In the third stage, the infection becomes chronic. The organisms may enter the blood stream and then invade the heart and/or freely movable joints.
4. Chancroid is an acute, localized genital infection caused by a species of Bacillus. The infection is characterized by ulcer formation at the site of entry. Regional lymph nodes become painfully inflamed. The infection is self-limiting, usually lasting for weeks. It is auto-inoculating.
5. Lymphogranuloma venereum is an infectious disease of the lymph nodes and channels, which is caused by a species of Chalamydia. The initial lesion is a small papule or erosion at the site of entry. This is shortly followed by inflammation and ulceration of the inguinal and pelvic lymph nodes. The infection may become chronic. During the lymphatic involvement there are usually some systemic symptoms and signs. (See also Chapter 20.)

Nursing Care

Nursing care should be directed toward assisting the patient to attain, retain or regain proper reproductive functioning and to prevent or limit disease or injury caused by disorders of the reproductive organs.

COLLECTION, EVALUATION AND COMMUNICATION OF DATA

1. Patients should be interviewed, observed and examined to identify symptoms and signs of problems related to the reproductive organs and functions.
   A. In the female, problems may be indicated by:
      [1] Absence of secondary sex characteristics after the age of puberty.
      [2] Menstrual disorders.
      [3] Vaginal spotting or bleeding between menstrual periods, during pregnancy or after menopause.
      [4] Symptoms and signs of inflammation involving external genitalia and/or the groin.
      [5] Lesions of the external genitalia.
      [6] Discomfort in the pelvic region or lower back.
      [7] Drainage of feces or urine from the vagina.
      [8] Symptoms and signs of abortion (miscarriage).
      [9] Painful or difficult coitus.
      [10] Infertility or habitual abortions.
   B. In the male, problems may be indicated by:
      [1] Absence of testes in the scrotal sac.
      [2] Absence of secondary sex characteristics after the age of puberty.
      [3] Urinary problems, including retention, urgency, frequency, burning.
      [4] Abnormal urethral discharge.
      [5] Symptoms and signs of inflammation of external genitalia, testes, groin.
      [6] Enlargement of a testis.
      [7] Inability to retract or reduce the foreskin.
      [8] Sterility, impotence.
   C. Systematic patient evaluation is of especial importance when the patient:
      [1] Is newborn.
      [2] Is at the age of puberty.
      [3] Is pregnant, postpartum or has borne several children.
      [4] Is menopausal.
      [5] Is over the age of 50.
      [6] Has a diagnosed disorder involving the reproductive organs.
   D. The menses should be evaluated in relation to:
      [1] The patient's age.
      [2] The average length of the menstrual cycle, normal ranges for menstrual cycles and what is usual for the patient.
      [3] Normal ranges for length and amount of menstrual flow and what is usual for the patient.

       [4] Temporary minor discomforts that are commonly associated with the menstrual period.

    E. Data collected should be evaluated not only on the basis of a single deviation from normal (e.g., metrorrhagia) but also on the basis of combinations of symptoms and signs that are commonly associated with specific disorders of the reproductive tract and reproductive functioning (e.g., symptoms and signs of a miscarriage).

2. How, when and what data are communicated to the physician and/or other nursing personnel depend upon:
    A. Any immediate threat to the patient's life processes (e.g., symptoms and signs of a ruptured ectopic pregnancy).
    B. Any potential threat to the patient's life and well-being (e.g., symptoms and signs of pelvic inflammatory disease).
    C. Any particular implications for the physician in relation to:
       [1] The patient's progress or lack of progress toward recovery (e.g., a change in amount or character of vaginal discharge).
       [2] Making a diagnosis (e.g., new objective or subjective data).
       [3] The patient's physical and emotional responses to specific diagnostic procedures and therapeutic measures.
    D. Any particular implications for nursing care (e.g., in relation to special counselling needs).

PROMOTION OF HEALTH AND PREVENTION OF DISEASE/INJURY

1. Health teaching should be concerned with:
    A. Appropriate sex education.
    B. Personal hygiene in relation to:
       [1] Maintaining cleanliness of external genitalia (of particular importance in prepubertal and postmenopausal females).
       [2] Douching (proper methods and the avoidance of excessive douching or douching with potentially harmful solutions).
       [3] Menstruation.
    C. Prevention and control measures for venereal disease.
    D. The importance of periodic health evaluations throughout the life cycle (including pelvic examinations, Pap smears and examinations of the prostate gland).
    E. The importance of proper obstetrical care, prenatally, during labor and delivery and postpartum.
    F. The importance of obtaining prompt medical consultation when there is:
       [1] Vaginal spotting or bleeding between menstrual periods or after menopause.
       [2] Enlargement of a testis or symptoms of orchitis.
       [3] Undescended testes.
       [4] Appearance of lesions on external genitalia.
       [5] Any abnormal discharge from the vagina or urethra.
       [6] Pain in pelvis, testes, groin.
       [7] A possible miscarriage.

[8] Difficulty with urination (male).
  G. The importance of obtaining medical consultation when:
    [1] Secondary sex characteristics fail to develop within the expected age limit.
    [2] There are persistent or troublesome menstrual disorders.
    [3] Marriage is imminent.
    [4] There are problems related to achieving satisfactory sexual relations.
    [5] There is a possible pregnancy.
    [6] There are possible problems of infertility or sterility.
    [7] There are problems related to menopause.
2. Female patients should be protected from injuries to reproductive organs.
  A. The external genitalia should be properly cleaned.
  B. Vaginal irrigations should be performed properly, with gentleness, without force and using surgical aseptic technique, as indicated.
  C. Special precautions should be used in caring for patients receiving radium treatment, to prevent any movement of the applicator.
3. Male patients should be protected from injuries to reproductive organs.
  A. The external genitalia should be properly cleaned.
  B. Catheterization should be avoided whenever possible; when necessary, it should be performed properly, with surgical aseptic technique and great gentleness.

CARE OF PATIENTS WITH SPECIFIC PROBLEMS
INVOLVING REPRODUCTIVE ORGANS

1. When a patient has dysmenorrhea:
  A. Intrapelvic pressure may be reduced by:
    [1] Having the patient lie down.
    [2] Pelvic exercises or positions that favor venous return and/or a change in the position of the uterus.
    [3] Warm applications to the pelvic region.
    [4] Preventing or treating constipation.
  B. Counselling may be indicated.
2. When a patient has a possible rupture of a fallopian tube due to an ectopic pregnancy:
  A. This is a medical emergency. Preparations should be made for surgical intervention.
  B. Nursing measures for the treatment of circulatory shock should be started promptly. (See Chapter 1.)
3. When abortion is threatened or there is an incomplete abortion:
  A. The patient should be kept quiet in the horizontal position.
  B. Vaginal spotting or bleeding should be observed closely and reported appropriately. Profuse bleeding represents a medical emergency.
  C. Any expelled tissue should be saved for inspection by the physician.
4. When a patient has acute pelvic inflammatory disease, positioning should promote localization of the infection in the lower pelvic region.
5. When a male patient has a disorder that involves the scrotum, the testes or the spermatic cord, the scrotum should be kept well supported.

Chapter 20

Infections and
Infectious Diseases

Some varieties of microorganisms are capable of producing infection or infectious disease.

Microbiology

MICROORGANISMS AS INFECTIOUS AGENTS

1. There are many varieties of microorganisms; most are harmless, but some are infectious agents.
   A. True pathogens are virulent organisms that are capable of invading healthy tissues.
   B. Some parasitic microorganisms are not true pathogens but, when given the opportunity, are capable of causing infections. These organisms are classified as opportunists or secondary invaders.
   C. There are some nonparasitic microorganisms that do not invade healthy tissues but produce toxins that are capable of causing disease (e.g., the tetanus bacillus).
2. Some varieties of protozoa cause disease in man.
   A. Protozoa are single-celled animals.
   B. Some pathogenic protozoa pass through life cycles which affect their control and transmission.
      [1] Protozoa in the cyst form are resistant to drying.
      [2] Some protozoa multiply sexually in arthropod hosts.

C. Protozoan parasites can be found in the intestinal tract, the genitourinary tract, the blood, the skin and mucous membrane.

3. Many varieties of fungi cause disease in man; they include true fungi (yeasts and molds) and fission fungi (bacteria).

   A. Molds, yeasts and most bacteria must have organic substances as part of their food.

   B. Molds and yeasts cause mycotic diseases, which may be cutaneous or systemic.

      [1] A few fungi that live in the soil are capable of causing infection under special conditions.

      [2] Yeast-like organisms that are found as normal flora in the mouths and intestinal tracts of healthy persons may act as opportunists.

   C. Genera of families of bacteria that can be infectious agents include:

      [1] *Staphylococcus, Micrococcus.*

      [2] *Escherichia, Salmonella, Shigella.*

      [3] *Pasteurella, Brucella, Hemophilus.*

      [4] *Bacteroides, Streptobacillus.*

      [5] *Neisseria.*

      [6] *Streptococcus, Diplococcus.*

      [7] *Corynebacterium.*

      [8] *Bacillus, Clostridium.*

      [9] *Vibrio, Pseudomonas.*

     [10] *Mycobacterium, Actinomyces.*

     [11] *Treponema, Borrelia.*

     [12] *Rickettsia, Chalamydia.*

   D. Bacteria are capable of a very rapid rate of reproduction. Cell division may take place as rapidly as every 20 minutes.

   E. A few species of bacteria possess flagella which enable them to move about in fluid. The spiral structure of spirochetes enables these organisms to move.

   F. Many species of bacteria produce a protective mucoid coating (capsule), which increases their virulence.

      [1] Species of *Bacillus* and *Clostridium* give rise to resistant forms called endospores.

      [2] Endospores are resistant to drying, sunlight, boiling and disinfectants for prolonged periods of time.

      [3] When conditions become favorable, spores return to their vegetative forms again.

      [4] Pathogenic bacteria that form spores include those that cause tetanus, gas gangrene, botulism and anthrax.

   G. Some species of bacteria are strict anaerobes and are killed by the presence of free oxygen (e.g., the tetanus bacillus).

   H. Bacteria may undergo genetic mutations when exposed to sulfur drugs or antibiotics. This sometimes happens when the dosage of the pharmaceutical agent is inadequate or when the blood concentration level is allowed to fall because of delayed administration.

   I. Pathogenic bacteria in body tissues, secretions and excretions are more virulent than organisms growing outside the body.

   J. *Rickettsia* and *Chalamydia* are obligate parasites.

4. Many varieties of viruses produce disease in man.
   A. Viruses are particles of nucleic acid (either DNA or RNA) with protein coatings. They are capable of reproduction.
   B. Nearly all viruses are easily inactivated by heat. The viruses that cause infectious hepatitis and homologous serum hepatitis are exceptions.
   C. Viruses are obligate intracellular parasites that can cause many types of cellular changes. Disease-producing viruses cause:
      [1] Lesions of the skin and mucous membrane (e.g., chicken pox).
      [2] Respiratory diseases (e.g., pneumonia, influenza).
      [3] Diseases of nervous tissue (e.g., encephalitis, poliomyelitis, rabies).
      [4] Visceral disease (e.g., hepatitis).
   D. Although many disease-causing viruses become inactive in organic material outside the body within only a few days (at room temperature), the viruses that cause poliomyelitis and infectious hepatitis can survive for a number of days.

Control of Microorganisms

1. Most pathogenic microorganisms are mesophilic. They grow best between the temperatures of 25°C. and 45°C. (86°F. and 113°F.).
   A. Low temperatures inactivate microorganisms but are rarely fatal.
   B. Boiling at 100°C. (212°F.) for 10 minutes inactivates or kills:
      [1] All bacteria not in spore form. (Mature spores can resist boiling for hours.)
      [2] Bacterial toxins (except staphylococcal enterotoxin).
      [3] *Rickettsia* and *Chalamydias*.
      [4] Pathogenic yeasts and molds (not in spore form).
      [5] Many viruses. (The viruses of hepatitis can resist boiling for at least 30 minutes.)
      [6] Helminths and their ova (not classified as microorganisms).
   C. All living organisms, including endospores, can be killed by exposure to moist heat at a temperature of 121°C. (250°F.) for 15 to 20 minutes.
2. All microorganisms need moisture for growth. Although drying inhibits the growth of microorganisms, it is not a reliable way of killing them.
3. Cleanliness (freedom from dirt and organic material such as food or body discharges) inhibits the growth of microorganisms.
4. If there is ample exposure, direct ultraviolet rays will kill many types of pathogenic microorganisms. Minutes or hours of exposure to sunlight may be necessary.
5. Chemicals that interfere with the life processes of microorganisms may kill them or inhibit their growth and reproduction.
   A. Bacteria and viruses vary in their resistance to different chemical disinfectants.
   B. Most pathogenic bacteria are inhibited by a pH environment below 5.5 or above 8.5.
6. Disinfection is a process in which the most susceptible pathogenic, nonsporing forms of microorganisms are destroyed.
   A. Disinfection may be accomplished by boiling or by chemicals.
   B. Raw milk can be disinfected by pasteurization (heating).
   C. Water can be disinfected by proper chlorination.

7. Bacteriostasis is a process in which the growth and reproduction of microorganisms are prevented. Bacteriostasis may be accomplished by cold, drying and chemicals.
8. Sanitization involves cleaning and disinfection so that objects are freed from organic material and pathogenic microorganisms.
9. Sterilization is a process through which all microorganisms are destroyed. Sterilization may be accomplished by incineration, autoclaving, prolonged boiling and dry heat.
10. The effectiveness of various methods of disinfection and sterilization depends upon:
    A. Characteristics of the physical or chemical agent being used, i.e.:
       [1] The nature and concentration of chemical being used.
       [2] The penetration and intensity of radiation being used.
       [3] The temperature and type of heat being used.
    B. The time allowed for the process.
    C. The nature of the material being treated. (The presence of organic material on objects interferes with disinfection and sterilization.)
    D. Characteristics of the microorganisms to be killed or inhibited.
    E. Numbers of microorganisms present.
    F. The contact of the agent with the microorganisms.

Sources of Disease-Producing Microorganisms

1. Sources of infectious agents include man, animals, arthropods, plants and the soil.
2. The major source of infectious agents that cause communicable diseases is a person who is discharging living organisms.
3. "Carriers" are persons who do not actually have clinical manifestations of an infection but may be sources of pathogenic organisms.
4. Some microorganisms regularly present on or in the body are primary invaders, secondary invaders and opportunists.
    A. Microorganisms are always present on the outer surfaces of the body and in cavities and tubes that have direct connection with the external environment.
       [1] Regularly present on the skin are varieties of *Staphylococcus* and *Corynebacterium*.
       [2] The nose, mouth and throat contain many types of microorganisms, including varieties of *Streptococcus, Corynebacterium, Borrelia, Staphylococcus, Neisseria, Lactobacillus* and yeasts.
       [3] The external genitalia have normal flora, including *Mycobacterium smegmatis* and *Corynebacterium*.
          a. The vagina normally has many organisms present, including varieties of *Lactobacillus* and *Trichomonas*.
          b. Various fecal organisms can also be found on the external genitalia, especially on that of the female.
       [4] Microorganisms found around the anal area include varieties of *Mycobacterium, Escherichia, Lactobacillus, Clostridium* and enterococci.
    B. The colon has a luxuriant growth of many varieties of microorganisms, including *Escherichia coli* (and coliform group), *Bacteroides, Clostridium, Streptococcus fecalis* (and enterococci), *Lactobacillus, Pseudomonas, Proteus, Enta-*

moeba and enteroviruses. Feces is composed largely of dead and living microorganisms.

  C. The nasal passages are constantly contaminated by inhaled air, but they do not normally favor the growth of any organisms.

  D. Microorganisms do not regularly colonize in the stomach, urinary bladder, uterus, trachea or lungs; these organs are normally free from bacterial growth.

  E. The remaining tissues of the body, including the blood, are normally free from microorganisms.

  F. When normal flora are destroyed, opportunists are more likely to cause infection.

Transmission of Microorganisms

1. Organisms may be transmitted from the source to a susceptible host directly (and usually immediately) by:
   A. Contact with an infected part of the body or discharges which contain the infectious agents.
   B. Direct spray of droplets from the nose and/or mouth onto mucous membrane.
   C. Direct contact with microorganisms that are contained in a substance such as soil.
2. Organisms may be transmitted from the source to a susceptible host indirectly by:
   A. Inanimate vehicles, including:
      [1] Contaminated objects (fomites).
      [2] Contaminated water, food, milk.
      [3] Contaminated biologic products such as blood or plasma.
   B. Vectors.
      [1] Common arthropod vectors include ticks, mites, lice, fleas, mosquitoes and flies.
      [2] Vectors may carry microorganisms on parts of their bodies or in their gastrointestinal tracts.
      [3] Vectors may be required for the reproduction and/or cyclic development of some microorganisms before they become infectious agents for man. The microorganisms may then be transmitted during biting or by discharges deposited on the skin.
   C. Air.
      [1] Droplet nuclei are tiny residues remaining from the evaporation of larger droplets sprayed from the nose and/or mouth. These nuclei can remain suspended in the air for long periods of time.
      [2] Dust containing pathogenic microorganisms may arise from contaminated floors, furniture, bedding or may come from dry soil.
3. Each communicable disease is transmitted in one or more rather definite ways, determined by:
   A. The way in which the pathogen leaves the source (portal of exit).
   B. The portal of entry for each type of pathogen.
   C. The ability of the pathogen to survive outside the host.

SOME SPECIFIC PATHOGENIC BACTERIA

1. *Salmonella typhosa* causes typhoid fever.
   A. Typhoid fever is a systemic disease that may affect a number of body structures. There is lymph tissue involvement, especially in the lower intestinal tract. The organisms are found in the blood early in the disease and in the feces and urine after the first week.
   B. The portal of entry is the mouth.
   C. The reservoir is man, both individuals who have the disease and carriers.
   D. The organisms may be transmitted by direct or indirect contact with the feces or urine of a patient or carrier.
      [1] The principal vehicles of transmission are contaminated food and water.
      [2] Flies may act as vectors.
   E. The organisms can live in moist feces and in ice for several months.
2. Species of *Salmonella* cause salmonellosis.
   A. Salmonellosis is an acute gastroenteritis. The organisms can be found in the blood and in the feces.
   B. The portal of entry is the mouth.
   C. The reservoir is man and domestic and wild animals.
   D. The organisms may be transmitted by contaminated water and food, in eggs, in meat and meat products and in poultry.
3. Species of *Salmonella* can cause paratyphoid fever.
   A. Paratyphoid fever is a systemic disease similar to typhoid fever. The organisms can be found in the blood, feces and urine.
   B. The portal of entry is the mouth.
   C. The reservoir is man, both individuals who have the disease and carriers.
   D. The organisms may be transmitted by direct or indirect contact with the feces or urine of a patient or carrier.
      [1] Principal vehicles for transmission are contaminated water and food.
      [2] Flies may act as vectors.
   E. The organisms can live outside the host for weeks or possibly months.
4. Species of *Shigella* cause shigellosis (bacillary dysentery).
   A. Shigellosis is an acute intestinal disease. The organisms are in the intestinal tract and can be found in the feces.
   B. The portal of entry is the mouth.
   C. The reservoir is man, occasionally domestic animals.
   D. The organisms may be transmitted by direct or indirect contact with the feces of a patient or carrier.
      [1] The principal vehicles of transmission are contaminated food and water.
      [2] Flies can act as vectors.
   E. The organisms can live outside the host for weeks, possibly months.
5. The *Vibrio comma* causes cholera.
   A. Cholera is an acute intestinal disease. There are profuse watery stools and vomiting, which cause rapid, severe dehydration and acidosis. The organisms can be found in the feces and vomitus.
   B. The portal of entry is the mouth.

    C. The reservoir is man.

    D. The organisms are transmitted by direct or indirect contact with the feces or vomitus of a patient.

        [1] The principal vehicles of transmission are contaminated water and food.

        [2] Flies may act as vectors.

6. Species of *Brucella* cause brucellosis (undulant fever).

    A. Brucellosis is a systemic disease characterized by a fever which may be continual, intermittent or irregular. The organisms can be found in the blood, bone marrow or other body tissues or in body discharges.

    B. The portal of entry may be the mouth or skin.

    C. Reservoirs include cattle, swine and sheep.

    D. The organisms may be transmitted directly by contact with or by ingestion of products from infected animals.

7. *Pasteurella tularensis* causes tularemia.

    A. Tularemia is an infectious disease in which there are chills and fever, often an ulcer at the site of entry and inflammation of regional lymph nodes. The organisms can be found in the blood and in lesions.

    B. The portal of entry is usually the skin.

    C. Reservoirs include wild animals (e.g., rabbits and other rodents) and wood ticks.

    D. The organisms are inoculated into the skin with blood or tissue of infected animals, by discharges from infected flies or ticks or through bites of infected ticks, deer flies and other insects.

    E. The organisms are able to survive in dead bodies for extended periods of time.

8. *Pasteurella pestis* causes plague.

    A. Bubonic plague is the most common form. Lymph nodes become acutely inflamed. There is usually severe septicemia and petichial hemorrhages. Pneumonic plague is a respiratory disease and is usually fatal. The organisms can be found in lesions, the blood, spinal fluid and in respiratory discharges.

    B. The portals of entry include the skin, the mouth and the respiratory tract.

    C. Reservoirs are wild rodents and persons with the disease.

    D. The organisms may be transmitted directly by respiratory discharges (in pneumonic plague) or may be airborne. They may be transmitted by contact with infected animals. Bubonic plague is transmitted by the bite of infective fleas (e.g., rat fleas).

9. *Bordetella pertussis* causes pertussis (whooping cough).

    A. Pertussis causes acute inflammation of the trachea, bronchi and bronchioles. The organisms can be found in the upper respiratory tract.

    B. The portal of entry is the respiratory tract.

    C. The reservoir is man.

    D. The organisms may be transmitted by direct contact with discharges from the respiratory tract.

10. *Corynebacterium diphtheriae* causes diphtheria.

    A. Diphtheria is an acute disease of the upper respiratory tract. It can be serious in infants and young children when the larynx becomes involved. The organisms can be found in the nasopharynx.

B. The portal of entry is the respiratory tract.

C. The reservoir is man, both individuals with the disease and carriers.

D. The organisms may be transmitted directly, by contact with respiratory discharges, or indirectly, by contaminated milk.

11. *Neisseria meningitidis* causes meningococcal meningitis.

A. Meningococcal meningitis is an acute inflammation of the meninges. There is severe headache and stiff neck. There may be delirium and coma. The organisms can be found in the blood, spinal fluid and in the nasopharynx.

B. The portal of entry is the respiratory tract.

C. The reservoir is man, both individuals with the disease and carriers.

D. The organisms are transmitted by direct contact with respiratory discharges.

12. *Neisseria gonorrheae* causes gonococcal diseases.

A. Gonococcal diseases include gonorrhea (see Chapter 19); gonococcal vulvovaginitis in young females; and gonorrheal ophthalmia neonatorum. The organisms can be found in the exudates produced by the inflammatory process.

B. The portals of entry are the mucous membrane of the genitourinary tract and the conjunctiva.

C. The reservoir is man.

D. The organisms are transmitted by direct contact.

E. The organisms are fragile and live only for a brief time when exposed to the air and dried.

13. Types of *Diplococcus pneumoniae* cause pneumococcal pneumonia.

A. Pneumococcal pneumonia is an acute pulmonary disease. The organisms can be found in the sputum.

B. The portal of entry is the respiratory tract.

C. The reservoir is man, both individuals with the disease and carriers.

D. The organisms are transmitted by direct and indirect contact with respiratory discharges.

14. Group A hemolytic streptococci cause scarlet fever, septic sore throat, upper respiratory infections, erysipelas and puerperal fever. These organisms may act as opportunists, causing wound infections and infections of other body tissues.

A. The organisms may be found:

[1] In the respiratory tract during scarlet fever, septic sore throat and various respiratory infections.

[2] In the skin in erysipelas.

[3] In the uterus in puerperal fever.

[4] In the inflammatory exudates from infected wounds or infected body tissues.

B. The portals of entry include the respiratory tract, the skin and the mucous membrane of the female reproductive tract.

C. The reservoir is man, both individuals with infections and carriers.

D. The organisms may be transmitted directly, by contact with discharges from infected body tissues, or indirectly, by milk, dairy products or food that has been contaminated by discharges.

E. Streptococci are pyogenic organisms.

15. Various strains of *Staphylococcus aureus* can cause many types of infections.

    A. Staphylococcal infections may be local or systemic. They include impetigo, pimples, boils, abscesses, osteomyelitis, pneumonitis and septicemia. The organisms can be found wherever the infection exists.

    B. The portals of entry are the skin and the mucous membrane, especially that of the respiratory tract.

    C. The reservoir is man, both individuals with infections and nasal carriers.

    D. The organisms are transmitted by contact with discharges from infected body tissues or from a nasal carrier. Air transmission is thought to be important.

16. Some strains of *Staphylococcus* produce an exotoxin that can cause severe gastroenteritis if ingested in sufficient quantity. The production of exotoxin may occur in improperly refrigerated foods that have been contaminated by organisms from infected persons.

17. The toxin produced by *Clostridium botulinum* causes botulism.

    A. Botulism is a serious disorder of the nervous system caused by ingestion of the toxin.

    B. The organisms are saprophytes and are found in water, soil and the intestinal tracts of animals, including fish.

    C. Foods most likely to be contaminated by these organisms are inadequately processed fruits and vegetables or fish.

    D. The organisms are anaerobic, gas-producing spore-formers.

18. The toxin produced by *Clostridium tetani* causes tetanus.

    A. Tetanus is an acute disorder that affects nervous tissue and is characterized by painful, severe muscle spasms.

    B. The toxin is produced by the organisms that grow anaerobically at the site of entry.

    C. The reservoir is the intestinal tracts of animals and man.

    D. Tetanus spores are introduced into the body through wounds contaminated with soil, dust, or animal or human feces.

19. Several species of *Clostridium* (including *Clostridium perfringens*) cause gas gangrene.

    A. Gas gangrene is tissue necrosis caused by gas bubbles and toxins produced by the microorganisms growing in injured tissue.

    B. The organisms are found in human and animal feces, in the soil and in wounds infected with these organisms.

    C. Spores are introduced into the body through wounds contaminated with soil, excreta or wound discharges from patients with the infection.

    D. The organisms are anaerobic, gas-producing spore-formers.

20. *Mycobacterium leprae* causes leprosy (Hansen's disease).

    A. Leprosy is a chronic systemic disease. Clinical manifestations include various types of skin and mucous membrane lesions and symptoms and signs of peripheral nerve damage. The organisms are found in the lesions they cause.

    B. The portal of entry is probably the skin and/or respiratory tract.

    C. The reservoir is man.

    D. The mode of transmission is not clearly established but probably involves direct or indirect contact with organisms from lesions or in nasal discharges. Transmission appears to require close contact for extended periods of time.

21. *Mycobacterium tuberculosis* causes tuberculosis.
    A. Tuberculosis is primarily a pulmonary disease, but there may be extrapulmonary involvement (e.g., lymph nodes, bones, joints and meninges). The organisms may be found in sputum, the stomach or body tissues that have been invaded.
    B. The portals of entry are the nose and mouth.
    C. Reservoirs are man and diseased cattle.
    D. The organisms may be transmitted by:
        [1] Direct or indirect contact with bacilli in the sputum of infected persons. The primary mode of spread is via the air.
        [2] Ingestion of unpasteurized milk or dairy products from infected cows.
    E. The organisms are capable of long survival inside or outside the host.
        [1] The organisms can remain encapsulated in the host (e.g., in the lungs or lymph glands) for many years.
        [2] The organisms can survive in sputum outside the body.
22. The spirochete *Treponema pallidum* causes syphilis.
    A. Syphilis is described in Chapter 19.
    B. The primary portal of entry is the mucous membrane of the external genitalia. An unborn child may be infected through the placenta.
    C. The reservoir is man.
    D. The organisms may be transmitted directly during sexual contact or transmitted to an unborn child via the blood.
23. The spirochete *Borrelia vincentii* is associated with Vincent's angina ("trench mouth").
    A. Vincent's angina is an ulcerative disease of the mouth and throat. The organisms are found in the lesions.
    B. Small numbers of these organisms are normally found in the mouth. They apparently are opportunists or secondary invaders when resistance is low or perhaps when a dietary deficiency exists.

Pathogenic Arthropod-Borne Rickettsia

1. Rickettsia are natural parasites of arthropods, such as fleas, lice, ticks and mites. They are usually found in the alimentary canals of these arthropods. The organisms are generally introduced into the human host by infection into the skin during biting or by rubbing or scratching the skin contaminated with fecal material from the infected arthropod.
2. Typhus-like fevers are caused by different species of *Rickettsia*.
    A. These diseases are characterized by high fever and a rash that has typical distribution.
    B. The typhus-like fevers may be classified according to their arthropod vectors. These include:
        [1] Louse typhus (classical or epidemic typhus fever). Man is the reservoir.
        [2] Flea typhus (murine or endemic typhus). Rats are the reservoir.
        [3] Tick typhus (Rocky Mountain spotted fever). Ticks and various wild animals are reservoirs.
        [4] Mite typhus (scrub typhus). Mites are the reservoir.

3. Q fever is an acute disease caused by *Rickettsia burneti*.
   A. The fever is usually accompanied by a pneumonitis.
   B. The reservoirs are ticks and domestic and wild animals.
   C. The organisms may be transmitted in dust, by direct contact with infected animals (including their hides and excreta) or by ingestion of unpasteurized milk from infected cows or goats.

SOME PATHOGENIC VIRUSES

1. The variola virus causes smallpox (variola).
   A. Smallpox is a severe systemic disease characterized by a progressive development of skin lesions: macules, papules, vesicles, pustules and scabs. Frequently there is hemorrhaging into the skin and mucous membranes. Classical smallpox (variola major) in an unvaccinated person has approximately a 50 percent fatality rate. The organisms are found in respiratory secretions and in the lesions.
   B. The portal of entry is usually the respiratory tract but may be the skin.
   C. The only reservoir is man.
   D. The virus is transmitted through direct or indirect contact with respiratory discharges or skin lesions.
   E. The virus is quite resistant to drying and can survive for days in crusts from lesions and in dust.
2. The varicella-zoster virus causes chickenpox (varicella) and herpes zoster.
   A. Chicken pox is a systemic disease characterized by skin lesions: macules, papules, vesicles and scabs. In herpes zoster, the skin lesions are localized to areas supplied by sensory nerves of specific dorsal root ganglia. The virus is found in the respiratory tract and in skin lesions before scabs form.
   B. The portal of entry is the respiratory tract.
   C. The reservoir is infected persons.
   D. The viruses are transmitted by direct or indirect contact with respiratory discharges or exudate from vesicles.
3. The virus of measles causes measles (rubeola).
   A. Measles is an acute and highly contagious disease manifested by fever, Koplik's spots in the mouth, coryzal symptoms and a typical rash. The virus is found in the nasal secretions and saliva before the rash appears. Later on, the virus can be found in the urine.
   B. The portal of entry is the respiratory tract.
   C. The reservoir is man.
   D. The organisms are transmitted by droplets or by direct or indirect contact with nasopharyngeal secretions and urine from the infected person.
4. The virus of rubella causes German measles (rubella) and congenital rubella syndrome in infants.
   A. German measles is a mild systemic disease of short duration. There is a diffuse macular rash. The virus is found in the nasopharynx, the blood and the feces.
   B. The virus appears to have an affinity for embryonic tissues. From 20 to 25 percent of the infants born to mothers who had German measles during the first trimester of pregnancy have severe congenital disorders, including cardiac defects, bone defects, cataracts, deafness and microcephaly.

C. The portal of entry is the respiratory tract.

D. The reservoir is man.

E. The viruses are transmitted primarily by direct or indirect contact with naso-pharyngeal secretions and possibly by contact with the urine and feces of infected persons.

5. The virus of mumps causes mumps (contagious parotitis).

A. Mumps is characterized by inflammation of the parotid glands and sometimes the gonads, particularly of the male. The virus may also invade the central nervous system. The organisms can be found in saliva, blood, urine and cerebrospinal fluid.

B. The portal of entry is the nose and throat.

C. The reservoir is man.

D. The virus is transmitted by direct or indirect contact with infected saliva before, during and after the appearance of symptoms and signs in the infected person. The virus may also be transmitted by contact with infected urine.

6. Three major types of influenza virus are known at present.

A. Influenza is an infectious disease of the respiratory tract. It is characterized by fever, headache, muscle aching and cough. Often there are coryzal symptoms. The organisms can be found in nasopharyngeal secretions.

B. The portal of entry is the respiratory tract.

C. The reservoir is man.

D. The virus is transmitted by direct and indirect contact with nasopharyngeal discharges from an infected person.

7. There are many rhinovirus types and adenoviruses known to cause the common cold or cold-like illnesses.

A. Colds and cold-like illnesses are inflammations of the upper respiratory tract. They often predispose to bacterial complications, such as sinusitis, otitis media, laryngitis and bronchitis. The virus is found in the nasal discharges and saliva.

B. The portal of entry is the respiratory tract.

C. The reservoir is man.

D. The viruses are transmitted by direct or indirect contact with nasopharyngeal discharges from infected persons.

8. Viral hepatitis includes both infectious hepatitis and serum hepatitis.

A. Hepatitis virus A causes infectious hepatitis, which is also referred to as epidemic viral hepatitis.

[1] The virus appears to be in the gastrointestinal tract, the urine and the blood. Organisms may also be found in nasopharyngeal secretions.

[2] The portal of entry is the mouth, although the virus may be injected into the blood.

[3] The reservoir is man.

[4] The virus is thought to be transmitted by direct and indirect contact with feces or urine from an infected person. The virus can also be spread by inoculation into the blood via contaminated blood or parenteral equipment.

B. Hepatitis virus B causes serum hepatitis or homologous serum jaundice. The infection does not occur in epidemics.

[1]   The virus is found in the blood.

[2]   The portal of entry is the bloodstream.

[3]   The reservoir is man.

[4]   The virus is transmitted by parenteral inoculation of blood (or blood products) from an infected person or by contaminated equipment (e.g., needles, syringes, intravenous sets).

C.   The viruses that cause hepatitis are unusually resistant to boiling. They are able to survive more than 10 minutes of boiling.

9. Infectious mononucleosis is caused by a virus.

A.   Infectious mononucleosis is an acute disease characterized by irregular fever, pharyngitis, cervical lymphadenopathy, enlargement of the spleen and lymphocytosis.

B.   The portal of entry is probably the mouth.

C.   Man is probably the only reservoir.

D.   The actual mode of transmission is unknown, but it is thought to be direct and through the mouth.

10. Types of poliovirus cause anterior poliomyelitis.

A.   Infection with the poliovirus may be nonapparent or may involve paralytic or nonparalytic disease.

B.   Poliomyelitis is an acute febrile disease, in which the motor cells of the anterior horns of the spinal cord are invaded; occasionally, the medulla oblongata is also invaded. There may or may not be permanent nerve damage. The virus is found in the feces and in the pharyngeal secretions.

C.   The portal of entry is the gastrointestinal tract.

D.   The reservoir is man, most often persons with inapparent infections.

E.   The virus is transmitted by direct contact with pharyngeal secretions or feces from an infected person.

11. The virus of rabies causes an encephalitis that is almost always fatal.

A.   The reservoirs include many wild and domestic animals: dogs, cats, foxes, coyotes, skunks, raccoons and bats.

B.   The portal of entry is through a break in the skin.

C.   The virus is transmitted by the saliva of infected animals, usually during biting.

12. Specific viruses cause different types of mosquito-borne viral encephalitides (e.g., Eastern equine, Western equine, California and St. Louis encephalitis).

A.   In viral encephalitides the brain, spinal cord and meninges may be invaded. There is a high fever and symptoms and signs of injury to the central nervous system. The disease varies greatly in its severity and progression.

B.   The true reservoir is unknown.

C.   The viruses are transmitted by infected mosquitoes. The mosquitoes acquire the infection from birds, rodents and sometimes horses.

SOME PATHOGENIC YEASTS AND MOLDS

1. Cutaneous mycoses (dermatomycoses) include the ringworm (tinea) infections.

A.   The infections may involve the scalp and hair (tinea capitis); the feet (tinea pedis or epidermophytosis ["athlete's foot"]); the groin and the nails. The

organisms are found in the lesions they cause (e.g., vesicles, scales and fissures).
   B.   The organisms are easily spread by direct or indirect contact with scales or discharges from lesions.
  2. Systemic (or deep) mycoses affect internal organs and are caused mostly by fungi that live in the soil as saprophytes.
   A.   *Coccidioides immitis* causes coccidioidomycosis, a pulmonary infection in which fibrosis and calcification of lesions may occur. The fungus is transmitted primarily by inhalation of spores from dust, soil or dried plant growth.
   B.   *Histoplasmosis capsulatum* causes histoplasmosis, a pulmonary infection. The fungus is transmitted by inhalation of spores in dust.
  3. *Candida albicans* causes candidiasis (or monaliasis).
   A.   The organism is yeast-like and found normally in the mouth and intestinal tract. Under favorable conditions (e.g., macerated tissues, tissues whose normal flora have been reduced by antibiotic therapy), the organisms can cause infection.
   B.   Infections include oral thrush, vaginitis and skin lesions of various types.
   C.   The fungus is transmitted by contact with saliva, vaginal secretions, skin and feces of carriers or infected persons. Oral thrush in the newborn is acquired during birth from organisms in the mother's vagina.

SOME PATHOGENIC PROTOZOA

  1. *Entamoeba histolytica* causes amebiasis.
   A.   Amoebiasis may be mild, causing intestinal discomfort with bouts of diarrhea and constipation; or the condition may be severe, causing an acute or chronic dysentery.
   B.   The protozoal forms (trophozoites and cysts) are found in the feces.
   C.   The portal of entry is the mouth.
   D.   The reservoir is infected persons.
   E.   The protozoa are transmitted directly and indirectly by feces of infected persons, mainly by contaminated water, vegetables and hands. Flies may also transmit the infection.
   F.   Cysts, under moist conditions, can survive many days outside the host.
  2. Species of the genus *Plasmodium* cause malaria.
   A.   Malaria is characterized by periodic cycles of chills and fever. The organisms are found in the blood.
   B.   The portal of entry is the skin.
   C.   The reservoir is man and infected mosquitoes.
   D.   The protozoa are transmitted by bites of infected female anophiline mosquitoes or may be transmitted by injection of the blood of infected persons, via transfusion or contaminated parenteral equipment.
  3. *Trichomonas vaginalis* causes trichomoniasis.
   A.   Trichomonal infections occur mostly in women and cause inflammation of the vagina, with production of a typical exudate.
   B.   The reservoir is man.

C. The protozoa are transmitted by direct and indirect contact with the vaginal discharge (urethral discharge in men).

SOME PARASITIC HELMINTHS

1. Some species of *Nematoda* (roundworms) and *Platyhelminthes* (flat worms) are common parasites of man. Some live in the intestines; others in the blood and other body tissues. Although the adult worms are not microscopic, the eggs are.
2. Male and female pinworms live in the ileum.
    A. The gravid female migrates to the perianal region, where she lays her eggs.
    B. If the eggs are ingested, they hatch in the intestine and develop into adult worms.
    C. The eggs may be found on contaminated parts of the body, fomites, in dust particles and in the air.
3. The intestinal hookworms live in the small intestine.
    A. Eggs that are laid are passed in the feces.
    B. Larvae hatch from the eggs and grow in the soil.
    C. After approximately 7 days, the larvae are able to penetrate the skin of a new host.
    D. The larvae then pass through the blood to the respiratory tract, where they are swallowed. The adult forms develop in the small intestine.
4. The large intestinal roundworms cause ascariasis.
    A. The adult worms live in the intestinal tract.
    B. The female worm lays eggs, which are passed in the feces.
    C. After about 3 weeks, the eggs, if ingested (e.g., from contaminated food, drink or fingers), reach the intestines where the larvae are liberated.
    D. The larvae penetrate the intestinal mucosa and travel through the lymphatics to the blood vessels, and, by the circulation of the blood, reach the lungs.
    E. After reaching the lungs, the larvae migrate up the respiratory tract, are swallowed, and develop into adult worms in the small intestines.
5. The trichina worm causes trichinosis.
    A. The adult worms live in the intestinal tract.
    B. The females produce larvae that are capable of encysting in muscle tissue.
    C. Man becomes infested by ingesting the flesh of carnivorous animals that contain encysted larvae (e.g., hogs).
    D. The ingested larvae develop in the intestines, and larvae produced by the female encyst in muscle tissue.
6. The source of tapeworms that infect man is man himself.
    A. The adult tapeworm lives in the small intestine and produces eggs, which are passed through the feces.
    B. If animals ingest these eggs (e.g., steer, hogs or fish), the eggs develop in the small intestines; the developed embryo passes through the blood to muscles where it encysts.
    C. Viable encysted forms, when ingested by man, develop to adult forms in the small intestine.
    D. One type of tapeworm that infests man needs no intermediate host; the eggs are immediately infective for the same or another person.

Pathology*

1. An infection is a process wherein an infectious agent (primarily microorganisms, but helminths are included) gains entrance into the body and grows and multiplies. There may or may not be apparent clinical manifestations.

2. An infectious disease is a pathologic condition that results from an infection. Clinical symptoms and signs are apparent.

3. Communicable diseases are illnesses caused by specific infectious agents (or their toxic products) that are transmitted from a reservoir to a susceptible host. Transmission may be direct or indirect.

   A. The time or times during which infectious agents can be transmitted from an infected person to another person or to an animal vector or from an infected animal to a person vary with the different communicable diseases. These are known as periods of communicability.

   B. Most diseases cannot be transmitted during the early incubation period (that period of time between exposure to the infectious agent and the appearance of the first clinical symptoms and signs) or after recovery.

   C. Some diseases can be transmitted over long periods of time or possibly intermittently, if the infectious agents remain in the body and are able to gain access to the outside.

   D. In arthropod-borne diseases, there are two periods of communicability:

      [1] The period of time in which the infectious agents are in the blood or other body tissues and can be transmitted to the vector.

      [2] The period of time in which the infectious agents are in the arthropod host and can be transmitted to man.

4. Symptoms and signs of infections include those associated with inflammation. (See also Chapter 14.)

   A. Local symptoms and signs may include:

      [1] Swelling, redness, pain, heat and loss of function. (Pain may include such physical discomforts as sore throat, burning with urination, painful respirations, intestinal cramping or headache.)

      [2] Sneezing, watery discharge from nasal mucosa or coughing.

      [3] Lesions of the skin and mucous membrane. (See Chapter 13.)

      [4] Vomiting, diarrhea.

      [5] Production of inflammatory exudates.

      [6] Enlargement and tenderness of regional lymph nodes.

   B. Systemic symptoms and signs may include:

      [1] Lassitude, malaise, headache.

      [2] Anorexia, nausea and vomiting.

      [3] Lesions of the skin and mucous membrane (e.g., macular rash).

      [4] Fever with associated symptoms and signs. (See Chapter 9.)

      [5] Generalized lymph node enlargement and tenderness.

5. Symptoms and signs of specific infectious diseases vary with the tissues invaded by

---

* Because of their effects upon specific body structures and functions, some infections and infectious diseases have been considered in preceding chapters.

the specific microorganisms (or injured by their toxins) and with the body's inflammatory responses to the injurious agent.

6. Prodromal symptoms and signs of many of the communicable diseases include those listed under #4B, above.

Nursing Care

Nursing care should be directed toward the prevention and control of infections and infectious diseases.

1. Patients should be interviewed, observed and examined to identify local and/or systemic symptoms and signs of infections and infectious diseases.
   A. Systematic evaluation is of especial importance when the patient:
      [1] Is an infant or small child.
      [2] Is known to have been exposed to an infectious disease and is not properly immunized.
      [3] Is likely to have been exposed to an infectious disease and is not properly immunized.
      [4] Has an unhealed wound.
      [5] Is a food handler.
   B. Indications of actual or possible infection or infectious disease should be reported promptly.
2. Individual resistance to infections should be promoted by providing and encouraging:
   A. Proper nutrition.
   B. Proper exercise.
   C. Adequate rest and sleep.
   D. Proper care of the skin and mucous membrane.
3. Routine immunizations for infants and children should be encouraged and provided.
4. Immunizations against communicable diseases for which vaccines are available should be encouraged and provided when there is likelihood of contact with specific infectious agents (e.g., during epidemics, when there is a polluted water supply or in preparation for travel to different parts of the world).
5. When active immunization is not possible and there is known or suspected contact with infectious agents, available passive immunization should be encouraged.
6. All food, water, milk and ice should be clean, prepared in a sanitary manner and properly stored.
   A. Thorough hand-washing should precede the preparation or service of food and drink.
   B. No individual with known respiratory or enteric infections should be allowed to handle food, milk, water or eating and drinking utensils.
   C. Raw fruits and vegetables should be thoroughly washed before eating.
   D. Unpasteurized milk or dairy products should not be used.
   E. Milk should be kept properly refrigerated at all times.
   F. Ice and ice equipment should be maintained in a clean condition.
   G. Foods that spoil easily or provide a good culture media (e.g., meats, poultry,

creamed foods, custards) should be kept properly refrigerated and should be discarded if not eaten within a few days.

   H. Foods that are canned or frozen at home should be properly prepared and processed. Processed foods should not be eaten if there is a bad odor or if there are bubbles in the liquid.

7. Sexual contacts should be avoided when either person has a known or possible infection of the genitourinary tract.

8. Helminth and protozoal infections may be prevented by:
   A. Sanitary disposal of feces.
   B. Thorough cleansing of the hands following defecation and before eating.
   C. Avoiding direct contact with soil that is contaminated with feces (e.g., wearing shoes in areas where hookworm is prevalent).
   D. Thorough cooking of meat (especially pork), fish, shellfish.
   E. Avoiding eating, drinking or contact with food, water or vegetables that have been contaminated by human waste.
   F. Avoiding arthropod bites.

9. Persons who have sustained animal bites should have prompt medical attention.

10. All persons should be protected from infections and infectious diseases.
   A. Strict personal hygiene measures are essential.
      [1] The skin, hair, nails and exposed mucous membranes should be kept clean and free from excessive moisture.
      [2] Hand-washing is of utmost importance:
         a. Prior to handling food.
         b. Prior to eating.
         c. Following any activity in which the hands have come into contact with the external genitalia, the body discharges (e.g., respiratory discharges) or known contaminated areas, such as floors.
      [3] The hands and any unclean objects should be kept away from the mouth, nose, eyes, ears, external genitalia and any wounds.
      [4] Good dental hygiene should be encouraged and provided.
      [5] All objects used in or around the mouth should be clean (e.g., toothbrushes, drinking straws, eating utensils, drinking glasses).
      [6] Breast-feeding hygiene should be practiced to protect nursing babies from infections.
      [7] Eating, drinking and toilet articles should not be used in common with other persons.
      [8] Exposure to spray from the nose and mouth should be avoided whenever possible (e.g., when there is sneezing, coughing, laughing, vigorous talking).
      [9] The nose and mouth should be covered during coughing and sneezing, and proper techniques should be used in handling and disposal of tissues or handkerchiefs.
      [10] Clothing should be kept clean by sufficiently frequent and effective cleaning methods.
   B. The immediate environment (e.g., furniture, curtains, bedding, clothing, walls, floors, sinks, toilets) should be maintained free from dust, dirt and organic materials, such as food or body discharges.

C. Air currents should be controlled; good ventilation should be provided; overcrowding should be avoided.
D. There should be adequate provision for safe handling and sanitary disposal of all organic wastes (e.g., urine, feces, vomitus, respiratory secretions, drainage from wounds or body cavities).
E. Arthropods and rodents should be controlled.
F. Effective hand-washing should be done:
    [1] Before giving personal care to a patient.
    [2] After giving personal care to a patient.
    [3] After contact with infective or potentially infective organic material (e.g., respiratory secretions, saliva, feces, urine, blood or exudates).
G. All equipment used in patient care should be clean, i.e., free from dust, dirt and organic material.
H. Equipment used for different patients should be properly disinfected or sterilized after each patient use. Disposable equipment is desirable whenever possible.
I. Effective methods of disinfection and sterilization should be utilized.
    [1] All organic material should be removed from equipment prior to disinfection or the sterilization process.
    [2] If heat (dry or moist) is used, the equipment must be fully exposed to the temperature required and for the length of time required to destroy the particular type or form of microorganisms present.
    [3] If chemicals are used for disinfection, the equipment must be fully exposed to the required concentration of drug for the length of time required to destroy pathogenic microorganisms.
    [4] If ultraviolet radiation is used for disinfection, the exposure must be direct and for the length of time required to destroy pathogenic microorganisms.
J. Only sterile equipment and solutions should be used for patient care that involves parts of the body normally free of microbial growth.
K. Special cleansing techniques should be utilized in preparing the skin or mucous membrane prior to procedures such as incisions or catheterization.
L. Wounds should be protected from microorganisms and microbial growth.
    [1] Minor superficial wounds (e.g., abrasions) may be treated using clean technique, but wounds in general should be treated using surgical aseptic technique.
    [2] Accidental wounds should be thoroughly cleaned as soon as possible after they occur. When wounds are deep, difficult to clean thoroughly and/or likely to be contaminated (e.g., with microorganisms from the soil):
         a. Medical attention should be obtained promptly.
         b. Proper wound-cleaning and tetanus precautions should be provided.
    [3] The skin or membrane around open wounds should be kept clean and as dry as possible.
    [4] Wounds should be protected from possible contaminants, such as hair, lint, dust, respiratory secretions, fecal material.
    [5] Dry dressings should be reinforced or changed (if allowed by medical orders) when they become moist.

11. Specific isolation and precaution techniques should be carefully followed as ordered and/or indicated by a diagnosed infection or infectious disease.
    A. Precautionary measures to prevent the possible spread of infectious agents may be indicated by a patient's symptoms and signs prior to medical orders or a definite diagnosis.
    B. Isolation requirements should be determined by:
       [1] Where the infectious agents are in the host and their portal(s) of exit.
       [2] How the infectious agents can be transmitted from one person to another.
       [3] How the infectious agents are able to enter the body.
       [4] The nature of the microorganisms (e.g., highly resistant or fragile, true pathogens or opportunists).
       [5] The period of communicability.
    C. When a patient has a disease condition caused by microorganisms, the following must be considered contaminated and be cared for appropriately:
       [1] Anything that has direct or indirect contact with the organs or tissues of the body that contain the causative organisms.
       [2] Anything that has direct or indirect contact with organic substances that come from an infected part (e.g., exudates, feces, urine).
       [3] Anything that has direct or indirect contact with organic substances associated with the portal(s) of exit for the pathogenic organisms (e.g., respiratory tract, urinary tract, alimentary canal).
    D. Fomites should be burned whenever possible, but when contaminated articles must be reused, they should be kept separate, cleaned and properly disinfected (sterilized, if possible, and always if spore-formers are involved). Fomites should be cared for as soon after use as possible.
    E. The furniture and floors in the patient's area should be maintained free from dust, dirt and organic material at all times. Meticulous cleaning with disinfectant solutions should be done when the patient is no longer infective or has left the unit.
    F. Infective (or potentially infective) body discharges should be wrapped and burned when possible (e.g., tissues, soiled dressings, uneaten food), or disposed of into the sewer system. In some instances, disinfection of excreta is necessary before its disposal into a sewer system. Body discharges should be properly disposed of as soon as possible.
    G. Meticulous cleansing of the hands after patient care is absolutely essential.
    H. When a patient has an infectious disease and the infectious agents can be transmitted to others directly or indirectly by respiratory discharges or saliva, everything in the patient's immediate environment, including the air, must be treated as contaminated.
       [1] Protective gowns should be used.
       [2] Masks should be used. (Masks should be changed frequently and always when moist.)
       [3] A barrier to prevent the free circulation of air outside the unit (e.g., closed door) may be indicated in some airborne diseases.
       [4] Proper ventilation should be promoted to limit the numbers of droplet nuclei.

[5] Careful tissue technique should be used for coughing and sneezing. Tissues and other objects that contain or have come in contact with respiratory discharges or saliva should be handled with special precautions.

I. When a patient has an infectious disease caused by infectious agents that can be transmitted to others directly (by feces and/or urine or vomitus) and indirectly (by sewage, food, water or insect vectors): everything that comes into contact with the patient or with his potentially infective discharges must be treated as contaminated.

[1] Protective gowns should be used when giving personal care.

[2] Gloves may be desirable when giving direct care involving the alimentary canal or the external genitalia.

[3] The patient's hands should be washed thoroughly whenever they have been in contact with the external genitalia or anal region.

[4] A barrier to prevent the circulation of flies (e.g., closed door, screening) may be indicated.

[5] Excreta should be handled with special precautions promptly after elimination.

[6] Utensils in contact with excreta should be cleaned thoroughly and disinfected (sterilized, if possible).

J. When a patient has an infection and the infectious agents can be transmitted to others by direct contact with the infected area or discharges from it (e.g., an infected wound), everything that comes in contact with the area or with inflammatory exudates must be treated as contaminated.

[1] Protective gowns may be used when giving personal care and doing dressings.

[2] Gloves should be worn for wound care.

[3] Any soiled dressings should be promptly wrapped and burned.

[4] Any contaminated clothing or bedding should be handled with special precautions.

[5] The patient's activities should be controlled to prevent direct contact of the infected part or discharges with other persons.

K. When a patient has an infectious disease caused by infectious agents that can be transmitted by blood, special precautions must be taken with any equipment that comes into contact with the patient's blood (e.g., needles, syringes, laboratory test tubes). Disposable equipment is preferable.

PART III

Psychosocial Principles
and Nursing Applications

Introduction

Several points need emphasis before the reader considers the material presented in Part III. It cannot be stressed often enough that this material is *not* a complete outline of social science principles important to nursing. Although each revision of this text provided more complete science information, there is no pretense that every fact, principle or hypothesis that might be useful to the nurse in nursing care planning and implementation has been included. As noted elswhere, the brief social science statements of principles do not substitute for thorough study of areas in the social sciences, any more than the summary statements of anatomy and physiology principles in the Biologic and Physical Sciences portion of this book substitute for comprehensive courses in anatomy and physiology.

For example, in Chapter 9, "Sociocultural Influences on Behavior," the amount of possible information on the relationships between sociocultural influences and behavior is almost limitless. Thus, the material included in this volume relative to cultural groups and subgroups is intended to be representative of the *types* of information the nurse should seek about individual patients, and it is intended to remind the nurse of the extent to which both the patient's and nurse's behavior patterns are influenced by sociocultural factors.

In each revision of this book, the authors have attempted to keep the ever-expanding material within reasonable bounds by avoiding theories, however currently popular, and by emphasizing concepts and principles which cut across several theories and have been demonstrated through organized study. Yet, in each revision, chapters and sections were expanded in an attempt to keep pace with concurrent nursing practice concerns. At the time of this third revision, the following 3 areas were receiving increased attèntion and space in nursing and related science literature. Consistent with previous revisions and the general format used throughout the volume, new sections have not been set up for these areas of interest. Rather, statements of principle, fact, or hypothesis have been added to the appropriate existing chapters or sections.

Crisis Intervention: It will come as no surprise to students of crisis intervention theory that the bulk of material written on the subject reduces to less than a dozen straight-forward principles or hypotheses. Some of the principles related to crisis intervention appeared in previous editions of Part III. Additional statements have been added to appropriate sections, particularly to Chapter 6, "Growth and Development, Learning and Adaptive Problem Solving," and to Chapter 8, "Disturbances of Equilibrium."

Death and Dying: Death and dying is by no means a newly emerged set of circumstances! The amount of attention given to death and dying in current literature, curriculum content and continuing education workshops and seminars is, however, a good indicator of how inadequately workers in the health professions have related in the past to this particular aspect of human experience. As might be expected from the way in which the original study which produced this book was conducted, the first edition contained a number of statements regarding death and dying. The current revision expands on that beginning, particularly in Chapter 9, "Sociocultural Influences on Behavior."

The Process of Aging: As with death and dying, the current increase in literature on the process of aging represents an attempt to make up for previous neglect of a segment of our population rather than any newly developed area of knowledge. Material regarding the aging process has been interspersed throughout Part II, since, obviously, the aging process alters the behaviors discussed in every one of the chapters and sections. In some instances, there is no direct reference to older age groups, since a principle may have been so worded as to refer to the continuous changes occurring from birth to death. The point must be made, however, that education of health service personnel should include as much emphasis on specific facets of growth and development in later years as has been included on specific facets of growth and development from birth through adolescence.

It is of particular interest to note that Chapter 7, "Primary and Acquired Needs," is the most extensively developed of the social science chapters and has been so in all editions. It was originally due to the exceedingly large number of nurse-patient situations reported in the original study that described patient distress or satisfaction in the area of comfort and security, as associated with need satisfaction. Over the years, there has been no indication that patient concerns have shifted in any other direction.

In the original study, the most important single factor was the patient's need to cope successfully with a current situation—to know what was happening, what was expected of him and what action was required to resolve current problems. Second in importance was the patient's need for a situational definition—the need to know who and where he was and how he and others fitted into the current environmental picture. These two needs were demonstrated repeatedly in the incidents reported, and the extensive development of substatements in Chapter 7 represents the wide variety of situations in which these needs were depicted.

The material in Part III is organized into 10 chapters, containing the complete material from the original study and later abstractions from contemporary literature. It is presented in outline and simple-statement form, for the sake of clarity and brevity. Statements of science make up the major part of each chapter. At the end of each chapter, examples or guidelines for the application of science to nursing are presented. The nursing statements are examples, intended to demonstrate how social science material can be used by the nurse to make judgments and decisions; they are not complete reiterations of every statement of science in nursing principle form.

No attempt was made to designate the specific social science discipline or subdiscipline (i.e., psychology, sociology, anthropology) to which the concepts, principles, facts and hypotheses were most closely related. A cursory glance at the material would seem to indicate that the majority of statements are most likely related to psychology. A closer look reveals the interrelatedness of all 3 major social science areas as they apply to nursing.

Perhaps some discussion of terminology may offset negative mental sets about the particular wording consistently used throughout Part III. The terms "psychosocial equilibrium" and "psychological homeostasis" are used, even though they may be viewed with disfavor by some readers. "Equilibrium" and "homeostasis," when used in the biologic and physical sciences, can be defined with far greater scientific accuracy than when applied to social science material. But, relatively speaking, other terms would be equally difficult to define, would meet with equal disfavor from some readers and would be much less useful.

In Part III, the term "homeostasis" refers to the tendency of an organism to seek and maintain relatively stable conditions of existence. In the physical sciences, homeostasis has a restricted meaning, implying the *internal* stability of an organism as maintained by self-regulatory mechanisms. As used in Part III, the term has been expanded to include psychological and social factors that influence human stability and the individual and collective actions that a person may take to establish and maintain relative homeostasis. As for the term "equilibrium," the common dictionary definition was used. This definition implies a state of balance or even adjustment between opposing forces, influences or interests of any kind. As used in Part III, equilibrium and homeostasis are complementary conditions, toward which the human being strives in his attempts to exist in relative safety, comfort and satisfaction.

The term "principle" was used in the original study and in subsequent revisions, even though its use may be somewhat controversial. In common practice, this term has been used rather loosely to denote any currently believed "fact" or idea, with or without scientific validation. In the science fields, "principle" has a much more restricted meaning. But in the area of social sciences, strictly scientific principles that have been proven by testing are few and far between!

In order to avoid controversy and negative reaction to perfectly useful material as much as possible, the terms "fact," "principle" and "hypothesis" have been used to designate social science material. The term "hypothesis" refers to any tentative theory or supposition provisionally adopted to explain facts and to guide in the investigation of others, or to something assumed or conceded for the purpose of guiding action. The science material in Part III includes statements at concept-, principle- or fact-level, including hypotheses when necessary. At any level, the statements are used in terms of guides to action. Their validity has either been scientifically demonstrated, or they represent man's best "educated guess" at this particular stage of understanding of human behavior.

For the third edition, a change in terminology designating a recipient of nursing or other health services was contemplated. The term "patient" is, in some areas of health services, being replaced by the term "client," for good though subtle reasons. This change is more often seen when the health services involve more social science than natural science principles, or when the service is rendered in settings where major emphasis is not on acute health care. Over the years, the way in which health services have been rendered has helped to give the term "patient" some very unintended connotations, usually not consciously recognized or admitted by those rendering the health service. If the reader will, for a minute, contemplate her own attitudes and expectations while applying the terms "patient" and "client" toward her own interaction with health professionals, perhaps some of the subtleties of these two terms will emerge.

The term "patient," unfortunately, carries with it a required giving up of some aspects of identity, a reduction in self-possession and participation in self-direction.To put it more bluntly, the way in which health professionals have used or misused their roles as givers of health services has given the term "patient" a dehumanizing quality. The term "client," on the other hand, carries with it the connotation that the recipient is purchasing a service and, if the way in which service is rendered is not satisfactory, can and will apply elsewhere. Somehow, health professionals who use the term "client" are less inclined to "take possession" of the recipient of services and more inclined to respect his individual rights to self-determination.

There are those who will argue that a change in terminology will not effect a change in behavior and that what is needed is concentrated effort toward recognizing and changing those attitudes and behaviors that do a disservice to the recipients of nursing ministrations. It is the authors' belief that the attitudes and behaviors surrounding the "patient" role are so ingrained and so subtle that nothing short of a change in terminology *as well as* concerted effort toward change will be effective.

Despite these considerations, the term "patient" has been retained for the third edition. The bulk of agencies offering health/nursing services still are predominantly concerned with acute care, and such agencies retain, at present, a firm grip on the term "patient."

In the original Commonwealth Study, certain assumptions and beliefs were used as a guide in the analysis of situations and the statement of principles. The major guiding assumptions or beliefs were:

Assumption: That the human being cannot survive as a psychologically healthy social being (even though he may physiologically survive) unless certain required conditions prevail. It is further assumed that these conditions include both internal (psychological) and external (sociocultural) factors, which have a reciprocal relationship.

Assumption: That the human organism functions as a total unit, implying that physiological homeostasis is affected by psychosocial factors, and that psychosocial homeostasis is affected by physiological factors.

Assumption: That the person who seeks attention for health problems, and subsequently receives nursing care for a disturbance of physiological function, requires and has a right to expect attention and care in the area of psychosocial function if he is to receive maximum benefit from medical and nursing care.

It was further held that a person in the situation described by the above assumptions comes within the province of nursing responsibility. Moreover, the nurse must necessarily have the understanding and the ability to assist the individual patient in achieving psychosocial equilibrium whenever equilibrium is disturbed or likely to be disturbed as a result of the situation. It is precisely in the area of care most closely related to the social sciences that the nurse is least likely to be guided by "doctor's orders" and medical or hospital policy. Probably the most uniquely *nursing* aspect of nursing care is the intelligent and creative application of social science principles.

Chapter 1

Perception

Psychological equilibrium (as well as physical survival) requires the ability to perceive and interpret internal and external data.

Social Science Principles

1. Perception of a given person, object or event is unique to the individual and depends upon a variety of factors:
   A. Perception is influenced by the nature of the stimuli.
      [1] A given stimulus tends to be more effective in shaping perception if it has one or more of the following qualities:
         a. Intensity.
         b. Repetitiveness.
         c. Isolation from other stimuli.
         d. Movement and change.
         e. Novelty.
         f. Incongruity.
      [2] Perception of a given object or event tends to be of better quality if aspects of the object or event occur or are arranged in meaningful, related groupings, to constitute a whole or a pattern.
      [3] Perception is less adequate if various aspects of the object or event are so divided as to demand division of attention among the various aspects.
      [4] Adequacy of perception is decreased or delayed if the stimuli or stimulus pattern is ambiguous.
   B. Perception is influenced by the nature and condition of the individual's perceptual equipment.

[1] Perception is influenced by the sensitivity of the individual's sensory equipment.

a. There is great individual variation (both constitutionally and developmentally determined) in sensory ability, with variation occurring among the several senses (e.g., one person may have particularly astute hearing but be less sensitive to taste or smell).

b. A person who is hypersensitive in any given sensory area will tend to react to environmental stimuli, regardless of his need to rest or attend to other stimuli.

[2] Perception is influenced by the individual's constitutional or developmental level ability to utilize cognitive equipment. (See Chapter 2.)*

[3] Perceptual equipment influences the automatic selection and organization of stimuli or stimulus patterns.

a. Perceptual equipment can tolerate an individually determined amount of stimulation at any given time.

b. When perceptual capacity is overloaded, attention shifts to less demanding aspects of a situation.

c. Perceptual attention to a given stimulus cannot be maintained indefinitely. When perceptual equipment becomes "tired" of a given stimulus, attention automatically shifts.

i. Ability to maintain perceptual attention for longer spans of time increases with age and practice; the young child is much less able than an adult to concentrate attention over a long period of time.

ii. In older age groups, ability to maintain perceptual attention for longer periods of time may be decreased.

d. When a given situation involves more separate parts than perceptual equipment can handle adequately, attention focuses on isolated aspects of the situation. (Unless later correction is made, recall of the perceived object or event may be distorted by such focusing of attention.)

e. Man has a natural tendency to organize perceptual data.

i. Man organizes incomplete perceptual data by "filling in" data to complete it.

ii. Man tends to organize perceptual data by finding meanings and relationships that provide adequate interpretation of the data and influence perception of subsequent data.

iii. Both the selection of data for attention and their organization are influenced by past experience and by the current psychological and physical state of the perceiver. (See C, following.)

iv. In general, perception is more likely to be complete and adequate if more than a single sense is involved.

C. Perception is influenced by the individual's current physiological and psychological states and his past experiences.

[1] An individual's physical size influences perception of objects, persons or

---

* Unless otherwise noted, all chapter references made in this Part III apply to those chapters also in Part III.

events. (A small person or a child perceives a large person differently than a person equally as large.)

[2] An individual's physical condition influences perception of objects, persons or events. (A physically handicapped person perceives objects in the environment in a way different from a nonhandicapped person; a person who is acutely ill perceives the environment in terms different from the person who is well; impaired hearing reduces the ability to test reality.)

[3] Perception is influenced by the individual's current state of need. The most strongly felt need is most likely to shape or direct perception. (See Chapter 7.)

[4] Perception is influenced by the individual's current emotional state. (See Chapter 5.)

[5] Perception is influenced by the individual's attitudes, opinions, values and current interests. (See Chapter 2.)

[6] Preoccupation with personal matters or other distracting influences interferes with adequate perception.

[7] Past experience influences an individual's "perceptual set," i.e., his tendency to organize and select perceptual data.

    a. Conflicting perceptual sets may interfere with adequacy of perception by causing inattention to some details, overattention to some details and distortion of some details or of the total situation in order to avoid unpleasant recognition of discrepancies.

    b. Perceptual set helps to determine what is perceived and how it is interpreted by setting up a state of anticipation of what will be perceived.

[8] The more ambiguous perceptual data are, the more their interpretation is influenced in the direction of need, desire or expectation.

[9] An individual's perceptual ability and characteristic ways of perceiving situations follow a pattern of growth and development.

    a. A certain amount of actual physical stimulation appears to be necessary to the normal maturation of sensory equipment and to the training of sensory equipment for use.

    b. In addition to physical stimulation, nonphysical stimulation of sensory equipment is necessary for adequate maturation of sensory equipment and its training for use.

    c. Even after maturation of sensory equipment, prolonged sensory deprivation may disrupt adequate utilization of perceptual ability, i.e., interfere with perception and interpretation of events.

    d. In older persons, a decrease in sensory acuity may promote an artificial sensory deprivation and social isolation unless preventive compensatory actions are taken.

    e. Structural changes due to the process of aging may result in impaired sensory ability, including impairment of perceptual ability.

[10] A person may have perceptual experiences without corresponding stimuli (e.g., dreams, hallucinations).

2. An individual's perceptions influence his behavior.
   A. An individual reacts to a situation or event as he perceives it, regardless of the reality of the situation or how the majority of other people see the situation.
   B. Perception of persons, objects or events (thus, behavior toward these persons or objects or in the situation) is susceptible to a number of errors or distortions. Such errors may involve one or more of the following:
      [1] Superficial observations.
      [2] Preconceptions.
      [3] Incorrect inferences.
      [4] Faulty memory.
      [5] Superstitions and prejudices.
      [6] Incorrect premises.
      [7] Rationalization.
      [8] Projection.
      [9] Certain errors in perception of people or events are particularly common. Such errors include:
         a. Tendency to oversimplify and reduce the total possible data about a person or event to the most quickly formulated generalizations (e.g., the use of stereotypes or categorizations made on the basis of 1 or 2 perceived characteristics, omitting other characteristics).
         b. Tendency to adhere to a stereotype or categorization once it is formed. Future data tend to be ignored or rationalized unless they fit the stereotype, in which case the data tend to be overemphasized.
         c. Tendency to project onto others characteristics common to oneself. (The need to eliminate possibly threatening differences.)

Nursing Care

The principles, hypotheses and facts related to perception can be used by the nurse to help patients maintain adequacy of perception.

1. The nurse can increase her understanding of the processes involved in perception in order to better understand the patient and herself and to therefore guide her behavior toward wiser judgments.
2. The nurse can increase her knowledge and understanding of the individual patient and his life circumstances in order to anticipate how he will perceive a specific situation. She can attempt to determine through observation:
   A. The patient's general sensory ability, by comparing and contrasting his ability to expected norms, in order to detect any deviations from those norms. (She notices such things as photosensitivity, poor eyesight, hypo- or hypersensitivity to auditory stimulation, hypo- or hyperesthesias, decreased ability to taste or smell, hypersensitivity to odors.)
   B. The patient's general developmental level as it might affect perception (e.g., intellectual ability in general, typical cognitive styles as demonstrated by the patient, educational level which might indicate concept development, age as an indication of possible perceptual level).

    C. The patient's current physical and psychological state (e.g., emotional state, type of illness and/or physical disability, current need state insofar as it can be determined, currently demonstrated attitudes and opinions).

3. Using her knowledge of the processes of perception, the nurse can guide her observations of the patient and his situation to determine any errors, omissions or distortions of perception and/or any ways in which data may have been presented that would decrease adequacy of perception.

4. After observation of the patient and his situation, the nurse can use information gained in order to make decisions for action that will increase or ensure adequacy of perception. For example, she can:

    A. Control her own behavior in the presence of patients who are small (e.g., children) or physically handicapped, in order to avoid behavior that might be perceived as threatening or that might be distorted because of a handicap.

    B. Regulate perceptual data presented to the patient in accordance with his ability to attend to details or to specific kinds of data (e.g., adjust for confusion, preoccupation, gross need states, hyper- or hyposensitivity in any given area).

    C. Regulate perceptual data presented to the patient in accordance with his emotional state (e.g., decrease demands on attention if the patient is particularly tense or anxious; introduce necessary new information when he is less tense; manipulate the environment to avoid depressing perceptions if the patient is already depressed; attempt to avoid anger-producing situations when they would interfere with perception).

    D. Control or influence the presentation of stimuli for most effective perception by:

        [1] Regulating the quality of the stimuli (e.g., providing adequate amount of information, with optimal degree of intensity, repetitiveness, novelty).

        [2] Presenting perceptual data in organized forms most conducive to adequate perception and interpretation (e.g., showing meaningful relationships and whole patterns rather than bits of isolated information; reducing the number of diverse parts of a situation needing attention).

        [3] Avoiding ambiguity and vagueness in the presentation of perceptual data.

        [4] Avoiding the "overloading" of stimulus patterns beyond the patient's ability to be attentive.

    E. Either avoid the introduction of perceptual data that will cause increased conflict or tension because of preexisting attitudes and beliefs or not pressure the patient to change his ideas simply because he has been presented with "facts."

    F. Obtain feedback from the patient to determine his adequacy of perception. Use feedback to plan the correction of errors, fill in gaps in data and correct distortions.

    G. In working with infants and young children, especially if they are isolated from parents and other children, the nurse should plan for adequate physical contact and/or sensory stimulation.

    H. In working with adults who must be isolated for long periods, provide sensory stimulation through such means as reading, radio or television, handcrafts, conversation with hospital personnel, and so forth.

I.   In working with older persons who have decreased sensory ability, provide for compensatory perceptual experience through such avenues as hearing aids or speaking in louder tones, presenting visual material in larger print uncomplicated by shadows or shading, increasing light levels in rooms, being careful not to avoid social contact with persons who have difficulty in communicating due to decrease in sensory ability.

J.   Be alert to any indications that perceptual experiences are not based on objective stimuli and regulate nursing behavior accordingly (e.g., avoid ridiculing the patient; see that protective measures are taken if hallucinations may cause irrational behavior; decrease environmental stimuli that may promote illusions).

5. The nurse should, in her observation of patients and interpretation of their behavior, be alert to clues regarding perceptions that might influence behavior. For example, she can:

A.   Obtain feedback from the patient regarding exactly how he sees a situation.

B.   Obtain any necessary additional information from the patient that might indicate perceptual set or errors in perception that may be influencing his behavior (e.g., superstitions, preconceptions, lack of information, past experiences, use of stereotypes).

6. The nurse must be alert to her own behavior, including her perceptive behavior, in order to determine how she may be perceived by the patient, how her perceptions may influence her actions in relation to the patient and how she can alter her behavior to the best interests of the patient.

Chapter 2

Cognition, Attitudes, Opinions and Beliefs

Psychological equilibrium is influenced by and complexly related to cognitive function, including opinions, beliefs and attitudes.

Social Science Principles

1. Psychological equilibrium is influenced by cognitive function.
   A. In general, psychological equilibrium is enhanced if the individual is able to think clearly and rationally.
      [1] For an individual who is confused, frequent reorientation is necessary to decrease confused behavior and prevent or decrease fear caused by the confused state.
      [2] The attention span of the confused person is usually short and easily interrupted.
      [3] Extremes of emotion and tension may interfere with rational thinking and behavior.
      [4] Extremely distorted thinking, such as occurs in delusion, may result in a corresponding illogical behavior. (An individual who has delusions acts on the basis of those delusions, regardless of the apparent reality of a situation or any attempts to convince him of the falsity of his ideas.)
   B. An individual's psychological state, including cognitive function, ideas, beliefs and attitudes, influences his physiological function.
      [1] Conscious and unconscious cognitive processes, in conjunction with other aspects of psychological function, can cause the subjective experiencing

of psychological symptoms where no physiological pathology can be demonstrated (e.g., pain, anesthesia, paresthesia).

[2] Conscious and unconscious cognitive processes, in conjunction with other aspects of psychological function, can have substantial influence on physiological functioning (e.g., paralysis, convulsive seizures, blindness, nausea and vomiting, increased pulse rate).

[3] There is some degree of general muscular tension always present during thinking.

    a. The more vivid the imagery of thinking, the greater the muscular tension.

    b. Thinking about certain kinds of activities causes muscular tension in those muscles involved in the activity being imagined.

2. Cognitive function is influenced by a variety of factors.

  A. The physical environment has a substantial influence on individual cognitive function (e.g., distracting features in the environment; events or objects that focus attention and direct the train of thought).

    [1] Through the process of developmental experience, an individual may learn to think better under certain environmental conditions (e.g., presence or absence of certain kinds of sounds or certain visual situations; varieties of physical position).

  B. An individual's physiological state has an influence on cognitive function (e.g., thirst, hunger, physical discomfort, pain, endocrine balance).

  C. The cognitive process of remembering is subject to the same influences as perception.

    [1] Remembered material tends to be systematized, organized and reinterpreted in relation to the individual's unique fund of percepts, past knowledge, current needs and interests.

    [2] In the process of remembering, actual events frequently become so reorganized and reinterpreted that they are only vaguely literal and may be substantially distorted.

    [3] The process of aging appears to influence ability to remember.

        a. With considerable individual variation, the aging process decreases the ability to remember recent events.

        b. With considerable individual variation, the aging process seems to promote the ability to recall earlier life events. (See Chapter 6 for the use of the "life review" process in aging.)

        c. Presence of chronic disease in the older person, even when asymptomatic, tends to lower performance scores on psychometric tests, especially for tests involving memory. Older persons without disease do not seem to experience the same degree of lowered performance.

3. Development of cognitive ability follows a systematic pattern of maturation, based on both constitutional ability and maturational experiences.

  A. The adequate development and functioning of cognitive equipment requires varied perceptual stimulation.

  B. Some cognitive styles develop in the process of maturation and experience.

    [1] An individual may develop rigid patterns of thinking, making it difficult

for him to change ideas, attitudes, beliefs and concepts even when objective conditions demand it.

  a. The person who utilizes primarily rigid thinking patterns most often was subjected to restrictive, punishing experiences during his formative years.

  b. The person with rigid thinking patterns seems to have other personality characteristics which either promote rigid thinking, correspond to rigid thinking or are reinforced by rigid thinking. These characteristics include: little initiative, excessive submission to authority, poor personal insight, feelings of insecurity, low self-esteem and self-acceptance, greater dependence on support from others and greater susceptibility to threat.

[2] An individual may develop flexible patterns of thinking, making it easier for him to adapt to new ideas and change concepts when objective conditions warrant change.

  a. The person who utilizes primarily flexible thinking patterns most often was subjected to permissive, autonomous experiences encouraging independence during his formative years.

  b. The person with flexible thinking patterns seems to have other personality characteristics which either promote flexible thinking, correspond to flexible thinking or are reinforced by flexible thinking. These characteristics include: unrestricted use of initiative, the ability to organize, self-reliance, goal direction and motivation, relatively good personal insight, acceptance of self but with ability to control impulses, adequate sense of self-esteem and of personal adequacy, less susceptibility to threat and ability to tolerate ambiguity.

[3] Some individuals tend to develop thinking patterns that make it easier for them to conceptualize in concrete, specific, literal terms, and others develop thinking patterns that make it easier for them to conceptualize in abstract terms.

[4] Persons in older age groups appear to demonstrate greater rigidity and concreteness in thought patterns, but this apparent tendency may be misleading. For example, the apparent rigidity may be the result of emphasis on accuracy as opposed to speed and novelty.

C. Ability to conceptualize develops relatively slowly. (For example, the child usually attributes life to nonorganic objects.)

  [1] The development of conceptualization requires communicative contact with others.

  [2] Concrete concepts are more easily grasped, both in the child and the adult. The development of concrete concepts precedes the development of abstract concepts.

  [3] Abstract conceptualization is either interfered with or impossible in some forms of mental handicap (e.g., mental retardation and brain damage and apparently in schizophrenia).

  [4] Persons in older age groups tend to be less able to acquire new or altered concepts.

4. Attitudes, beliefs and opinions seem to have certain characteristic features.
   A. It is unsafe to assume that people having the same attitude or opinion regarding a given object, person or event have the same cognitive content to support that attitude or opinion.
   B. Attitudes, opinions and beliefs may not always be supported by systematic reasoning; they may be vague, poorly defined or not consciously based on logical reason.
   C. All the attitudes, opinions and beliefs of a given person may not be consistent with each other. Some attitudes may conflict but be held in isolation from each other. (See Chapter 8.)
   D. Attitudes, opinions and beliefs are more likely to give force to behavior motivation and be resistant to change if:
      [1] The reasoning behind the attitude, opinion or belief is clearly defined.
      [2] The feeling or emotion associated with the attitude, opinion or belief is extreme.
      [3] The attitude, opinion or belief is consistent with the individual's other attitudes, opinions or beliefs.
      [4] The attitude, opinion or belief is approved of by the groups with which the individual identifies.
   E. An individual's attitudes, opinions and beliefs exert substantial influence on his behavior.
      [1] Attitudes, opinions and beliefs that consistently guide or motivate behavior are most resistant to change.
         a. A person whose attitudes, opinions and beliefs have strong emotional overtones resists suggestions for change, including "not hearing or seeing" data that would suggest change. There is a tendency to avoid contact with new or opposing ideas.
         b. When a person consciously commits himself to an attitude, opinion or belief, the commitment itself serves as a further barrier to change.
         c. When a person receives support for his attitudes, opinions and beliefs from others he perceives as significant, he is less likely to change.
      [2] Attitudes, opinions and beliefs may be used to organize experience and give meaning to behavior.
      [3] The expression of attitudes, opinions and beliefs may be used to gain position in desired social groups.
      [4] Attitudes, opinions and beliefs influence perceptual experience by directing attention, by shaping the interpretation of data to fit the attitudes, opinions and beliefs, and by guiding the "selectiveness" of perceptions.
   F. Attitudes, opinions and beliefs are formed in the process of growth and development.
      [1] Most attitudes, opinions and beliefs are culturally determined, the earliest and strongest determinants being the family group and the child-rearing practices of parents.
      [2] The growth and change of attitudes, opinions and beliefs occur slowly as a result of several factors:
         a. Change in group identity.

   b. Enforced changes in behavior.
   c. New learning through information or different experiences with the object, person or event in question.
   d. Perceived changes in the object, person or event in question.
   e. Use of reason in the presence of one or more of the above factors.

Nursing Care

Constructive nursing care in relation to cognition and attitudes, opinions and beliefs can be achieved by the nurse in the following ways.

1. The nurse should increase her understanding of cognitive function and the relationship of opinions, beliefs and attitudes to physiological and psychological well-being.
2. The nurse should orient her observations of the patient to determine the patient's:
   A. Clearness and rationality of thinking.
   B. Deviations from accepted "normal" cognitive function.
   C. Emotional states that might influence rational thinking.
   D. Environment, as it might influence cognitive function.
   E. Physiological state, as it might influence or be influenced by cognitive function.
   F. Individual thinking habits or styles of thinking.
   G. Age, in relation to thinking and attitudinal behavior.
   H. Demonstration of attitudes, opinions and beliefs as they relate to illness, care and treatment, hospitalization.
   I. Factors in the environment that might influence or be in conflict with opinions, ideas, attitudes and beliefs.
3. The nurse must use her knowledge of cognitive function and the formation of attitudes, opinions and beliefs, and their influences on behavior, as well as her observations of the individual patient, as a basis for planning nursing approach and intervention.
   A. When interacting with a confused person, the nurse should:
      [1] Avoid ambiguity and multiplicity of stimuli.
      [2] Not demand immediate responses involving reasoning and/or prolonged attention.
      [3] Provide frequent reorientation; make simple directive statements or requests.
      [4] Provide environmental support for orientation (such as written signs, objects the person may recognize).
      [5] Promote frequent patient contact with calm, supportive people.
   B. When interacting with a person under emotional strain or in an exaggerated emotional state, the nurse should:
      [1] Avoid demands on reasoning abilities; avoid increasing tension or the exaggeration of emotion.
      [2] Provide emotional support when problem solving is unavoidable.

[3] Create distractions from emotions or tension-causing factors while problem solving is in progress.

[4] Give clear and simple directions requiring less work in thinking.

C. If a person is delusional or irrational, the nurse should:

[1] Avoid arguing with him or ridiculing his ideas.

[2] Not introduce problems or environmental factors that would come into
direct and open conflict with delusional content.

[3] Not attempt prolonged reasoning or expect that reasoning is possible while
the person is irrational.

[4] Provide adequate observation and other safety measures to prevent the
person from harming himself or others.

[5] Provide unobtrusive reminders of reality that do not demand choice between delusional content and reality.

[6] Give kind, firm, simple direction when direction is necessary but may be
in conflict with delusional or irrational ideas.

D. For the person who demonstrates functional physiological states or subjective
symptoms unsupported by pathology, the nurse should:

[1] Avoid drawing attention to the symptom or state; showing rejection,
hostility or ridicule; or providing secondary gains by giving sympathy and
attention to his symptoms or state.

[2] Provide opportunity for the person to function normally without drawing
attention to any inconsistency between his symptoms or state and normal
function.

[3] Give emotional support while the person mentally and verbally works
through problems related to his symptoms or state.

[4] Give good physical nursing care to relieve discomfort regardless of cause
of symptoms.

[5] Give attention and emotional satisfaction for behavior or achievements not
related to his condition.

E. If a person is acutely ill and/or in need of large amounts of rest for recovery,
the nurse must avoid demands on cognitive function and not expect optimal
cognitive function.

F. The nurse should provide the best possible climate for cognitive function,
including:

[1] Keeping the environment conducive to optimal cognitive function (e.g.,
controlling distracting factors; avoiding thought-directing events that
interfere with the problem at hand; introducing thought-directing events
conducive to the problem at hand).

[2] Reducing physiological discomfort or need states that interfere with
adequate cognitive function (e.g., do not ask the patient to concentrate on
an important problem if he is hungry, thirsty or in pain).

[3] Providing needed information; asking thought-provoking questions;
providing a supportive and nonjudgmental attitude while the person
verbally works through problems.

[4] Acting as a sounding board, asking helpful questions and providing

information as the person attempts to remember and correct his memory for greatest accuracy.

[5] If the person is isolated from others for long periods or is a child away from family and peers, providing the opportunity for development and adequate function of cognitive faculties by planning varied perceptual stimulation; allowing him communicative contact with others and the opportunity to assist in planning his own care and solving his own problems; and adjusting demands on cognitive function to the individual's developmental level and/or handicap state.

[6] Avoiding conflicts with the individual's particular style of thinking:

   a. Avoid demands on the person who demonstrates rigid thinking patterns (and associated personality characteristics) to adjust to new ideas and routines unnecessarily, particularly if the person is in an unusually stressful situation.

      i. Increase emotional support when illness and hospitalization place increased demands on the person for adjustment to new ideas, situations or circumstances.

      ii. Provide for successful experiences with new ideas, situations or behavior, and for ego-building experiences in general. (Avoid actions that would lower self-esteem and the ability to use flexible thinking patterns.)

      iii. Prevent reinforcement of rigid thinking habits and associated personality characteristics by avoiding punitive and/or restrictive attitudes and practices.

   b. Avoid demands on the person who demonstrates flexible thinking habits and associated personality characteristics to conform to rigid rules and regulations, unless absolutely necessary. The nurse can foster flexible thinking habits by:

      i. Allowing maximum participation of the patient in planning his own care.

      ii. Providing reasons and information regarding actions that must be required.

      iii. Providing nonjudgmental supportive attitudes as the person thinks through problems caused by illness or health-related events.

      iv. Avoiding rejective or hostile attitudes if the patient finds solutions to problems that do not necessarily fit with the nurse's preconceived ideas.

   c. Avoid demands for abstract thinking if the individual has a "concrete" orientation to problem solving. (Provide concrete, specific and literal information and interpretations; avoid ambiguous and highly abstract generalizations.)

   d. Expect that the person who is very ill or very threatened may regress and need more specific information coming from the environment. Also, expect a greater need for specifics among those who are mentally retarded, schizophrenic or suffering from brain damage.

G. Make use of the individual's existing attitudes, opinions and beliefs whenever possible to effect optimal therapeutic care.

[1] Avoid assumptions about the individual's attitudes, opinions and beliefs until they have been assessed through communication with the individual concerned.

[2] Avoid criticism or rejection of the person whose attitudes, opinions and beliefs are different from one's own.

[3] Avoid, unless necessary for optimal health care, increasing tension or conflict for the individual by avoiding pointing out conflicts among his attitudes, opinions and beliefs or behavior.

[4] Avoid, unless necessary for optimal health care, demanding behavior of the individual that would be in conflict with his existing attitudes, opinions and beliefs.

[5] Attempt to show relationships between new behavior necessary for the person to acquire and his existing attitudes, opinions and beliefs.

H. When new attitudes, opinions or beliefs are necessary for optimal physical and/or mental health, the nurse should make use of what is known about attitude, opinion and belief formation to effect change with the least amount of psychological discomfort. For example, she should:

[1] Provide adequate information as the basis for changes.

[2] Promote the reasoning process in relation to change.

[3] Point out the relationship of changed attitudes, opinions and beliefs to valued goals or known motivations.

[4] Provide contact with persons who may be held in high esteem who have the desired attitudes, opinions or beliefs. (Contact may be through reading, movies, etc., as well as actual contact.)

[5] Provide supportive and pleasurable or rewarding experiences that reinforce the new attitude, opinion or belief.

4. The nurse should examine her own thinking habits, attitudes, opinions and beliefs, in order to determine how they may influence health care or her own development as an increasingly effective professional person.

Chapter 3

The Integrative Function: Development of Self-Concept

Psychological equilibrium requires adequate integration of all aspects of the individual's psychological processes.

Social Science Principles

1. Integrative processes are usually seen as a function of the "ego" or "self." Such terms as "ego integrity" and "personality integrity" are frequently used to denote the individual's total psychological integrative processes.
2. The "self," as experienced by the individual, is an organized and enduring perception, involving integrated processes of perceiving, feeling and thinking.
   A. Included in the concept of self is the concept of body image. (Body image is one of the earliest self-concepts to be developed.)
      [1] Physiological changes occurring in the normal process of growth and development usually necessitate changes in body image (e.g., physical growth spurts and maturation during adolescence and the alterations in size, shape, structure and function that accompany aging).
      [2] When body image must be changed as a result of unexpected physiological changes (surgery, injury), the total concept of self is threatened, resulting in psychological tension or anxiety.
      [3] Body image is usually so firmly established that any necessary changes are accomplished slowly (e.g., after amputation, imagined body image still retains the absent limb for some time, including the physical sensation of its presence; a person who has been very heavy for a long time and has

lost much weight continues to walk, act or use mannerisms appropriate to his previous weight.)

B. The concept of self exists in relation to one's total psychological environment, including what one sees as the world or worlds in which he may function.

[1] Changes in one aspect of a person's psychological environment necessitate readjustment of the total concept of self and self-function.

[2] Gross changes in self-concept necessitated by changes in psychological environment are usually accompanied by increased stress, tension, uncertainty and loss of a sense of direction.

C. The concept of self includes a culturally determined self or ego ideal (the concept of what one ought to be), against which the individual measures his actual behavior and achievement.

3. The concept of self is acquired through the process of growth and development.

A. Development of self-identity follows a characteristic order of development:

[1] Sense of bodily self.

[2] Sense of continuous self as separate from others and from the environment.

[3] Sense of self-esteem.

B. The infant has no sense of "self" as separate from the environment. Sense of self develops slowly over the first 5 to 6 years of life, the most rapid growth occurring after the acquisition of language.

C. During the early stages of developing self-identity, fantasy and reality merge and separate on an uneven course. By the age of 4 to 6 years, the child still occasionally merges fantasy with reality (as with imaginary playmates) but can identify other "selves."

D. During the first few years of self-identity development, the child is ego-centered, seeing the world as existing for his benefit and without any purpose separate from himself.

E. Between the ages of 4 to 6, the child develops the concepts of:

[1] Self-extension (e.g., "I" as a separate person, with "my" as object of ownership).

[2] Self-ideal (e.g., what "I" should or ought to be and do).

F. Between the ages of 6 and 12, the child gradually develops the ability to use his self as a mediating instrument to cope with the world rationally (e.g., he learns to think and to think about thinking).

G. Further development of adequate integrative function during adolescence is marked by:

[1] Increased efforts at conscious self-identity, characterized by the demonstrated need to be a separate self, apart from the peer group.

[2] Confusion and contradiction, particularly in some societies, caused by the need to become a definite separate self and at the same time retain identification with peer groups.

[3] Prolonged sensory deprivation may result in disturbance of self-concept or the sense of self. Ego identity requires constant reminders that the self is

separate from others, as provided by contact with the environment (e.g., being referred to by name, being reacted to as a separate and autonomous organism, experiencing reactions from the environment that indicate other, separate individuals and objects).

[4] Adequate personality integration requires some degree of satisfaction of basic primary and acquired needs. (See Chapter 7.)

[5] Adequate personality integration and/or ego function requires that an individual participate with and be accepted by other individuals and groups of individuals.

    a. Ego integrity requires that an individual be able to identify with other individuals.

    b. Adequate self-concept requires that the individual have the opportunity to learn and subsequently achieve satisfaction in practicing sociocultural roles.

[6] One of the methods by which individuals learn the sociocultural limits for ego function is through identification with other individuals.

[7] One of the methods by which the individual learns the sociocultural limits for ego-determined behavior is through "reality testing."

[8] A person who has acquired flexible methods of adaptation adjusts to life situations with greater ease and satisfaction than one whose methods are rigid and uncompromising.

4. If self-concept or ego integrity is disrupted, disorganization of personality results. (See Chapter 8.)

Nursing Care

**The nurse can increase and maintain effectiveness of nursing
care in relation to integrative function in the following ways.**

1. She can increase her knowledge of human psychological integrative processes in order to understand patient behavior and needs and to understand her own behavior as it relates to health care.

2. The nurse can guide her observations of patients and their environment to determine:

    A. How the individual sees himself, particularly in relation to his illness and/or hospitalization. (She should observe for expressions of self-doubt, self-assurance, autonomy; orientation toward family, friends, hospital personnel, work roles; ability to adapt to hospital experiences and health-promoting procedures.)

    B. Any indications of disturbance of integrative function, particularly if illness and/or hospitalization requires changes in self-concept (e.g., evidences of increased anxiety, confusion and doubt; depression; refusal to participate in necessary therapeutic procedures that will alter either body image or social image; regression to earlier forms of integrative function).

    C. Indications of the individual's stage of growth and development of ego struc-

ture and function. (In working with children, is the child's integrative behavior appropriate to his chronological age?)

D. Factors or situations in the environment or caused by illness and/or hospitalization that might disrupt integrative function (e.g., experiences the patient
might be subjected to, such as attitudes of hospital personnel, family and
friends; therapeutic procedures that might lower self-esteem and/or sense of
individuality and autonomy; isolation procedures that might be destructive to
self-concept).

3. The nurse should use both her knowledge and observations to guide health care
planning in order to maintain integrative function at an optimal level and/or to
assist in further development of integrative function. She can, for example:

A. Provide opportunity for the individual who is sustaining a change in body
image or social image to talk with supportive, nonjudgmental, informed persons, in order to gradually incorporate change and its implications for future
living (e.g., allowing questions and discussion of possible future behavior,
expression of feeling about changes).

[1] If possible or necessary, provide positive experiences in relation to
changes (e.g., observation of others who have benefited from similar
changes; opportunity to experiment successfully with the "new" self in
a protected environment).

[2] Avoid unnecessary demands for adjustment to life situations until the individual has had an opportunity to "get used to" his altered self-concept.
(The nurse must not push the person faster than he is able to develop.)

B. Through attitudes, information and positive experiences, provide opportunity
for the patient to adjust changes in his self-concept to his previous concept
of ideal self (e.g., if changes are in conflict with previous ego ideal, provide
positive experiences to help the patient alter his concept of "ideal").

C. Adapt health care of children and adolescents to provide for maximum
growth and development of integrative processes.

[1] Allow maximum autonomy consistent with age level and physical or
psychological safety.

[2] Provide consistency in attitudes of health occupations personnel toward
the individual, including attempts to avoid conflict with parental attitudes, unless parental attitudes are deemed actually harmful.

[3] If appropriate to age level, provide reasons for nursing actions and required patient behavior, requesting cooperation rather than blind compliance with rules.

[4] Provide adequate sensory experiences and contact with the environment.

a. In direct contact with the child, communication should point out "self-
hood" and extensions of self, as well as relationships of self to environment.

b. Provision should be made for maximal opportunity to interact with
other children and objects, consistent with health requirements.

[5] Avoid punitive, rejecting and rigid attitudes and behavior in general, particularly when the child or adolescent experiments with limits of self-
direction.

[6] Alter her attitudes and behavior to the most constructive degree, reflecting respect for the individual and approval of self-directed actions and variations in adaptive behaviors; showing warmth, caring, and patience with uncertainty, fear and inconsistent changes in direction.

[7] Increase contact with parents or known and trusted persons, who can affirm ego identity, particularly when self-concept is threatened by illness and/or hospitalization. (Attitudes should reflect faith in the *continuous* existence of the child as a cared-for and esteemed person, regardless of permanent or temporary disruptions of usual existence.)

D. Provide supportive nursing care whenever integrative function and structure are threatened. For example, the nurse can:

[1] Increase efforts to help the patient retain his individual indentity and sense of worth.

[2] Increase positive contacts with hospital personnel, family and friends (e.g., assign the patient to the most "person-oriented" staff rather than the most "task-oriented" staff).

[3] Increase efforts to permit verbal expression of fears, uncertainties and disturbing emotions in the presence of warmly supportive people, who can accept the patient's feelings without needing to deny the validity or necessity of such feelings.

[4] Increase efforts to avoid additional demands for change and/or conformity to behavior that might be inconsistent with the patient's self-concept.

4. See Chapter 8 for additional nursing actions.

Chapter 4

Communication

Psychological equilibrium requires that the individual have adequate means for communication with others and for self-expression.

Social Science Principles*

1. Communication between individuals takes place in a variety of ways.
   A. Every culture provides a symbolic means for communication between individuals and groups of individuals.
   B. In order for symbols to be used effectively in communication, they must be mutually understood.
   C. Nonverbal behavior is an essential part of the communication process.
   D. The total complex of interactive and interrelationship behavior constitutes continuous communication between individuals and groups of individuals (i.e., an understanding of communication processes requires an understanding and analysis of all interactive behavior).
2. Communication is influenced by a variety of internal and external factors.
   A. Communication between individuals is influenced by the relationship that exists between them (i.e., communication is influenced by the perceptions that the message sender and the message receiver have of each other).

* Most of the information pertinent to communication is included in other chapters. For example, an understanding of communication processes would be impossible without first understanding perception—the first step in message reception is, after all, perception. At the same time, the learning and use of language symbols is central to the development of cognitive function, but language symbols cannot be learned apart from cognitive function. And, the complex relationships developed in the satisfaction of human needs would be literally impossible without communicative interaction. Therefore, in a sense, all the material in other chapters is a part of the human communication process. This chapter contains only those few generalizations not already included in other chapters or those generalizations needed to show relationships between the concept of communication and concept statements included in other chapters. It does not include either validated principles or current theories about abnormal patterns of communication found in mental illness.

[1] The more a person is trusted or viewed as a prestige person, the more likely others are to accept his communication as valid and acceptable without alteration.

[2] Messages received from persons perceived as less trustworthy or of less prestige tend to be discredited or distorted.

[3] If the communicator is liked but the message has negative or unpleasant connotations, the message tends to be distorted or "rationalized" to fit with the opinion held about the communicator.

[4] Reception and interpretation of a given message is influenced by the degree of expertness assigned to the message sender.

[5] Reception and interpretation of a given message is influenced by what the recipient believes to be the intent of the message sender (e.g., persuasion, evasion, kindness, harm).

[6] Message-sending and -receiving is influenced by stereotyped categorization or perception of each other by sender and receiver (e.g., a patient's stereotyped perception of "social worker," or a nurse's stereotyped perception of "psychotic").

B. In addition to the relationship of the communicators, reception and interpretation of messages is influenced by a variety of factors, such as:

[1] The situation in which communication takes place, which includes:

a. What the recipient perceives as expected behavior in response to the communication (i.e., what the message requires him to do, such as act in support of the message or reinterpret the message to others in his own words).

b. The presence of others in the situation (e.g., when other people are present who might inhibit response or cause response to be altered because of known attitudes or later consequences of response to the communication).

c. Concentration of attention on environmental events and distracting influences in the environment.

d. The general tone or atmosphere of the environment (e.g., a schoolroom as opposed to a kitchen).

[2] The internal state, personality characteristics and other factors relative to the individuals involved in the communication.

a. Preoccupation with personal matters and/or the presence of thoughts regarding emotionally charged subjects may interfere with an individual's ability to receive, interpret, respond to and send messages.

b. A message is more likely to be received if its content is personally desired or pleasing or if it fits existing attitudes, ideas and beliefs.

c. A message is more likely to be ignored or distorted if its content has negative connotations for the recipient or if it does not fit preexisting attitudes, ideas and beliefs.

d. The educational level of the recipient of messages influences the effectiveness of various types of communication media.

i. An individual with a higher level of education tends to make more adequate use of written communicative material.

ii. An individual with a lower level of education tends to respond more efficiently to aural and visual communication media and less efficiently to printed words alone.

e. Message reception and interpretation are subject to the same processes as perception in general (e.g., omission of data to simplify complex messages, selective attention to details, filling in of data to complete percepts or concepts in order to form whole patterns).

f. Message reception and interpretation are influenced by the appeal of the message to emotion versus cognition (i.e., if the message has elements evoking fear, the reception and interpretation of the message is different than if it appeals primarily to reason).

g. The interpretation of communicative symbols is limited to meanings made possible by the experience of the recipient, regardless of any possible meanings those symbols might have for others.

h. Message reception and interpretation are influenced by the individual's need, interest or motivation state (e.g., a message relative to a need state is more likely to be attended to if the need existed prior to the message).

i. Message reception and interpretation are influenced by social and personality characteristics of recipients and senders (e.g., a chronically anxious, insecure person attends to and interprets messages differently than an individual who has a stable self-concept, characterized by high self-esteem and an ability to tolerate threat). Current literature suggests that:

   i. Persons who are consistently hostile and aggressive or who are consistently withdrawn from interactions with others are less easily influenced by persuasive communication.

   ii. Persons who are capable of vivid imagery tend to respond empathically.

   iii. Persons who have lower self-esteem and higher dependency levels are more easily influenced by persuasive communication.

j. Communication is altered by an individual's physiological or psychophysiological state (e.g., state of consciousness, ability to hear or see, reaction to medications such as sedatives, toxic states).

k. Communication is influenced by the perceptive and cognitive ability of the individual (his current emotional state, his integrative abilities, and so forth).

l. A reciprocal relationship exists between learning and communication (i.e., much of human learning is not possible without adequate communicative ability, and adequate communication depends on learning).

[3] Reception and interpretation of messages are influenced by the way a message is organized for presentation (i.e., the order of presentation of parts of the message, the relationship of the message to environmental events).

3. Problems in communication frequently arise because of inattention to certain characteristics of message-sending and reception, for example:

A. The content and intent of messages, as well as reception and interpretation of messages, depend upon the frames of reference of the individuals involved.

B. Difficulty in transmission and reception of messages may be increased if the participants in communication use specialized verbal symbols, form a personal compression of complex ideas into single symbols or use vague symbols or ambiguous generalizations.

C. Difficulties in communication occur because of individual assignment of values to symbols used and the assumption that others involved in communication assign the same values to those symbols.

D. Problems in communication often arise because participants in the communication process draw inferences from inadequate data.

E. Difficulties in communication are increased because a given communicative symbol usually has both a denotative meaning and a connotative meaning. Although the denotative meaning may be the same for all individuals, the connotative meaning may vary widely from individual to individual (e.g., a cross may be, in the dictionary sense, the same to several people but have quite different emotional or evaluative meanings for people with different religious backgrounds and experiences).

F. Difficulties in communication are increased because messages may have both a literal meaning and an underlying or subtle meaning not obvious in interpretation of the actual symbols used.

[1] A mother, while visiting a neighbor, may observe her own child doing something that displeases her. She may say, "Johnny, I think it's about time we went home." The message may have both literal meaning, in terms of time of day and length of visit, and subtle meaning, such as "You, Johnny, have committed a social error, and you're going to catch it when you get home."

[2] The same characteristic of messages or symbolic conventions may facilitate communication and interpersonal relationships. For example, "Good morning, how are you?" is usually a symbolic communication that does not require a literal answer but carries with it the intent to convey interest in the individual and a desire to begin communication.

G. Difficulties in communication (and therefore in responsive relationships) occur if the verbal message is not consistent with the nonverbal message, regardless of the intent of the communicator.

H. Difficulties in communication occur if the message is overloaded (carries more content than the recipient can take in), disorganized, ambiguous or has too many diverse elements. (In general, communication is subject to the same difficulties as perception.)

Nursing Care

Effective nursing care depends largely upon the nurse's effective use of communication skills and knowledge.

1. The nurse should increase her knowledge and understanding of the process of communication and of the relationship of communication processes to all other psychological functions.

2. A nurse should guide her observation of the patient and his environment and obtain feedback from the patient, in order to determine:
   A. The individual patient's personality characteristics, sociocultural background and educational and intellectual developmental levels, as they influence communication in general.
   B. Factors in the environment that may influence specific communication.
   C. Frames of reference of the patient in relation to specific communications.
   D. Current physical and psychological states that might influence specific communication.
   E. Characteristics of various relationships that might influence specific communications (e.g., nurse-patient relationships, patient-doctor relationships).
   F. Indications that problems exist in communication in general, that specific communication processes are ineffective or that the patient's communication patterns deviate from normal.

3. The nurse can use her knowledge of the communication process and her observations of a specific patient to plan nursing interventions. She can:
   A. Avoid use of specialized language symbols, vague referents, or language symbols outside the patient's experience, in communicating with the patient.
   B. Be careful to obtain feedback from the patient to determine the actual message he has received.
   C. Attempt to correct misinterpretations and distortions of messages, as determined through feedback.
   D. Be alert to nonverbal communicative behavior of the patient, and of her own nonverbal behavior, which might have unintended meaning for the patient.
   E. Avoid discrepancy between verbal and nonverbal messages.
   F. Attempt to establish a relationship of trust that will facilitate effective communication.
   G. Avoid communicative responses to the patient based on stereotyped perceptions (i.e., get to know the patient as an individual, not as a typed representative of some sociocultural group).
   H. Use her knowledge of the role of emotion, perception, and motivation in the organization and presentation of communication to allow for maximum communication effectiveness.
   I. Avoid giving important messages when the patient is in an unreceptive state (e.g., when the patient is upset, semiconscious, sedated, highly distracted).
   J. Alter communications to fit the patient's current state and current environmental situation.
   K. Alter the environment when possible or necessary in order to achieve maximum benefit from communication efforts.
   L. Plan for patient learning experiences that will increase communicative ability when necessary or appropriate.
   M. Alter health care situations which would isolate the individual from communicative or other sensory experience.

Chapter 5

Emotional Behavior

Emotion is a basic psychological experience common to man; it has a wide variety of effects, both constructive and nonconstructive, on total psychological equilibrium.

Social Science Principles

1. Emotion is demonstrated or reflected in subjective feeling states, emotion-generated behavior and adaptive changes.
   A. Emotions are related to situational events. Certain situations tend to evoke certain feelings and are usually sought or avoided, depending upon the total physical and psychological state.
      [1] Joy is a desired and usually sought emotional experience accompanying tension release or goal achievement.
      [2] Anger is an uncomfortable and usually avoided emotional experience accompanying the accumulation of tension or goal frustration.
      [3] Fear is an unpleasant and usually avoided emotional experience accompanying danger to the life of the organism or damage to it, especially when the individual perceives himself as unable to avoid or eliminate the threat.
      [4] Grief is an unpleasant and usually avoided emotional experience accompanying loss of something valued.
      [5] Pride is a pleasant and usually sought emotional reaction to goal achievement in accord with ego ideals.
      [6] Shame is an unpleasant and usually avoided emotional reaction to goal failure, when the goal was important to the maintenance of self-esteem.
      [7] Embarrassment or self-consciousness is an unpleasant and therefore

avoided emotional reaction to perceiving oneself as an actual or potential object of criticism, dislike or ridicule.

    a. Criticism is usually interpreted and felt to be a sign that one is inadequate, incompetent or unworthy.

    b. Embarrassment or self-consciousness may interfere with the clarity of rational thought and action.

[8] Loneliness is an unpleasant and usually avoided emotional experience accompanying real or perceived isolation from other human beings. (Identification of oneself with other individuals or groups of individuals is necessary to decrease or eliminate loneliness.)

[9] A given group of similar or related emotions sustained over time is referred to as a "mood" (e.g., sadness, happiness, anxiety).

B. The expression of feeling or emotion may be achieved through a variety of behavior and adaptive reactions. In addition to the commonly recognized vocal and nonvocal expressions and the psychological and physiological manifestations of emotion, there may be:

[1] Energy generated by an emotion that must be repressed, which tends to be expended in disguised, indirect ways.

    a. Feelings that cannot be directly expressed toward the object or the individual engendering the feeling may be displaced onto other symbolic or convenient objects or individuals.

    b. Illness and/or physical symptoms (physiological phenomena) may be used as a method of expressing unconscious feelings.

[2] Crying, usually an effective form of behavior for relieving tension or expressing emotion that cannot be otherwise expressed.

[3] The presence of strong emotion that alters cognitive function (e.g., anger may interfere with rational problem-solving; various emotions may lead to impulsive rather than reasoned behavior; exaggerated fear may lead to confusion and irrationality).

[4] A prevailing mood, which influences all other psychological experiences, including perception, cognition and motivation.

C. Emotional experience is related in complex ways to total physiological and psychological function. In addition to the above statements (#B):

[1] Experiencing emotion to any degree requires expenditure of energy.

[2] Emotional reactions influence and are influenced by nervous system function, and physiological correlates to emotion can be demonstrated.

[3] Emotional reactions and their physiological correlates, when sustained over a period of time, can result in physiological structural changes (e.g., hypertension, ulcerative colitis, gastric ulcers).

[4] The experiencing of an unpleasant emotion or mood usually has negative effects on total physiological and psychological function (e.g., promotes disequilibrium: profound and prolonged depression may be accompanied by general metabolic retardation, cognitive confusion and dullness).

[5] The experiencing of pleasant emotion or mood usually has positive effects on total psychological and physiological function (e.g., promotes equi-

librium: a state of joy or happiness tends to be accompanied by a feeling of physical well-being, energy, motivation toward constructive action, ability to sustain problem-solving efforts).

[6] An individual who experiences pleasant emotions at reasonable intervals over time is more likely to be able to adapt to frustrations and other unpleasant emotions than an individual who rarely experiences a pleasant emotion.

2. Emotional experiences are influenced by a variety of circumstances.
   A. Environmental situations or changes influence emotions. In addition to situations cited in all of #1, above:
   [1] Emotion may be controlled or manipulated by diverting one's attention from events causing the emotional reaction.
   [2] Emotional states may be altered by environmental stimuli, such as object colors and arrangements, introduction of pleasant or unpleasant sounds, introduction or removal of objects having agreeable or disagreeable associations.
   B. Emotion or feeling may be altered by changing one's perception of an object or event (e.g., introducing new elements, pointing attention to isolated aspects of an event, fostering mental rearrangement of data, seeing examples of different reactions to the same event by different people).
   C. Emotional reactions are influenced by ideational content and cognitive processes.
   D. Any given emotion tends to be blunted or decreased if sustained over time (e.g., fatigue occurs with overstimulation and sameness).
   E. Emotion tends to be contagious, i.e., to be transmitted to others in the environment.
   F. Emotion is influenced by the individual's physiological state (e.g., in addition to statements under #1C, above, exhaustion and malnourishment are usually accompanied by depression).
   G. Verbalization of problems causing tension and emotion in the presence of a nonjudgmental but receptive listener may temporarily or permanently reduce the degree of emotion or tension.

3. Some varieties of emotional experience are learned in the process of growth and development, and others are thought to be basic (innate) or primitive emotions.
   A. Anger, fear and a general sensation of pleasure are thought to be basic or primitive emotional reactions to appropriate stimuli.
   B. Self-appraising emotions are thought to be learned through interaction with others and experiencing approval or disapproval. (Such emotions include shame, pride, guilt.)
   [1] Self-appraising emotions, along with the learning of attitudes and values used for self-appraisal, tend to be influenced by the reactions of others, even after the basic emotion has been learned (e.g., the expression of criticism, disapproval or disgust by others tends to arouse shame or guilt, even when the adult, through conscious self-appraisal, may know that the attitudes are unjust or not well-founded).

[2] Negative self-appraising emotions may be generated by internalized attitudes and values when behavior fails to be consistent with such values, regardless of external approval.

[3] Experiencing vague or ambiguous disapproval may result in a feeling of guilt unattached to a specific object or event. As a result, the individual tends to feel that he is a "bad" person rather than that he has committed a wrong act.

    a. If the child, in the process of growth and development of self-concept, is continuously subjected to ambiguous attitudes that label him as a "bad" person, he will be less able to function with self-assurance, autonomy and freedom from restrictive unattached guilt.

C. Differentiation of basic primitive emotional reactions into specifically identifiable subcategories occurs as a result of interaction with others (e.g., general pleasure is differentiated as joy, love, sensory pleasure, and so forth, through identification with others and the variety in experiences causing the reactions).

Nursing Care

**In order to plan nursing care that is consistently therapeutic, the
nurse should implement her knowledge of emotional behavior.**

1. The nurse should increase her understanding of emotional processes and their relationships to health and well-being.

2. The nurse can guide her observations of the patient and his environment in order to determine:

    A. The patient's current emotional state: as related to a specific event, as part of a prevailing mood or as emotional reaction patterns typical of the specific patient.

    B. The effect of events necessitated by illness and/or hospitalization on the patient's emotional state.

    C. Aspects of the environment that will most likely cause specific emotional reactions.

3. The nurse should utilize both her knowledge of emotional processes and her observations of the individual patient to plan nursing interventions. For example, she should:

    A. Promote situations, experiences or events that increase pleasurable emotions.

    B. Attempt to control or eliminate unnecessary situations, experiences or events that increase unpleasant emotions.

    C. Intervene if a specific emotion is detrimental to health care, for example:

        [1] Avoiding emotion-producing actions if the patient needs total energy for physical restorative processes.

        [2] Using distraction or environmental manipulation to alter existing undesirable emotions or moods.

        [3] Introducing new ideas and accompanying discussion which will alter mood or emotional reaction, eventually altering the patient's perception or his emotion- or mood-producing life situations.

[4] Decreasing anger or other undesirable emotions before the patient is required to take rational action or make problem-solving decisions.

[5] Actually controlling impulsive or irrational behavior caused by emotion if the emotion cannot be reduced and rationality restored in time to prevent harm to the patient or others.

[6] Through her knowledge of the nervous system and physiological correlates of emotion, attempting to prevent the experiencing of emotions detrimental to specific health conditions (e.g., avoiding anger for hypertensive patients, excitement for coronary patients).

D. Attempt to induce the mood or emotional reaction most consistent with the achievement of other desired goals (e.g., helping the patient to feel comfortable, pleased with himself and his surroundings, oriented toward pride-producing action before introducing a new idea or action that will require effort; reducing or preventing the experiencing of disgust, anger, fear, embarrassment before meals or in relation to elimination procedures).

E. Provide for adequate expression of emotion in the most direct fashion, consistent with patient safety and well-being (e.g., allowing the patient to express anger, fear and frustration, without guilt, punishment or retaliation).

F. Avoid demonstrating emotional reactions that might negatively influence the patient but attempt to demonstrate moods and emotional reactions that might positively influence the patient.

G. When planning patient care, take into account and be aware of the patient's physical condition (including reactions to medications) that might influence mood or emotional reactions (e.g., the patient who has been physically exhausted by therapeutic procedures and who has been without food for several hours will be in no "mood" to assimilate new information about sodium-free dietary restrictions).

H. In caring for children, organize nursing care to promote healthy experiences and the expression of emotion, for example:

[1] Avoiding demonstrations of ambiguous, generalized disgust, criticism or rejection. (If criticism is deemed necessary, it will be most constructive if specifically related to isolated behavior that is objectionable and can be changed.)

[2] Allowing and promoting a full range of emotional experience and expression consistent with health and well-being, including social well-being (e.g., anger can be safely expressed in some ways, but it must be controlled to prevent destruction. Any emotion and its expression can be considered "normal" and/or permissible, if the expression is consistent with safety of others and goals of self).

[3] Planning for experiences that will elicit expressions of approval from others (thus stimulating pride and self-assurance).

[4] Avoiding experiences that cause unnecessary shame and embarrassment; making provision for supportive attitudes when shame and embarrassment cannot be avoided.

4. The nurse should examine and evaluate her own emotional reactions to determine possible effect, on nursing actions.

Chapter 6

Growth and Development, Learning and Adaptive Problem-Solving

Maintenance of psychological equilibrium requires that the individual have the opportunity for positive growth and development experiences, for learning in general and for the acquisition of adaptive problem-solving behavior in particular.

Social Science Principles

1. Patterns of behavior are learned in the process of growth and development.*
    A. The development of behavior reflects maturation through growth, as well as the cumulative effects of learning through experience.
        [1] Overall physical and mental growth curves run parallel courses, with the rate of growth showing a drop at puberty.
        [2] Growth and development follow an uneven course; not all aspects of function mature at the same rate at the same time.
        [3] Gross, general patterns of behavior precede differentiated behavior, with structure and function becoming increasingly differentiated (e.g., the in-

---

* Where appropriate, growth and development principles have been included in other chapters. For example, some growth and development aspects of perception, cognitive function, and integrative function have been included in the appropriate chapters for more expedient organization of material.

fant demonstrates total organismic reaction rather than differentiated emotional response to situations normally calling for differentiated response).

[4] In cortical development, sensory and motor areas develop first, and association areas develop later. (Simple conditioning may be possible at relatively early ages, while complex percepts and problem-solving functions are impossible until later.)

[5] At adolescence, physical and intellectual growth decelerates, except for the accelerating development of the sexual system.

[6] When an individual must give up behaviors of one stage of development prior to or during progress to a higher level of development, disequilibrium occurs, with its concommitent stresses. (See Chapter 8.)

[7] Success or lack of success in achieving the tasks of one stage of development affects the success or lack of success in achieving tasks of later stages of development (e.g., failure to develop trust in early stages of development interferes with development of autonomy and initiative in later stages of development.)

B. According to the best of current knowledge, various emotional experiences seem to have certain effects on growth and development.

[1] Evidence collected to date indicates that single or isolated traumatic events do not usually result in major or lasting effects on personality.

[2] Excessive degrees of anxiety and insecurity experienced in connection with need satisfaction and training practices seem to result in the belief, continuing into adult life, that people cannot be trusted.

[3] Parental attitudes seem to have substantial influence on subsequent adult behavior.

   a. The child who receives little affection, satisfaction of dependency needs, warmth or tenderness is likely to progress toward maturity more slowly, to experience more problems in adjustment, to be more apathetic and less able to exercise independent action and to have a more slowly developed and less definite sense of self.

   b. Rejection by parents seems to cause insecurity and self-devaluation. Rejection-induced insecurity and self-devaluation may result in hostile, negativistic, rebellious behavior; apathy, indifference and withdrawal from relationships in general; and an inability to give and receive affection freely.

   c. Maternal overprotection seems to produce behavior that interferes with adult adaptation.

      i. Indulgent maternal overprotection may cause selfishness, egocentrism, irresponsibility and low frustration-tolerance levels.

      ii. Dominating maternal overprotection may cause submissiveness, obedience, inadequacy, lack of initiative and passive dependence.

   d. Excessively severe discipline may cause an overdeveloped need for social approval, feelings of self-condemnation, and displaced hostility from parents to society in general.

   e. Inconsistent or insufficient discipline may cause inadequate development of self-control, vacillation in decision-making, and inability to work within highly structured social institutions.

f. Excessively strict moral standards may cause rigidity, guilt-producing conflicts, or generalized rebellion against moral restrictions.

g. When parental demands for achievement are started early, and the rewards for achievement are in the form of parental affection rather than material objects, the child is more likely to develop strong and lasting drives toward achievement.

h. Parental attitudes of consistent warmth and openness are more likely to help the child develop ability to relate to peers in a friendly, responsive way.

i. Greater dependency needs may be experienced in both early and subsequent stages of development if parental attitudes are rejective, overly rigid and restrictive during feeding and weaning phases of development.

j. Parental imposition of independent behavior before the child is ready to move toward independence is likely to produce anxiety and over-concern regarding independence as an adult.

[4] Prolonged separation of the child from parents and home (as in hospitalization) produces different effects on different children, depending upon the child's age and his relationship to his parents.

a. Prolonged separation is more likely to produce emotional and intellectual retardation in development if the child is between 3 months and 5 years old than if at other ages (e.g., less satisfactory peer or extrafamily relationships, delayed ability to express or experience affection, slower speech and cognitive development).

b. Up to the age of 5, the child who has had a better and closer relationship with his mother seems to suffer most from prolonged separation.

c. After the age of 5, the child who has had a better and closer relationship with his mother seems to suffer less from separation (e.g., can tolerate it better).

[5] Isolation, whether imposed by self or others, tends to promote personality disintegration at any age, with decreasing ability to maintain adequate psychological function or to achieve optimum growth and development.

C. Prevailing cultural attitudes may either impede or accelerate growth and development in several areas.

[1] For the adolescent, inconsistencies in social attitudes and demands may cause increased conflict, retarding adequate adjustment (e.g., in some societies, the adolescent is encouraged to accept adult attitudes and responsibilities and, at the same time, prohibited from any attempts at adult sexual behavior and independent life decisions).

[2] Identical child-training practices favored by different cultures may have different effects on children (e.g., the particular practice seems to have less definite effect than the significance of the practice for the child—that is, his perception of what the practice means in terms of his relationship to his parents).

[3] Role diffusion in a complex society may cause inability to develop, without anxiety or conflict, a clear self-concept. (Conflict due to role diffusion

may be particularly acute during adolescence, when the individual must identify and harmonize a variety of sociocultural roles to form a coherent self-identity.)

    [4] In order to live comfortably within sociocultural limits of behavior, the individual must have the opportunity to learn accepted roles, rules and codes of conduct.

        a. One of the methods by which individuals learn sociocultural limits for behavior is through testing and exploring the environment to determine results of specific behaviors (i.e., "reality testing").

        b. Individuals learn sociocultural limits of behavior through identification with others.

        c. Individuals learn sociocultural limits of behavior by having authority figures impose and enforce the limits.

        d. Personal definition and acceptance of a social role is learned through contact with a social environment in which the person has the opportunity to see and practice the designated role.

D. Any given age or stage of growth and development may be influenced by (defined by) the society in which the individual lives.

    [1] Contemporary historical events occurring during any given stage of growth and development may alter the outcomes of that particular stage (e.g., development of attitudes and values due to major wars, depressions, major social movements, major scientific or technological advancements that alter life styles.)

    [2] The process of growth and development is influenced by individual interaction with social, cultural and biologic factors to produce uniquely individual results.

2. Psychological equilibrium requires that the individual have and be able to utilize the ability and opportunity for learning.

A. Learning is influenced by a variety of internal and external factors.

    [1] Behavioral learning is most likely to be effective if the learner has the opportunity to try out the new behavior.

        a. For task-involved learning to be effective, practice should include as many sense experiences as possible.

        b. For ego-involved learning to be effective, practice should include behaviors that are motivated by goals, motives, interests and self-concept.

    [2] Disturbing emotional factors may interfere with effective learning. In extremely tense or traumatic situations, an individual may need frequent repetition of what is to be learned or repeated successful experiences before learning takes place.

    [3] A behavior that obtains an adequate response in one situation is likely to be repeated in similar situations.

        a. Once a person has learned a response to a given situation, he tends to generalize that response to other situations (e.g., if the situation or certain parts of the situation are similar, the first response will be in accord with past learning).

      b. When a behavior no longer obtains expected results, the behavior tends to disappear. An unreinforced behavior disappears slowly or rapidly, depending on the strength of the original stimulus and the amount of emotion involved in original learning.

[4] First impressions are likely to be the most lasting impressions, tending to shape or influence subsequent impressions.

[5] In complex learning, acquisition is more effective if separate parts of a whole are studied intensely and later put together to form a whole made up of related parts.

[6] Acquisition of knowledge (memorization) is influenced by a variety of factors.

      a. Boredom, fatigue, exaggerated emotional states and negative motivation decrease efficiency of acquiring knowledge.

      b. Information encountered at the beginning and end of a learning period is more likely to be learned with ease than information encountered in the middle of a learning period.

      c. Information that has meaning in the life context of the individual is more efficiently learned.

      d. Acquisition of knowledge generally proceeds more rapidly if it is distributed and spaced over time rather than in long, uninterrupted sessions.

      e. Active participation or motion by the learner assists the process of memorization (e.g., speaking, writing, moving objects, as opposed to reading alone).

      f. Acquisition of knowledge is facilitated if material is grouped into meaningful units.

[7] The changing of concepts or perceptions may be facilitated by the separation of parts from a whole for concentrated attention.

[8] The changing of concepts or perceptions may be facilitated by the addition of new information or experience that necessitates reinterpretation or reorganization of originally held concepts or perceptions.

[9] The learning of motor skills or cognitive skills is influenced by a variety of factors, including:

      a. Repeated performance, necessary to the acquisition of a complicated motor skill.

      b. The opportunity to practice many variations of the basic skill (i.e., concentrated repetition of a single aspect of a skill, or one basic variation of a skill, tends to limit future adaptation of the skill to different situations).

[10] What a person learns in a given situation depends upon what he perceives.

B. Retention of learning is influenced by a variety of factors.

[1] Retention of information or other learning is more stable if the original learning experience was efficient.

[2] Retention of learning is more stable if ego involvement was high in the

original learning (e.g., if learning was consistent with beliefs, values, ideals or accompanied by high motivation).

[3] In general, recent learning tends to take precedence over remote learning, as far as recall of details is concerned.

C. Motivation is prerequisite to optimal learning.

[1] Learning is facilitated when an individual sees the relationship between what he is learning and his personal needs and problems.

[2] If an individual is able to recognize or experience for himself what he is able to do, learning is likely to be more effective.

[3] Comfort in the learning situation is increased if motivation for learning is positive (rewarding) rather than negative (punishing).

[4] Change in behavior may be motivated by the anticipation of desirable conditions that will result from the new behavior.

D. Learning is influenced by the individual's stage of growth and development.

[1] Individual differences in maturation, experience, and constitutional capacity have a substantial influence on learning (e.g., what is learned, rate of learning).

[2] The acquisition of new behavior partially depends upon the individual's physiological and psychological readiness to learn.

    a. Attempts to learn by going through learning steps (even when the individual is not yet "ready" to learn) may increase the speed of learning, because learning is itself a skill procedure.

    b. Conversely, forced and repititious attempts to learn before the individual is physiologically or psychologically ready, may set up resistance to the future learning of a particular skill.

    c. With advanced age, sensory abilities are less acute, and complex perceptual capacities are decreased, influencing the ability to learn and the efficiency of learning.

    d. It is believed that older people may have more difficulty in learning new tasks because increased security needs require continuance of long-practiced habitual patterns in order to maintain ego integrity. Older people will be aided in learning new skills if these skills are related to or incorporated in well-established habit patterns.

    e. With increased age, there tends to be a need for increase in time required to accomplish complex sensorimotor tasks.

    f. Commonly used intelligence tests may be misleading for older people; while it is generally believed that there is a decline in IQ test performance with age, subscores for verbal abilities in otherwise healthy persons show little or no decline with age, while subscores for performance tests show decline due to decreased speed of response or slower performance.

    g. While the reasons for decline in short-term memory in older persons are not yet clearly understood, the decline does seem to interfere with new learning.

    h. Some studies suggest that decreased learning ability in older age groups may be more a function of decreased performance speed than of actual decreased learning ability (i.e., if the learner has opportunity for self-pacing, learning is more effective).

    i. Some studies seem to indicate that possible decrease in learning ability in older age groups is less a function of the aging process than it is of a combination of factors: state of health, previous education, individual differences.

3. Psychological equilibrium is directly influenced by the ability to adapt to a variety of life situations, which involves both conscious and unconscious problem-solving processes.*

  A. Creative problem-solving usually runs an erratic course, including changes and shifts in perception and discontinuity of conscious effort.

  B. Ego involvement tends to increase the amount of effort sustained in problem-solving activities.

  C. Problem-solving is influenced by the individual's ability to utilize imagery (e.g., the more ability a person has for vivid mental imagery, the more likely he is to "see" relationships and to visualize alternatives without having to experiment with actual materials).

  D. The way in which a problem is presented may determine the way in which it is solved (e.g., initial presentation may provide a perceptual "set" that directs thinking, either promoting or preventing possible alternatives.)

  E. Successful problem-solving requires a fund of previously acquired knowledge and/or experience.

  F. Previous problem-solving patterns may interfere with new approaches to current problems.

    [1] Problem-solving tends to be more difficult when solutions require the application of the familiar in an unfamiliar way.

    [2] When a given solution to a problem has been learned to be associated with a specific situation, the individual will have more difficulty in adapting that solution to other situations.

    [3] Preconceptions and previously learned concepts or ways of relating concepts tend to limit novel interpretations of data and creative solutions to problems.

    [4] If previous learning has been generalized and/or abstract, it is less likely to inhibit new approaches to problem solutions (e.g., if learning has been in the form of specific procedures or formulas, it will be less useful in creative problem-solving).

  G. Physiological and psychological changes occurring as a result of the aging process tend to decrease ability to cope with life situations (problem-solve).

    [1] Concurrent with the aging process and the decreasing ability to problem-solve, life situations in many societies increase the number and severity of problems that must be dealt with (e.g., an increase in normal number of loss situations, a decrease in physical and social resources.)

---

* As with growth and development, much of the material related to adaptive behavior has been incorporated in other chapters, particularly Chapters 7 and 8. The following statements are mostly generalizations relevant to creative problem-solving.

[2] Concurrent with the aging process, the tendency toward increased ability to recall earlier events may have a positive or negative influence on problem-solving.

    a. Reevaluation of earlier life events ("life review") may have a positive influence on problem-solving through resolution of old conflicts, arriving at acceptance of current status, preparation for death.

    b. Reevaluation of earlier life events may have a negative influence on problem-solving if it serves to intensify old conflicts or give rise to excessive anger, bitterness, despair, depression.

[3] In older age groups where chronic disease is present, even though asymptomatic, there tends to be a decrease in ability to pursue a task goal and to pursue an ordered sequence of thought. These functions seem not to be affected in older persons who are healthy.

[4] In older age groups, experiencing of social loss tends to decrease ability to pursue task goals or ordered sequences of thoughts.

[5] In otherwise healthy older persons, a consistent and organized daily living pattern tends to prolong ability to adapt to life situations.

[6] Increased incidence of illness and/or physical disabilities in older age groups tends to further decrease ability to cope with ordinary and/or unusual stress situations.

[7] The process of aging, with or without accompanying illness or disease, slows general reaction time. This slowing of reaction time is exaggerated if aging is accompanied by social or environmental loss.

H. A person who cannot tolerate ambiguity will have more difficulty with creative problem-solving.

[1] The more rigid the person is, the less he can tolerate "unknowns" and unexplained phenomena (e.g., he will tend to generalize or categorize too quickly, to organize material with insufficient data or to draw hasty conclusions in order to have the problem "solved").

[2] The more rigid the person is, the more he tends to avoid new and novel ideas and interpretations of data and untried solutions that might fail.

[3] A person, otherwise flexible but currently under unusual threat or discontinuity of life style, may react with greater rigidity in problem-solving situations than would be usual for him.

I. Highly creative problem-solving, although dependent upon adequate levels of intelligence and a fund of knowledge and experience, equally depends upon certain personality characteristics.

[1] The individual who is secure in his self-concept, who is less dependent upon authority and more independent in arriving at decisions and judgments, who is less likely to perceive situations in predetermined ways and who has a sense of humor usually demonstrates a better ability to arrive at creative solutions to problems.

[2] The more creative person tends to be less afraid of being wrong or of being criticized for his problem solutions.

[3] In general, the person who demonstrates creative ability tends to show more evidence of psychological well-being than the less creative person.

Nursing Care

The nurse should increase her knowledge and understanding of processes of growth and development, learning and adaptive problem-solving in order to accomplish optimal nursing care.

1. A nurse should make observations of the patient and his environment in order to determine:
   A. The patient's growth and development level, particularly for a very young child.
   B. Any apparent problems or incongruities in the growth and development process.
   C. Individual learning needs necessitated by illness and/or hospitalization.
   D. Individual problems requiring adaptive problem-solving.
   E. Environmental or circumstantial influences that may interfere with growth and development, learning and/or adaptive problem-solving.
   F. Child-parent relationship patterns that will influence growth and development, learning and problem-solving.
2. A nurse should plan nursing care in accord with both her knowledge of processes and her observations of the patient and his environment. She can:
   A. Gear expectations for behavior of the individual (child, adolescent, adult or older adult) to his particular level of development, including allowance for regression during stressful illness and/or hospitalization.
   B. Prevent or avoid situations that would increase negative effects on growth and development of the child or adolescent. For example:
      [1] Planning nursing intervention to avoid increasing anxiety and insecurity in relation to need satisfaction and training practices.
      [2] Avoiding demonstrating attitudes that the child might interpret as rejective.
      [3] Providing, if possible, sources of counsel for parents who demonstrate nonconstructive or actually destructive attitudes and child-rearing practices.
      [4] Avoiding open conflict (in front of the child) with parents regarding differences in opinions regarding child-rearing practices and attitudes.
      [5] Avoiding judgmental behavior toward parents regarding child-rearing practices based on inadequate data or superficial observations (e.g., if any specific practice differs in result from culture to culture or subculture to subculture, the practice itself may not be detrimental).
      [6] Avoiding the exaggeration of conflict for the adolescent (e.g., allow maximum desired autonomy consistent with safety without making demands for performance based on the nurse's preconceived expectations for behavior).
      [7] Avoiding punitive or rejective attitudes when the adolescent attempts to test social attitudes and role behaviors, providing a rational, nonjudgmental and reasoned sounding board for testing ideas and behaviors (e.g., provide a climate accepting adolescent inconsistencies in behavior, which vary from childlike to adult behaviors while under stress).

    C. Plan nursing interventions in accord with growth and development principles relative to other aspects of behavior. (See other chapters.)

3. The nurse should plan nursing care in accordance with both her knowledge of learning principles and of the individual patient, his circumstances, needs for learning and environmental influences on learning. (See Social Science Principle #2, this chapter. These statements are explicit enough to be directly applicable, provided the situation has been adequately analyzed).

4. The nurse should plan and implement nursing actions that promote adaptive problem-solving, whenever possible, or that prevent interference with adaptive problem-solving. She can:

    A. Increase supportive behavior for the patient who is faced with problems to be solved under stress.

    B. Avoid excessive demands for problem-solving by the patient under extreme stress.

    C. Avoid any interference with the patient's adaptive problem-solving efforts by remaining nonjudgmental, patient and nonrejecting of novel solutions that might not have occurred to her (i.e., the patient is most likely to find solutions suitable to his total life situation, regardless of how desirable other solutions may seem to the nurse, who has different life circumstances).

    D. Assist the patient less likely to see alternative solutions to visualize possibilities (e.g., if the patient lacks needed information or has been restricted to narrow ranges of choice, discussion with informed and supportive persons may help increase the possible alternative solutions).

    E. Organize the presentation of problems in such a way as to maximize use of previous experience and minimize problems associated with previous learning (e.g., present the problem in a novel way if previous learning will interfere; relate problem to past experience if relationship will promote problem-solving).

    F. Present problems in such a way as to draw on maximum motivation and ego involvement.

    G. Assist persons in older age groups to use the "life review" process to aid in positive adaptation.

5. The nurse can utilize principles of learning to guide the development of her own professional and personal competence.

6. The nurse can utilize principles of learning and of adaptive problem-solving to guide leadership activities and interactions with auxiliary staff for improvement of patient care.

Chapter 7

Primary and Acquired Needs

There are some psychological and psychosocial needs which may be considered common to all people and for which there must be some degree of satisfaction if the individual is to maintain psychological and psychosocial equilibrium.

Social Science Principles

1. In order to achieve and maintain psychological equilibrium, a person must have satisfying relationships with other human beings, both individually and in groups.
   A. The feeling of being cared for or about by another person or persons is necessary for psychological homeostasis.
      [1] The attitudes and actions of others that indicate the individual is worthy of attention, assistance or concern contribute to a feeling of being cared for or about.
      [2] The physical presence of those who are affectionally important reassures the individual that he is cared for.
   B. The awareness that one is not alone is basic to psychological homeostasis. The feeling of aloneness is decreased by:
      [1] The sharing of experiences with others.
      [2] The knowledge that one's behavior, experiences or feelings are not unique but are common to or shared by others.
      [3] Effective interaction and communication with other individuals.
      [4] The feeling that one is understood by others.

C. The approval of others in one's sociocultural environment is necessary for the psychological homeostasis of the average person.

[1] Approval from others may be elicited by contributing valued actions, materials or beliefs or by otherwise conforming to group standards.

[2] A feeling of being approved by others is achieved by being regarded or reacted to with positive, as opposed to negative, attitudes. The value of the attitude is determined by the culture in which one lives.

[3] A feeling of being approved by others is increased if one's presence or participation in social groups is sought.

[4] Assurance of approval by others is achieved by conforming to social conventions established for interpersonal relationships.

[5] An individual who receives inadequate evidence of approval or of his positive value may seek demonstrations of caring by others in a variety of ways, such as:

    a. Negative behavior which elicits punishing attention.

    b. Any activity that will gain attention, regardless of its positive or negative social value.

D. Acceptance by others of one's self and one's individual differences is necessary for psychological homeostasis for the average person.

E. In order to experience satisfying relationships with others, the average individual must be able to feel that he will not be harmed as a result of the relationship.

[1] If an individual experiences a feeling of acceptance and esteem in relation to other individuals or groups of individuals, he is better able to tolerate criticism or correction with a minimum of discomfort.

[2] In general, opportunities for satisfying relationships with others are increased if the individual is able to see others as trustworthy and capable.

    a. Trust and confidence in others is acquired through experiences in which the individual is not harmed or by which he benefits.

    b. Trust and confidence in others is enhanced by the demonstration of concern and interest of others in the individual's welfare.

[3] An individual who is suspicious, fearful or distrustful of others may be threatened by interpersonal relations and may be unable to experience security and satisfaction in individual or group relations until fear is decreased or remedial learning takes place.

F. The achievement of satisfying relationships with others is influenced by the psychobiologic structure and function of the organism. These factors include the following:

[1] Perceptual ability and learned patterns of perception, which involve:

    a. Perception of one's own role and the role of others in relationships.

    b. The ability to examine and evaluate one's own behavior in relation to others.

    c. The ability to perceive oneself correctly; knowing one's own capabilities and limitations.

[2] Self-concept and ego function.

    a. Positive self-esteem contributes to the achievement of satisfactory relationships with others.

b. The ability to accept one's self and one's own capabilities and limitations contributes to the achievement of satisfactory relationships with others.

c. Any mutilation or basic change in body structure will influence the individual's concept of himself and his relationships with others.

[3] The ability to communicate effectively.

[4] Behavior in relation to thinking patterns, attitudes, opinions and beliefs.

[5] Ability to experience and appropriately control emotion.

G. The achievement of satisfying relationships with others is influenced by sociocultural factors.

[1] If satisfactory interpersonal relationships are to be achieved and maintained, there must be a mutual recognition of culturally established roles, with behavior appropriate to those roles. (See Chapter 9.)

[2] In every society or culture there are established rules and codes of conduct to which the individual must adhere, in order to be approved and accepted by others. (See Chapter 9.)

[3] In order to live comfortably within a given sociocultural structure, an individual must have the ability and opportunity to learn the accepted roles, rules and codes of conduct. (See Chapter 6.)

[4] A single individual may function satisfactorily in a variety of roles.

[5] An individual is likely to respond to others in a given social situation in a manner similar to the one by which he is approached or in accord with his perception of the response expected of him.

2. The achievement and maintenance of psychological equilibrium is enhanced if the individual has a sense of self-esteem.

A. Satisfying relationships with others are necessary to the development and maintenance of self-esteem.

B. The development and maintenance of self-esteem depend upon one's ability to function in accordance with the internalized standards, beliefs and values that have been acquired from the sociocultural environment.

[1] In most North American cultures, self-direction and independent action are highly valued forms of behavior.

[2] In some cultures, maintenance of individuality is necessary for a sense of self-esteem.

[3] A sense of self-esteem may be increased or decreased due to one's identification with a particular sociocultural group and the status of that group within the total social structure.

C. Repeated failures tend to decrease self-esteem and foster development of the expectation that one will fail or be inadequate.

3. In order to achieve and maintain psychological equilibrium, the individual must have an adequate means of self-definition and situational definition (i.e., he must know, to his own satisfaction, who he is, where he is, and what his goals are.)

A. A sense of personal identity may be enhanced by the recognition (by oneself and others) of the person's individuality in relation to others.

B. Adequate personal and situational definitions require a knowledge and understanding of what the individual perceives to be the facts about himself and the situation.

[1] Knowledge of the facts about a situation requires adequate perception of factors in the situation.

[2] In addition to factual knowledge about a situation, an individual may be helped to achieve an adequate personal and situational definition through beliefs and convictions (e.g., for some individuals, a belief in a supreme being or deity provides a means of personal and situational definition.)

C. Adequate self-definition is partially achieved through identification with and sharing of experiences with other individuals and groups of individuals.

D. Adequate personal and situational definition requires clarity of perception of one's role and status in relation to others.

E. Adequate situational definition requires that the individual be aware of the behavioral limits in a situation.

F. Development and maintenance of an adequate personal and situational definitions require the establishment of familiar and consistent sociocultural patterns.

G. For some individuals, the possession of material objects provides a symbolic means of identification.

4. In order to establish and maintain psychological equilibrium, the average individual attempts to achieve a feeling of safety and comfort in life situations.

A. A feeling of safety and comfort is engendered if the individual feels he is able to cope with life situations successfully (i.e., control the situation and himself in such a way as to prevent harm).

[1] The ability to handle life situations in a socially approved manner requires a knowledge of and ability to act within the sociocultural limits of the situation.

[2] The ability to handle life situations with success is most probable when there is a clear perception of the factors inherent to each situation, including the goal to be reached.

a. One of the factors contributing to the clarity of perception of a situation is the possession of factual knowledge.

b. Clarity of perception is increased if one is able to identify one's own feelings, attitudes, limitations and capabilities.

c. Clarity of perception may require the opportunity to experience the actual situation, in addition to or rather than hearing a verbal description of the situation.

d. Clarity of perception may be increased by verbal exploration of the situation in the presence of an informed and supportive person.

e. Inconsistency, confusion and multiplicity of demands may contribute to a lack of clarity of perception.

[3] An individual is more likely to achieve a feeling of comfort and safety in coping with life situations if he has an understanding of action to be taken and possesses the skills and abilities necessary for the action.

a. Security in life situations is likely to be increased as the individual gains more experience (skill) in coping with specific situations or variations of a situation.

b. The acquisition of skills necessary for successful action requires the opportunity for adequate learning experiences.

[4] For some individuals or in some situations, a feeling of comfort and safety requires that the individual maintain control of himself and the situation, regardless of the actual necessity for such control.

   a. In most North American cultures, individuals experience anxiety if deprived of the opportunity or right to make decisions regarding self and personal property.

   b. Frustration of one's efforts toward a specific goal constitutes loss of control over the situation.

   c. Dependence upon others imposed by illness constitutes loss of control.

   d. For some individuals a feeling of comfort and safety is achieved through controlling or manipulating the environment and the people in it, above and beyond self-control.

[5] A feeling of comfort and safety in handling life situations may be achieved by the establishment of familiar routines, behavior patterns and environmental circumstances which have been previously experienced as safe and comfortable.

   a. A feeling of comfort and safety in coping with life situations is enhanced if the individual previously has had similar experiences in which he has not been harmed.

   b. Any interference with or change in normal physiological and/or psychological functioning is likely to cause psychological disequilibrium, because: it may be perceived as a threat to life; it may require new, unknown patterns of behavior; unknown consequences may be feared.

   c. To the extent that illness, hospitalization, advancing age or other health-related events disrupt previously established behavior patterns, the individual will experience psychological disequilibrium.

[6] A feeling of safety and comfort in a specific situation may be increased by positive preparation before the situation occurs, which may include:

   a. Increasing one's knowledge about the event.

   b. Changing one's perception of the event. (See Chapter 1.)

   c. Verbalization of the event in the presence of a supportive person.

   d. The opportunity for vicarious successful experiences, through discussion with someone who has lived through the event successfully.

   e. An opportunity to learn skills that will be needed for mastery of the situation.

[7] Disturbances of physiological or psychosocial equilibrium that result in exaggerated emotional reactions or mental dysfunction decrease the individual's ability to cope successfully with life situations.

   a. Internal and external confusion interfere with an individual's control of his own behavior.

   b. In extremely threatening situations, an individual may need constant repetition of successful experiences before tension can be decreased sufficiently to allow successful coping with a situation.

   c. A high degree of apprehension may interfere with the ability to successfully cope with a situation.

   d. Clarity, simplicity and lack of threat in the way others approach a confused person facilitate cooperation between the confused person and others in the environment and give a feeling of comfort and safety to the confused person.

B. Feelings of comfort and safety in a situation may be increased by identification with others who have experienced the situation without harm.

C. Comfort and safety in a situation may be increased by the possession of material objects that symbolically represent safety and comfort.

D. A feeling of comfort and safety may be achieved through relationships with others.

   [1] A feeling of comfort and safety may be achieved through feeling able to depend upon and/or cooperate with others.

      a. Cooperation between individuals depends upon adequate communication between the individuals involved.

      b. In a situation where the individual must depend upon others, a feeling of safety and comfort is based on the assurance that help is available for the satisfaction of basic needs of self and dependents.

      c. An individual may be helped to feel safe and comfortable in a dependent situation if he receives a positive interpretation of ongoing events. (Feelings of safety and comfort are further increased if the positive interpretation is unsolicited.)

      d. The achievement of a feeling of comfort and safety through dependence upon or cooperation with others requires that the individual be able to trust and have confidence in others. Confidence in others is likely to be increased if:

         i. The individual receives assurance that important matters pertaining to self will be considered confidential.

         ii. The individual is assured that others are capable of carrying out tasks assigned or entrusted to them.

         iii. The individual is assured that others have a genuine concern for the health and welfare of persons dependent upon him.

         iv. There is consistency of attitude and behavior demonstrated by those on whom the individual must depend.

         v. An individual has had repeated experiences involving trustworthy and honest people.

         vi. The suspicious or doubtful person receives a realistic interpretation and encouragement from someone outside the situation whom he trusts.

      e. The person who is suspicious, doubtful or fearful will react with increased suspicion and fear if others in the environment show doubt and lack of control.

   [2] A feeling of comfort and safety may be achieved through mutually sharing responsibility with others whom one trusts or for whom one cares.

      a. The inclusion of an individual's family in a situation may increase the feeling of safety and comfort by the sharing of responsibility within the family group.

      b. In a threatening situation, an individual may receive the greatest support from a member of the family or from some individual with whom a close affectional bond exists.

[3] A feeling of safety and comfort may be achieved through relationships with others who realistically indicate that the individual will not be harmed or allowed to come to harm.

    a. Psychological support and assistance may be given through the attitudes and behaviors of others in the situation.

        i. The suspicious, doubtful or fearful individual can frequently be helped to feel safe and comfortable in a situation if others are, or appear to be, calm, self-assured and in control of the situation.

        ii. An attitude of objectivity on the part of others in a situation may help the individual to feel safe and comfortable.

        iii. In some situations, setting limits or giving firm directions will be helpful in assisting a person to feel safe, comfortable and competent.

        iv. A feeling of comfort and safety may be enhanced by the presence of a warm, understanding person.

        v. Realistically based approval and the encouragement of others contribute to a feeling of safety and comfort in a situation.

        vi. An individual's feeling of security may be increased if he is made to feel welcome in strange or unfamiliar surroundings.

        vii. Physical care procedures may be used as a means of giving emotional support and may help in the establishment of positive interpersonal relations.

    b. Actions by others, motivated by the anticipation of an individual's needs, tend to increase one's feeling of safety and comfort.

    c. If an individual experiences a feeling of acceptance and esteem in relation to other individuals, he will be better able to tolerate criticism, correction or guidance from those individuals with a minimum of discomfort.

[4] A feeling of comfort and safety in life situations requires that the individual experience a feeling of approval and acceptance by others.

[5] For most individuals, feelings of comfort and safety in life situations follow feelings of relatedness to others.

E. The ability to communicate one's needs is prerequisite to a feeling of safety and comfort. (See Chapter 4.)

F. A feeling of safety and comfort may be achieved through religious beliefs and practices.

G. A feeling of safety and comfort requires the absence of threat to the life and integrity of the organism.

[1] The presence of persons who are in ill health or who are diseased may constitute a threat to the life of other individuals, either through fear of contracting the illness or through the symbolic implications the illness may have.

[2] The presence of hostility in the environment may have implications of potential danger.

[3] Any interference with or change in normal physiological and/or psychological function is usually perceived as a threat to the life or integrity of the organism.

[4] Any use of physical force by one person upon another may constitute (symbolically or realistically) a threat to the integrity or life of the organism.

[5] Illness and hospitalization realistically or symbolically imply an existing or potential threat to the life and integrity of the organism.

[6] The presence of dead or dying persons in the environment usually produces anxiety, particularly if the individual is himself in a state of impaired health.

5. Above and beyond basic or primary needs and the most strongly inculcated secondary or acquired needs, a person will be motivated toward "self-actualization."

A. Self-actualization involves demonstrating drives in the direction of adaptation, reproduction, creative invention, growth toward potentials.

B. The individual tends to seek new experiences, explore environmental or personal possibilities, and know and understand that which is not necessary to merely survive comfortably.

6. Above and beyond basic or primary needs and the most strongly inculcated secondary or acquired needs, a person will be motivated toward seeking stimulation and novelty.

A. The individual exhibits interest in mental and physical exercise and stimulation (e.g., he shows interest in puzzles and problems, games requiring physical and mental challenge and other activities that are experienced as pleasurable, above and beyond mere necessity).

B. The individual tends to respond to novel or changing stimuli as opposed to familiar stimuli.

C. The individual tends to spend energy seeking varieties of experience, even in relation to otherwise satisfactory situations.

7. Above and beyond basic or primary needs and the most strongly inculcated secondary or acquired needs, man seems to be motivated toward activities that are experienced purely as pleasurable, including that which is referred to as aesthetic appreciation.

A. The individual who is provided with (or able to acquire) a reasonable amount of purely pleasurable experience, tends to exhibit a more positive outlook on life in general and is better able to tolerate necessary unpleasant experiences.

8. The needs of an individual at a given time vary according to internal and external factors, such as the following:

A. The constitutional and life-experience altered nature of the organism.

B. Membership in a specific sociocultural group.

C. Past experiences, particularly those associated with growth and development.

D. Current life situations.

[1] Illness or hospitalization disturbs the individual's total pattern of need satisfaction.

[2] Certain needs of the individual are intensified by physical illness.

[3] Certain needs of the individual are more difficult to satisfy if he is physically ill or hospitalized, and the frustration of needs adds to the problems of adjustment to illness and/or hospitalization.

[4] Inherent in illness or hospitalization are potentially traumatic elements or problem situations, to which the individual must make some form of adaptation. (See Chapter 6.)

[5] At any given time, those needs which are most intense take priority over those creating less tension. Those needs most closely related to actual survival and to survival of ego integrity usually take precedence over other needs.

[6] All human needs are interrelated; a disturbance in one area of function causes reactions in other areas of function.

    a. Persistent lack of satisfaction of psychological needs appears to be correlated with physiological reactions, and vice versa.

    b. Psychological comfort and well-being are partially dependent upon physiological comfort and well-being, and vice versa.

E. A behavior that obtains an adequate response (reduces a need) in one situation tends to be repeated in similar situations.

Nursing Care*

To plan for and implement therapeutic nursing interventions effectively, the nurse should use her knowledge of primary and acquired needs.

1. The nurse should increase her knowledge and understanding of human needs and their relationship to physiological and psychological equilibrium.

2. The nurse should guide her observation of patients in order to determine:

  A. Needs the patient may be experiencing but which he cannot satisfy by independent action under circumstances of illness and/or hospitalization.

  B. Factors in the environment that are actually or potentially interfering with need satisfaction.

  C. Evidences of unusual need states (e.g., behavior that might indicate chronic unmet needs for acceptance and approval or satisfying relationships with others).

  D. Individual patterns of and preferences for behavior and activities that satisfy specific needs.

  E. Evidences that frustration of need-satisfying behaviors not specifically related to illness and/or hospitalization is interfering with therapy goals.

3. The nurse should use both her understanding of the function of human needs as they relate to total equilibrium and her observations of the patient to plan individual patient care. For example, she will use basic principles regarding needs and need satisfaction to:

---

* As in Chapter 6, unnecessary reiteration of each principle has been avoided. The following statements are examples directing the nurse's attention back to science content.

A. Plan care to increase the patient's feeling of being genuinely cared for, particularly by those upon whom he must depend.

B. Organize care to prevent exaggeration of feelings of aloneness.

C. Demonstrate attitudes of approval and acceptance.

D. Regulate her relationships with patients to increase the feeling of comfort, safety and satisfaction in the relationship, thus allowing the patient to make maximum use of the relationship for therapeutic purposes.

E. Adapt nursing care to accommodate the individual patient's abilities and limitations in relation to need satisfaction.

F. Avoid activities that tend to decrease or disturb the patient's stable concept of self and his self-esteem; increase activities that foster the development of a stable and constructive concept of self and maintenance of self-esteem.

G. Provide opportunities for adequate self- and situational-definition by patients under her jurisdiction; encourage others involved in patient care to do likewise.

H. Avoid activities that increase fear regarding safety, integrity and comfort, and plan activities that increase feelings of safety and comfort.

I. Use her knowledge of need as a motivation for behavior to effect therapeutic goals (e.g., present necessary but unpleasant therapy procedures or desired activities in such a way as to capitalize on need motivation).

J. Devise comprehensive plans for care that include satisfaction of the individual's needs for self-actualization, stimulation and pleasurable experiences.

4. The nurse should examine, evaluate and regulate her behavior in relation to her own needs and methods of need satisfaction, in order to avoid nontherapeutic activities while implementing patient care.

Chapter 8

Disturbances of Equilibrium

The individual organizes and integrates his world to prevent destruction or disruption of function. He develops elaborate systems of behavior (thinking, feeling and acting) to preserve ego integrity and thus his ability to cope successfully. Severe disturbances of equilibrium may result in noticeably deviant and/or nonconstructive behavior systems.

Social Science Principles

1. Frustration of efforts toward goals evokes a number of responses.
   A. Moderate or tolerable frustration may have a constructive effect.
      [1] Tolerable frustration serves to intensify goal-directed behavior.
      [2] Successful efforts to eliminate frustration-creating barriers tends to increase one's sense of adequacy and ability to cope.
      [3] Tolerable frustration tends to focus attention and organize problem-solving behavior.
   B. Intolerable and/or continuous frustration may have destructive effects.
      [1] Continuous failure to remove frustration-creating barriers tends to cause a sense of inadequacy and failure.
      [2] Ambiguous frustration (when the barrier is unidentified) tends to cause diffuse or random reactions, generally unsuccessful.
      [3] Continuous frustration usually leads to anxiety. (See Social Science Principle #3, below.)

C. Objectified frustration-creating barriers (causes outside of self) tend to provoke less anxiety than barriers arising internally.

D. Frustration accompanied by punishment tends to produce rigid, nonadaptive behavior, which may endure as a chronic reaction when the frustration-creating barrier no longer exists.

E. When goal-directed behavior is accompanied by or results in inconsistent reward or punishment, neurotic behavior may result.

F. When goal-directed behavior is accompanied by both reward and punishment at the same time, neurotic behavior may result.

2. Psychological equilibrium requires the development of and ability to utilize psychological mechanisms for warding off anxiety and for adapting adequately to life situations.

A. By definition,* a crisis situation constitutes a threat to psychological equilibrium. What constitutes a crisis event varies from person to person, dependent upon individual perception.

[1] In a crisis event, habitual coping mechanisms are inadequate to handle the situation.

[2] Attempts to restore equilibrium, disturbed by crisis events, may result in either personality disorganization (with concomittent retardation of psychosocial growth) or in promotion of maturation.

a. When a crisis event results in promotion of maturation, the individual gives up preexisting behavior patterns and acquires new, more effective behavior patterns.

b. In the process of giving up old behavior patterns and acquiring new ones, some behaviors may occur that have the appearance of personality disintegration. Crisis theorists believe that such behaviors are a reasonable part of reintegration, not to be considered maladaptive.

c. An individual who achieves growth through crisis resolution must be able to consider and select new alternatives to problems, necessitating availability of information and resources out of which new alternatives may be derived.

[3] Crisis situations may be defined as situational or developmental.

a. Situational crisis events are those occurring by chance or by accident during the life process (e.g., loss of job).

b. Developmental crisis events are those that must be expected or anticipated during the life process (e.g., transition from childhood to adolescence, marriage).

B. Any disturbance of psychological equilibrium causes a primary reaction of anxiety, fear, apprehension or tension.

[1] Anxiety is commonly accompanied by physical reactions, such as tremor, loss of appetite, perspiration, sleeplessness, increased pulse rate and so forth.

[2] Gross or continuous anxiety may be accompanied by disturbances of physiological function, such as endocrine system changes, alterations of autonomic nervous system responses or circulatory system reactions.

* Gerald Caplan, *Principles of Preventive Psychiatry* (New York: Basic Books, Inc., 1964), p. 56.

[3] Some forms of behavior are nonspecific indications of threats to psychological equilibrium, the causes of which must be determined by further investigation.

a. Attempts to manipulate or control the external environment (in excess of control necessary for safety) may be an indication of an individual's attempt to dissipate or alleviate anxiety.

b. An individual may rely on hostility, dependence or withdrawal as methods for handling anxiety-producing and/or problematic situations.

c. Regressive behavior is a common reaction to threatening situations.

d. An attitude of suspicion, doubt or mistrust may be an indication of underlying anxiety or insecurity.

e. Excessive demands for attention may indicate psychological disequilibrium.

f. Excessive complaints or dissatisfaction in a situation may be an indication of underlying anxiety.

g. Hostility may be a general indication of threats to ego integrity, frustration or emotional stress.

h. Withdrawal may be a general indication of frustration, traumatic experiences in interpersonal relations or threats to ego integrity.

i. Illness and/or physical symptoms may be used as a method of gaining attention, responding to a crisis situation or expressing unconscious feelings or conflict.

j. Activities that are primarily used to meet physical needs (e.g., eating) may be used as a symbolic means for attaining emotional satisfaction, resolving unconscious problems or relieving general tension.

k. Atypical or (to the observer) unexpected behavior may indicate disequilibrium in some area of the organism's function.

l. Continuous states of anxiety, even though unconscious, may result in physiological pathology because of the effect on nervous system function (e.g., ulcers, hypertension).

[4] Some forms of behavior are more specific indications of psychological disequilibrium, leading to easier determination of the specific cause.

a. An individual who is threatened by interpersonal situations tends to withdraw from social interaction in order to prevent or avoid greater psychological discomfort.

b. An individual who is in a state of gross disequilibrium is more likely to experience an exaggerated emotional response to minor environmental disturbances than an individual whose equilibrium is relatively stable.

c. An individual experiences feelings of inferiority or inadequacy if he is unable to live up to personal or social expectations.

d. An abrupt change of subject usually indicates an area that is either emotionally charged or that the individual is fearful of exposing.

e. Undesirable forms of behavior often indicate an individual's need for and attempts to obtain a positive response from others.

C. Any given activity or adaptive mechanism may be considered normal or healthy in one situation and abnormal or unhealthy in another, depending upon circumstances and cultural definition.

D. Adaptive mechanisms are not usually consciously selected but occur as a result of growth and development experiences.

[1] In general, there are no specific mechanisms for specific situations; the individual "selects" the mechanisms best adapted to his situation and his general pattern of adaptation.

[2] Adaptive mechanisms, when not used to excess, have constructive benefits.

a. Adaptive mechanisms decrease or alleviate anxiety, leaving ego integrity intact.

b. With anxiety under control, the individual is able to live with conflict or threat while he seeks realistic solutions to his problems.

c. Creative and/or socially constructive work may result from the use of some mechanisms.

d. Excessive use of mechanisms to avoid anxiety or frustration may prevent the development of the ability for constructive problem-solving.

[3] As a result of the aging process, both physiological and psychological defenses may become less effective.

[4] A number of adaptive (defensive) mechanisms have been identified and described.

a. Negativism: A person who fears loss of individual identity or loss of autonomy may react continuously and automatically with counter-suggestions or negative responses, even when the suggestion is in accord with his best interests or his own original beliefs and ideas.

b. Displacement: If the original object of a feeling, thought or action is seen as too powerful or is socially disapproved of or if the real object is unconsciously obscured, a person may direct the feeling, thought or action toward another (permissible) object.

c. Somatization and Conversion: A person's ideas and convictions can cause him to experience subjective physiological symptoms where no physiological pathology can be demonstrated. Unconscious conflicts may be converted to physical manifestations, such as functional paralysis or blindness.

d. Projection: Unpleasant or anxiety-producing impulses may be avoided by literally transferring such impulses, ideas, feelings or actions to others. Such cognitive distortion leaves the person unaware of the trait in himself; thus he remains free of anxiety, guilt or shame.

e. Identification and Incorporation: The process of seeing oneself as similar to or like another, or of idealizing another and wishing to emulate, has several functions:

i. Identification may help a person to successfully relate to others without anxiety.

ii. Identification is extensively used in learning one's role and function in life situations.

iii. Identification can be used to dilute the intensity of one's own guilt or negative reactions by providing an acceptable climate for his reactions.

    iv. Identification is extensively used to reduce feelings of loneliness and isolation.

    v. The incorporation of ideas, attitudes and attributes of others may reduce the threat of others, provide a way of "possessing" others or help to retain a sense of autonomy while conforming.

f. Rationalization: When a given thought, feeling or action is seen as unacceptable, cognitive distortion of facts may occur to allow acceptable reasons for the thought, feeling or action.

g. Insulation and Isolation: When 2 or more ideas, feelings, attitudes or necessary actions are conflicting, a person may separate them into logic-tight compartments without recognizing their discrepancy.

    i. One form of insulation is "intellectualization"—the process of separating emotion from ideational content, as though the understanding of an event strips it of any threat to the person.

    ii. Another form is the attributing of feelings and thought to ambiguous "others," thus separating self from responsibility. This mechanism helps other mechanisms, such as projection, repression and fantasy, to be effective.

h. Repression: Undesirable, unpleasant or painful thoughts, feelings or experiences may be completely erased from consciousness, unamenable to conscious recall but still functioning as motivating forces or energy, causing anxiety.

i. Reaction-formation: Unacceptable impulses, ideas, feelings or desired actions may be first repressed, then transformed into actions in direct opposition to the original. This form of denial of the original impulse tends to result in exaggerations of behavior beyond what is reasonable for the circumstances.

j. Fantasy and Autism: A person who cannot cope with reality because of threats to self-esteem or ego integrity may withdraw from actual situations, substituting ego-enhancing and self-defensive fantasy.

    i. Fantasy may also be self-destructive in nature if the individual is experiencing guilt.

    ii. Fantasy and autism may provide substitute satisfaction through wish-fulfilling imagery.

    iii. Fantasy may be constructive if it leads to the creation of original approaches to problem situations.

k. Compensation and Overcompensation: An individual who experiences a sense of inadequacy may overcome the inadequacy by directly concentrating on the development of a specific skill (compensation) or by over-developing a particular ability (overcompensation).

l. Substitution and Sublimation: An individual who experiences inadequacy in one area or frustration of impulse or desire in one area may develop compensatory skill in a substitute area (substitution) or dissipate energy through some activity that has social approbation or significance (sublimation). Thus, ego integrity is maintained, guilt and inadequacy are avoided and satisfaction is experienced.

3. The removal, destruction or weakening of an individual's psychological defenses against anxiety by external forces or circumstances causes an increase in the anxiety experienced by the person and an intensification of his attempts to restore equilibrium.

   A. When defenses are threatened and tension increases, aggressive outbursts may serve to decrease tension and allow the person to direct his energy toward rational problem-solving or strengthening the defenses.

   B. When defenses are threatened, the individual usually demonstrates over-reactions and exaggerations of emotion rather than flexible attempts to use rational problem-solving.

   C. When defenses are threatened by anxiety-producing situations, distraction of attention may temporarily relieve the anxiety of allow the person to direct energy toward rational problem-solving.

   D. When defenses are threatened, the individual experiences a decreased ability to tolerate ambiguity.

   E. If adaptive mechanisms are unsuccessful, personality or ego disorganization may result.

      [1] Disorganization or disintegration of the ego is manifested by such general behaviors as incoherence of thought and communication, confusion, random and unrelated ideation, inability to adapt or cope with situations, lack of control of behavior and emotion, illogical and irrational behavior, emotional agitation and exaggerated outbursts, loss of sense of self or ego identity.

      [2] Impending disorganization or disintegration of the ego may result in the development of patterns of behavior aimed at controlling the anxiety but which leave the individual unable to participate normally in society (e.g., severe neurotic and psychotic behavior patterns, such as conversion reactions, schizophrenic reactions, hypo- or hyper-reactive states).

      [3] Impending disorganization or disintegration of the ego may result in the development of patterns of behavior that control the anxiety temporarily and allow the person to retain the appearance of rational control but are destructive in nature (e.g., alcohol and drug addiction, sociopathic behavior).

Nursing Care

The nurse can be of therapeutic assistance to the patient if she has a knowledge of principles related to disturbances of equilibrium.

1. The nurse should increase her knowledge and understanding of processes relative to preventing disturbances of equilibrium and restoring disturbed integrity.

2. The nurse should guide her observations of the patient in order to determine:

   A. Evidence of intolerable frustration, anxiety, defenses against anxiety and threats to adaptive defenses.

    B. The individual patient's particular behavior patterns for controlling threats to integrity.

    C. Environmental or circumstantial factors that would be likely to threaten ego integrity or disrupt adaptive defenses.

    D. Evidence of ego or personality disorganization and/or psychotic and neurotic behavior patterns.

3. The nurse should use her knowledge and her observations as a guide to planning constructive patient care. She can:

    A. Introduce or allow only that amount of frustration that would serve as positive motivation for problem-solving.

    B. Attempt to eliminate or control intolerable amounts of frustration.

    C. In working with children, avoid use of punishment and inconsistent reward in relation to patient behavior directed toward need or goal satisfaction.

    D. Avoid destruction of the patient's consistently used adaptive mechanisms.

    E. Provide for the relief of uncomfortable or painful symptoms associated with anxiety.

    F. Assist the patient to use rational and flexible problem-solving methods of adaptation whenever possible.

    G. Provide substitute behavior or mechanisms to control anxiety whenever a particular mechanism must be interfered with or disrupted.

    H. Avoid criticism, rejection, punishment or negative attitudes and judgments when the patient uses adaptive behaviors which she personally sees as undesirable.

    I. Provide external control when patient behavior indicates disorganization of personality or behavior that will be dangerous to himself or others.

    J. Support or strengthen constructive mechanisms and assist the patient to develop constructive mechanisms when development of mechanisms is necessitated by situations under her jurisdiction.

    K. Attempt to control the situation (including her own behavior), in order to prevent increasing threats to integrity or equilibrium.

    L. Seek consultation as necessary for herself in planning nursing interventions and for the patient when patient behavior indicates uncontrollable or intolerable anxiety, nonconstructive adaptive mechanisms used to excess and impending or actual personality disorganization.

    M. Record and report evidences of disequilibrium that may require medical intervention.

4. The nurse should examine and evaluate her own use of adaptive mechanisms in order to provide the patient with healthy examples for behavior and to avoid nontherapeutic nursing actions.

Chapter 9

Sociocultural Influences on Behavior

Social and cultural institutions exist as a result of the needs of man (individually and collectively) and are maintained for the preservation of man's psychosocial and psychobiologic equilibrium. The individual tends to seek satisfaction of his needs within his culture, through the channels that that culture has established for satisfaction of individual needs.

Social Science Principles

1. The society or culture in which an individual lives, grows and develops helps to determine the ways in which his needs are met and the direction some of his acquired needs will take. Cultures may provide alternative ways of satisfying a specific human need.
   A. Socialization takes place more rapidly in the process of growth and development if socializing agencies (home, school, peer groups) are consistent and in accord with one another.
   B. If there is a wide discrepancy or conflict between the socializing agencies, the individual tends to completely renounce one agency in favor of the other, renounce both agencies or exhibit maladaptive behavior.
2. Man, as a social animal, tends to seek approval and acceptance by society. He is required to behave in a prescribed manner, within given limits, in order to be approved or accepted.

A. In the process of growth and development, many cultural values become internalized to the extent that they are no longer regarded as sociocultural requirements but experienced as subjective ideas, attitudes, beliefs and needs.
B. Social role and socially acceptable behavior are learned through contact with the environment in which the individual is given the opportunity to see and practice the designated role.
C. Any given activity may be considered normal, healthy or permissible in one situation and abnormal, unhealthy or unacceptable in another situation, depending upon cultural definition.
D. Every society or culture has established rules and codes of conduct governing major aspects of social interaction.
    [1] Cultures differ in their conduct requirements regarding relationships of members of the same sex and members of the opposite sex. (For example, in some cultures, physical exposure, even when necessitated by illness or hospitalization, in the presence of a member of the opposite sex is not condoned except under specific circumstances. In some subcultures, physical exposure is not permitted in any case.)
    [2] Cultures differ in their requirements of conduct regarding roles of authoritative, subordinate and peer positions.
        a. Every known society demonstrates some form of behavioral differentiation regarding status or dominant role positions and activities.
        b. In many cultures, doctors are usually seen in a role of authority.
        c. In many cultures, authority figures are regarded with respect, awe, sometimes fear, frequently suspicion and resentment.
    [3] Every known culture has some culturally organized form of behavior associated with religion. The importance of religious beliefs and practices tends to be increased during times of stress and/or uncertainty.
    [4] Societies having more than one racial and/or religious group will have some systematized codes for behavior regarding role, status and intergroup relations between the groups. In addition, subgroups within the society as a whole develop additional customs, attitudes and practices regarding race and religious differences.
        a. In a society where there are multiple racial and religious groups, satisfactory interpersonal relationships may be interfered with because of preconceived ideas, misconceptions, and lack of knowledge of one group about another.
        b. Individuals who belong to minority or fringe groups within a society usually experience some feelings of insecurity or inadequacy by reason of belonging to a group that is not accepted as part of the major group.
        c. Behavior resulting from stereotyped prejudice is more likely to decrease when members of ethnic groups interact on a personal basis of equality, while sharing a common task or activity that does not emphasize ethnic differences.
    [5] Every society or culture has established rules and codes of conduct governing the roles and relationships of family members.
        a. In every society, certain types of parental behavior in childrearing practices are either condoned or disapproved.

[6] In every society or culture, there are established rules and codes of conduct governing voluntary physiological functions and physical appearance.
   a. In some cultures, the control of eliminative processes and associated procedures is governed by comparatively rigid standards.
   b. In some cultures, physical cleanliness and a neat appearance are socially approved attributes.

[7] In every society or culture there are established customs and beliefs governing attitudes and behaviors regarding illness and death.
   a. In some cultures, attendance at the bedside of a dying person by other specified individuals is socially approved or mandatory.
   b. In every culture, there are some physical conditions, states of health or disease processes that have negative connotations.
   c. Every organized religion has specific attitudes, beliefs and ritual practices associated with death.
   d. Absence of cultural support rituals for grief and mourning can contribute to prolonged depression and/or failure to achieve resolution.
   e. Individual and cultural attitudes toward death may impede or assist the individual to cope with the dying process.
      i. Cultures and/or individuals seeing death as a negative experience tend to ignore, deny or impede natural processes and thus interfere with the dying person's ability to cope (e.g., they may ignore, isolate, concentrate on carrying out physically oriented tasks in lieu of interpersonal attention).
      ii. Cultures and/or individuals that see death as an integral part of the total life experience can assist the dying person to integrate the dying process in a positive manner.
      iii. In addition to cultural attitudes, an individual's past and present relationship to the dying person may cause him to impede or assist the dying person to cope with tasks associated with dying (e.g., dependence on the dying person, guilt, inability to cope with the potential loss).
   f. Some social factors seem to influence attitudes toward or ability to cope with death.
      i. Some studies indicate that negative ideas about death are more common among those with little education than among those with higher levels of education.
      ii. Acceptance of death (vs. denial) appears to be greater in persons with religious conviction and in those who live with others than for nonreligious persons and those who live alone.
      iii. Ability to accept death and to work through the dying process in a positive manner seems to be decreased for persons who sustained a major change in life style or circumstances shortly before death (e.g., loss of spouse, removal from home to nursing home, removal from nursing home of consistent residence to another living situation).

[8] Every society or culture places positive or negative value on certain general attitudes, ideas, beliefs and their attendant actions and gives or withholds

approval of the individual according to how he conforms to those standards.

   a. Generally speaking, in North American cultures:
- *i.* Personal adequacy in handling problems, independence and self-control are highly valued attributes.
- *ii.* Self-direction and independent action are considered basic human rights.
- *iii.* Any action that is perceived by the individual as a threat to independence or freedom (the right to select action by free choice) is most likely to be resented and/or resisted.
- *iv.* Respect and consideration are considered basic human rights.

   b. In some cultures and subcultures:
- *i.* Personal privacy is highly valued.
- *ii.* The suppression of overt hostility is required.
- *iii.* Individual possession, ownership and subsequent disposal of material objects has significance and is governed by customs and laws.
- *iv.* Expression of emotion before strangers and/or demonstration of pain or unhappiness is disapproved.

[9] In the development of the above culturally determined attitudes, ideas, beliefs and practices, some that originally arose from a basic need have attained a significance sufficient to guide behavior even though the original need may no longer exist.

3. Changes in a society or culture may cause diverse reactions.

  A. When social changes are perceived by the individual or group as threatening to traditional values, change will be resisted or the individual or group will experience disequilibrium and/or disorganization.

  B. When social changes occur slowly or are seen as related to other existing values, there is less resistance, disorganization or disequilibrium.

  C. When social change is attempted by an agent, there will be more conflict and resistance if the communication between members of the society and the agent effecting the change is inadequate.

  D. When social change is caused by rapid industrialization, there may be a number of predictable results.

    [1] Family relationships may be disrupted because of changes in social roles of family members.

    [2] The individual may experience increased tension if the social change necessitates an increase in the number of social roles for which he has not been adequately prepared.

    [3] Possibilities for social mobility increase, furthering the disruption of family relationships and individual uncertainty and tension.

4. Every known society has some system of establishing membership in social class; mobility between classes is usually governed by certain rules or codes, and such mobility may result in a variety of reactions.

  A. In societies with a designated lower class, the motivation to move upward (improve the standard of living) seems to be less among members of the lowest possible class or classes.

  B. An individual learns, in the process of growth and development, to identify himself with a given social class and to conform to the practices peculiar to that class.

C. In North American culture, members of the lower class tend to accept physical and psychological suffering with resignation and little motivation to eliminate or avoid such suffering.

D. Lower-class parents tend to discourage more than minimal education in their children.

E. Child-rearing practices tend to differ from social class to social class within a society.

   [1] In North American culture, lower-class parents tend to be more authoritarian, use more physical punishment and less reasoning, provide less supervision, permit greater ranges of expression of feeling, permit less freedom of interaction between parents and children and put less stress on achievement.

   [2] In North American culture, middle-class parents tend to place importance on publicized "popular practices" in child-rearing, be less authoritarian but more concerned about conformity to social standards, permit greater freedom of interaction between parents and children but less freedom of expressions of emotion, and put more stress on achievement.

   [3] When parents change social class (more upward in social placement), they tend to exhibit greater tension, strictness, and demands on conformity to class behaviors in child-rearing practices.

F. Sudden or rapid shifts in social class membership tend to increase the general insecurity of family members because of uncertainty about how to behave in multiple new social roles.

G. In North American culture, members of the middle class tend to place greater importance on joining and being active in organizations; there is less motivation for such activity among members of the lower class.

H. In North American culture, members of the lower class tend to have a narrower range of interests and activities (not including hobbies or aesthetic experiences) than do members of the middle and upper classes.

Nursing Care

The nurse should organize and implement nursing care in accordance with sociocultural requirements for behavior.

1. The nurse should increase her knowledge of the influence of sociocultural requirements on behavior in general and her knowledge of the cultures and subcultures to which her patients might belong.

2. The nurse should guide her observations of the patient and his environment to determine:

   A. Evidences of the patient's identification with any specific sociocultural group or groups.

   B. Evidences of the intensity of the patient's need to adhere to specific socioculturally determined behavior or codes of conduct, even though health requirements might indicate a departure from that behavior or code of conduct.

   C. Patient behavior that indicates conflict between social role requirements of different groups to which the patient might belong.

D. Environmental influences or circumstances that might put the patient in a position of conflict with socioculturally determined values and practices (i.e., be a source of tension, embarrassment, loss of self-esteem).

E. Experiences necessitated by illness and/or hospitalization that will be difficult for the patient to adjust to, because of previously acquired sociocultural attitudes or codes of conduct.

F. Ways in which the patient's membership in sociocultural groups influence health practices and adaptation to altered states of health.

G. Evidences of difficulty in learning necessary role behavior in relation to group membership.

H. Indications that the patient is confused, uncertain or insecure about role expectations while in the hospital.

3. The nurse should utilize her knowledge and her observations to plan and implement nursing interventions for optimal patient physiological and psychological well-being. She should, for example:

A. Avoid conflict whenever possible between the patient's established socioculturally determined requirements for behavior and the requirements of health agencies (e.g., arrange for required dietary practices, religious practices, the maintenance of family interaction patterns).

B. Avoid disruption of the patient's identification with sociocultural groups, unless such identification is obviously detrimental to health and well-being (e.g., avoid demonstrating rejective attitudes, such as criticism, belittling or disgust when the patient demonstrates attitudes not in accord with the nurse's group identification).

C. Provide the patient with the opportunity to practice sociocultural roles when the learning of those roles is necessary for psychological equilibrium (e.g., in child care, promote the practice of behavior consistent with future role behavior).

D. Avoid placing patients in close proximity to other patients if such proximity will arouse negative feelings and tension (e.g., if the patient retains strong prejudice regarding some racial or religious group).

E. If prejudice or stereotyped reactions are detrimental to health and well-being, provide experiences to help decrease and eliminate such prejudice or stereotyping.

F. Avoid placing the patient in distressing or embarrassing positions relative to socioculturally acquired behaviors (e.g., avoid physical exposure, provide privacy for eliminative functions and the expression of emotion, if these are in accord with the patient's expectations for behavior).

G. Provide the patient with clear definitions of expected role behavior *as a patient*, whenever role requirements differ from his usual practices or whenever role requirements are unfamiliar to the patient.

H. Avoid hasty stereotyping of patients based on superficial observations.

I. Avoid pressuring patients to conform to a certain sociocultural role behavior, simply because the nurse favors those roles by virtue of her own identification.

4. The nurse should examine and evaluate her own sociocultural identification, role behavior and expectations in order to avoid nontherapeutic nursing actions.

Chapter 10

Small Group Behavior

Within organized groups, certain phenomena have been observed to occur predictably.

Social Science Principles

1. In the development of any group, if it is in association long enough, there occurs a differentiation of social roles of individual members.
   A. Eventually, if no one is appointed by external influences, a leader will emerge when perceived by the group as the person most likely to further group goals.
      [1] The particular member selected as leader depends on predominant personality types in the group, capabilities existing among members of the group and the group goal.
         a. A group in which authoritarian personalities predominate will tend to select a strong, directive leader.
         b. In less formal groups not requiring designated leadership, leadership may tend to rotate, depending on the activity at any given time.
      [2] Leaders of groups functioning under a higher authority (such as individual hospital unit groups under nursing service administration authority) tend to experience greater conflict because of conflicting perceptions of what constitutes "good" leadership (e.g., higher authority has one set of expectations of the leader, and group members have another set of expectations).
      [3] In democratic cultures, there tends to be a general suspicion and resentment of leadership dominance.

[4] "Authoritarian" leadership (where a leader directs but remains somewhat apart from membership in general) tends to produce group behavior that is:
   a. Either more aggressive or more apathetic than "democratic" leadership groups. The aggression is usually directed outward toward other groups or toward scapegoats in the group but not at the group leader directly.
   b. Demanding of attention from the leader.
   c. Disruptive and nonproductive when the leader is absent or does not assign tasks.
   d. Indicative of lower group morale.

[5] "Democratic" leadership (where action arises as a result of group discussion and decision with the leader fully participating) tends to produce group behavior that is:
   a. Less demanding of attention from the leader.
   b. Productively active in solving problems when the leader is absent or does not assign tasks.
   c. More supportive of group members in general, with less nonspecific aggressiveness and little need of scapegoats.
   d. Indicative of higher group morale.

2. In addition to the type of leadership, group morale, motivation and interaction are influenced by a number of factors.
   A. If group morale is low in general, the group tends to disintegrate under stress (e.g., form antagonistic subgroups; openly and subtly demonstrate hostility toward each other and the leader; be unable to concentrate on problem-solving or productive activity).
   B. If group members are predominantly individually competitive, group action tends to be less consistently productive.
   C. If group members are predominantly oriented toward cooperation, group action tends to be more consistently productive.
   D. If group members, including the leader, are predominantly interested in instigating innovations, differences or original adaptations, group action tends to be more consistently creative and productive in solving problems.
   E. If group members, including the leader, are predominantly rigid, rejecting newness, differences and untried ideas, group action tends to maintain the status quo or to look for ready-made solutions to problems.
   F. Individual and group morale are enhanced when there is a clear perception of the goal to be reached and the steps necessary to reach that goal. Demoralization results when ambiguity or confusion are excessive.
   G. When group interaction under conditions of equality are increased, individual members tend to increase shared values and norms and to like each other better, thus raising the level of morale and group unity.
   H. Group morale tends to be higher when group membership is stable. Stable groups tend to reject the introduction of new members, with rejective behavior increasing in proportion to the number of new members introduced.
   I. The less communication and interaction between related but separate groups, the greater the tendency toward conflict between those groups.
   J. When small group actions are imposed from outside, there tends to be less development of norms by the group; when actions of the group are determined

through group discussion, there tends to be the creation of ideal goals, with higher motivation to work toward those goals.

K. Group motivation toward changing goals or activities will be higher if potential changes are discussed freely in the group rather than imposed from outside by an authoritarian leader.

L. Group activity is more likely to be stimulated if group effort produces demonstrably valuable results (i.e., if there is realization of accomplishment).

M. Effective group action is influenced by a number of environmental and practical considerations.

    [1] Noise, interruptions, distracting movements and visual stimuli and physical discomfort decrease group efficiency.

    [2] Physical proximity and the position of members in relation to each other influence group interaction and efficiency (e.g., group interaction tends to be less effective if distance or position makes hearing difficult, if members are not facing each other, if members are crowded together in a small space, if the leader sits apart from the group).

    [3] The environment for meetings of small groups can be arranged for conduciveness to goal-directed activity (e.g., if writing or written materials are required, tables with materials can be present when members enter; if group action consists primarily of discussion, chair arrangement can suggest conversation and distracting materials can be removed).

    [4] Group members are likely to be irritated and thus less productive if prearranged meetings begin and end later than anticipated.

    [5] Effective group action is likely to be decreased if prearranged meetings coincide with other activities that members perceive as more important than group goals.

3. The actions of an individual within a group are influenced by a variety of factors.

A. In face-to-face group actions, the opinions, behavior, verbal and nonverbal expressions and prestige of each individual member will affect all members.

B. The reaction of group members (feedback) to an individual influences his subsequent behavior.

C. An individual who perceives himself as a member of a group (or desiring to be recognized as a member of a group) will have a stronger motivation to conform to group pressure than to deviate from it.

    [1] Within a group, an individual member will be more likely to retain individuality (demonstrate independent thinking and resist group pressure to conform when his own ideas and attitudes are not consistent with the group) if he has certain characteristics, such as:

        a. A higher than average level of intelligence.

        b. A predominantly original or creative approach to personal problem-solving.

        c. A high level of self-confidence and freedom from anxiety.

        d. A tendency to approach other people and events with tolerance, responsibility and comfort in relationships.

        e. An absence of such characteristics as passivity, dependence, and vagueness or instability in perception of self.

    [2] Conformity or nonconformity to group pressure is influenced by:

a. The individual's perception of the group and the group's position in the total cultural structure.

b. The nature of the problem to be solved or task to be accomplished.

c. The strength of the individual member's own convictions and what he foresees as the results of conforming or nonconforming actions.

d. Rewarding or punishing actions of the group toward conforming and nonconforming behavior (e.g., the group will provide support, reinforcement, security, encouragement, protection and rationale for behavior that is acceptable to the group and will provide punishment for deviant behavior by ridicule, dislike, shame and threat of expulsion).

[3] An individual who cannot tolerate authority tends to be a nonconformist in group behavior at all times, rather than only when his ideas conflict with group ideas (i.e., he tends to automatically reject group suggestion or pressure to conform, even when the desired behavior is in accord with his own original convictions).

4. Groups tend to stay in existence and be consistently of benefit to individual members and to the purpose for which the group was formed if certain conditions exist.

A. A basic factor in the continued existence of a group is that the interaction of group members continues to satisfy the desires and needs of its members.

B. Effective communication among group members is prerequisite to effective interaction and group continuity.

C. Effective group action requires that members be mutually compatible or that individual members be able to control behavior to avoid disruption (e.g., occasionally a group will be unable to function effectively unless a disrupting member is removed).

D. Cooperation and effective group action are facilitated if individual members feel mutual trust and goodwill.

E. Efforts to reach a given goal are more likely to be stimulated if individual members and the group as a whole feel that their efforts are appreciated or that they are contributing something of value.

F. Group stability is greater and interaction increased if members experience a sense of unity or cohesiveness. Conversely, group stability is decreased and interaction is less when there is dissention and/or individual competitiveness.

G. Group stability and effectiveness tend to increase when group activities are consistent with both necessary task goals and personal goals of individual members.

H. When an individual member of a group feels threatened by either group activities or other members of the group, that member will be less effective, tending to decrease the effectiveness of the group as a whole.

I. In task-oriented groups, a certain amount of personal-social discussion and interaction tends to relieve tension produced by task-oriented discussion and allows the group to return to work with greater comfort.

Nursing Care

The orientation of this book has been the basic sciences and their application to nursing care. There has been no attempt to include material appropriate to nursing specialization, such as, for example, psychiatric nursing. The chapter on small group behavior is, therefore, kept within the limits of appropriateness for actions of the average first-level nurse and does not pretend to include principles relative to psycho-therapeutic patient groups. Rather, the content of this chapter includes statements about behavior important to the nurse as she participates in work or professional groups.

The average nurse finds it necessary to actively participate in an increasing number of work-related groups. She almost certainly will be required to act as "team leader" in planning, organizing and implementing direct patient care. She will probably be re-quired to serve on task-oriented committees, such as procedure or policy committees, and she will most likely participate in in-service education discussion groups. It is hoped that she will also belong to and be active in professional organizations and serve on committees for those organizations. If she functions in any of the emerging expanded nursing roles, she will be called upon to work with community agency groups inter-ested in various aspects of health promotion.

The principle statements in this section are applicable to nursing action in groups of the type described. Nursing care implications for this chapter have not been outlined in the same manner as for other chapters, since these nursing actions are not directly related to individual patient care. The student or graduate nurse reader can find ready application of principle statements through observation and analysis of groups encoun-tered in daily experience. For example, the reader can, in remembering the last daily nursing care planning conference, evaluate the environment and the interaction to determine either interferences with group effectiveness or factors which increased group efficiency. She can, by reviewing principle statements, think of ways in which the meeting could have been made more conducive to effective action.

PART IV

A Guide to Use for Nursing Educators

During the process of developing the science and nursing care content presented in Parts II and III and during the study of teaching and evaluation methods in the first three years of the Commonwealth project, a number of imaginative ideas emerged on how the material in Parts II and III could be of value to other instructors of nursing or, possibly, to science teachers who work with nursing students. Although we offer the following suggestions, it is hoped and expected that instructors will discover many other helpful uses for this material.

In the discussion that follows, natural and social sciences have been separated to some extent, to allow for differences in content, and combined to some extent, to reflect that both underlie comprehensive nursing care. For the sake of organization and readability, the authors have organized this Part IV around a recognized method of curriculum development. This method advocates the following:

1. Definition of objectives, including content and behavior.
2. Planning of learning experiences to attain these objectives.
3. Selection and organization of learning experiences.
4. Evaluation of attainment of the objectives.

Definition of Objectives

It sounds ridiculously simple to say that one major objective of any nursing curriculum is developing the students' ability to perform effectively the nursing care of patients. But finding an answer to the automatically implied question "What is effective nursing care?" is anything but simple. Nowhere in nursing literature is there a comprehensive, universally agreed upon *and simple* statement that defines nursing or its effectiveness at various levels of practice. An attempt to answer this question leads naturally to a qualitative analysis of nursing care—an analysis that takes into consideration the major aspects of nursing, as well as the means for accomplishing nursing care to the desired end of patient well-being.

Because the life of an individual depends upon the maintenance of a constant internal environment (physiological homeostasis) and because in disease that internal environment is threatened and/or changed, the maintenance and restoration of homeostasis are primary nursing goals. Similarly, the well-being and adequate adjustment of the individual to life situations depends upon the maintenance of psychosocial homeostasis. Because illness and hospitalization, primarily due to a disturbance of physiological function or not, disturb the total pattern of the individual's satisfaction of psychosocial needs, the nurse must be concerned with the maintenance and the restoration of psychosocial homeostasis. The analysis of the nursing care of patients in terms of requirements of physiological homeostasis is essentially that material found in Part II. Part III comprises statements of nursing action related to the identified social science facts, principles and hypotheses that have direct bearing on the achievement and maintenance of psychosocial homeostasis.

If the statements of nursing care in these two sections actually do present major aspects of nursing care, one should be able to use them in the process of defining objectives, related to: (1) providing physical and psychosocial comfort; (2) providing essentials of life, such as oxygen, fluid balance and emotional security; (3) providing protection from traumatic chemical, physical, microbial or psychological injury; and (4) providing for the observation of deviations from normal physiological and psychosocial function and the appropriate communication of these deviations to other members of the health team.

Student learning objectives should contain two essential components: some indication of the behavior that is desired on the part of the nurse and some indication of an area of knowledge to which that behavior is related. Objectives concerned with the physical and psychosocial nursing care of patients can be stated readily in this manner, as they are in the chapter opening statements and nursing care statements in Parts II and III. Following are two examples of the development of unit objectives, in which a major objective was identified and analyzed to ascertain specific objectives inherent in it.

BIOLOGIC AND PHYSICAL SCIENCES

Major Objective: To perform nursing care that serves to maintain the body temperature within a normal range.

Preliminary Analysis
1. To identify signs and symptoms of abnormal body temperature.
2. To communicate effectively with other members of the health team relative to the signs and symptoms of abnormal body temperature.
3. To perform specific nursing activities to:
    A. Measure the body temperature.
    B. Lower an elevated body temperature.
    C. Elevate a low body temperature.

Continued Analysis

1. To understand normal regulation of body temperature (heat production, heat loss, physiological temperature-regulating mechanisms).
2. To understand possible causes of deviation in body temperatures (disease conditions that may affect heat loss, heat production or the temperature-regulating mechanisms).
3. To understand observable body responses to abnormal body temperature (e.g., peripheral vasoconstriction or vasodilatation, changes in heart action, chills and fever, sweating, delirium, convulsions, loss of consciousness).
4. To recognize signs and symptoms associated with abnormal body temperature and to understand when patients should be observed especially closely for those signs and symptoms.
5. To apply scientific knowledge in:
   A. Using equipment for measuring the body temperature.
   B. Adjustment of external environmental conditions.
   C. Adjustment of insulating materials.
   D. Adjustment of physical activities.
   E. Application of external heat.
   F. Removal of body heat.
   G. Administration of drugs to lower body temperature.
6. To report and record appropriately information about body temperature.

It should be noted that the major objective involves an essential factor of homeostasis; namely, that "there is a definite temperature range for efficient cellular functioning and proper enzymatic activity." The science and nursing care related to this requirement of homeostasis can be found in Part II, Chapter 9.

SOCIAL SCIENCES

> **Major Objective: To take action that will assist the patient to acquire or maintain the approval of others or to prevent disapproval from others in his sociocultural environment.**

Preliminary Analysis

1. To make observations regarding:
   A. Patient behavior that indicates that he receives adequate approval from others.
   B. Patient behavior that indicates a disturbance of psychological equilibrium due to lack of approval or to disapproval.
   C. Patient behavior that demonstrates the patient's attempts to acquire approval in satisfactory or unsatisfactory ways.
   D. Patient behavior that might cause disapproval or lack of approval.
   E. Factors in the patient's life situation that influence the receiving or withholding of approval or the demonstration of approval.
2. To analyze and interpret the observed data to determine:
   A. The relative satisfaction or dissatisfaction of the patient's need for approval in his current life situation.
   B. The sources of disturbance or interference with the satisfaction of the patient's need for approval.

    C. The necessity and/or feasibility of nursing action to help the patient satisfy his need for approval in his current life situation.

    D. The extent of nursing responsibility in assisting the patient toward satisfaction of his need for approval.

    E. The necessity and/or feasibility of referring the patient to other sources of assistance.

  3. To take specific nursing action aimed at:

    A. Removing, eliminating or changing factors in the current situation that cause the patient to feel disapproval or subject to a lack of approval.

    B. Providing an environment and/or experiences that will contribute to the patient's feeling of being approved.

    C. Providing the patient with psychological support as he works through adjustive problems relative to receiving approval or avoiding disapproval.

    D. Helping the patient to change behavior that interferes with receiving approval or causes disapproval.

  4. To communicate with other members of the health team regarding:

    A. Patient behavior that indicates a disturbance of psychological equilibrium due to lack of approval or to disapproval from others and the causes of the disturbance.

    B. A plan of care that will assist the patient in the satisfaction of his need of approval.

Continued Analysis

  1. An understanding of and ability to recognize human behavior that indicates a state of psychological disequilibrium due to lack of approval or to disapproval from others in one's sociocultural environment.

  2. An understanding of the dynamics of human behavior relative to the satisfaction of this particular need.

  3. An understanding of the relationship between psychological equilibrium and physiologic homeostasis, as demonstrated by lack of satisfaction of this need.

  4. An understanding of the sociocultural influences on the satisfaction of this need in general and in specific situations.

  5. An understanding of personality growth and development patterns that influence the satisfaction of this need.

  6. An understanding of and ability to function within the nursing role in the satisfaction of this need.

  7. A knowledge of additional sources of assistance in satisfying the patient's need and how to utilize these sources when necessary.

  8. An understanding of and ability to apply sociopsychological principles in establishing an environment that will:

    A. Eliminate or reduce sources of disapproval.

    B. Provide or encourage opportunities for the patient to receive approval from others.

    C. Provide the patient with psychological support and encouragement when he is working through potentially traumatic problems relative to approval or disapproval.

D. Assist the patient to learn new behaviors or modify behaviors that will contribute to a feeling of approval or the elimination of disapproval.

It should be noted that the major objective involves one of the subconcepts relative
to psychosocial homeostasis: "The approval of others in one's sociocultural environment is necessary for psychosocial homeostasis." The nursing care and underlying
principles related to this subconcept can be found in Part III, Chapter 7.

In both of the primary analyses of the above examples, major skills (observational,
technical and communicative) involved in the nursing care were identified, along with
a general description of the nursing content. The more specific objectives stated in the
continued analyses not only include reference to these major skills but also contain
some degree of information about the knowledge that underlies the effective performance of these skills and a more complete description of nursing activities involved in
attaining the major objective.

The skills, the knowledge and the specific nursing activities included in the previous examples are either stated or implied in the material contained in Parts II and III.
Of course, this material does not provide complete and final answers to the questions of
what skills and *what* knowledge should be taught to nursing students. It does, however,
provide a basis for determining some of the behaviors and some of the knowledge
toward which clinical nursing instructors should guide their students. Other objectives
similar to those presented here can be identified from further analysis of the material
in Parts II and III.

Planning Learning Experiences

The identification of learning experiences to help students attain the desired objectives stems quite naturally from a careful examination of the objectives. If understanding
is involved, the nursing student must have access, through such media as lectures,
laboratory sessions, informal discussions, textbooks and guided observations, to the
facts that are essential to the understanding. The same is true if the objective concerns
the application of scientific knowledge; the student should be given an opportunity to
learn the science material before or during the teaching of the nursing care that involves
the application of that material.

The scientific content identified in this study as important for a nurse to understand
and be able to apply can be used as a partial answer to the question of what science
should be taught. Identification of additional facts can be accomplished through the
analysis of specific observational and technical skills involved in physical nursing care
and through the analysis of specific diagnostic tests and therapeutic procedures in
which the nurse participates or which she should be able to interpret. Additional facts
also can be identified through the analysis of specific patient problems in the areas of
social and psychological adjustment, when such problems are encountered in the
nurse-patient situation.

The ability to identify significant signs and symptoms, the ability to apply facts and
principles of science in the performance of nursing care and the ability to perform
tasks with some degree of manual dexterity can be developed only through practice.
This implies that one responsibility of the clinical instructor is the planning of student
experiences so that problems requiring these skills are provided. Discussion of teaching

methods for the development of knowledge and skills is not within the scope of this book. However, some general considerations of the selection and organization of learning experiences utilizing the identified science material and associated nursing care is included.

One type of decision facing every clinical instructor in nursing concerns the choice of patients for students to care for during clinical practice. There are many factors to be taken into consideration in this selection process, for example: the individual learning needs of each student; the theoretical preparation of the student; and the need for new learning pertaining to a particular type of nursing problem. Now that the trend in nursing education is toward decreasing the time that students spend in the bedside practice of patient care and increasing the depth of any single experience, this selection process has become increasingly significant. The use of more effective teaching methods, with emphasis upon specific, selected learning goals, has shown that it is possible to shorten the length of time a student devotes to clinical experiences. The objectives for such learning experiences must be clearly defined, and the experiences themselves must be carefully planned.

Selection and Organization of Learning Experiences

Following are some examples of how the principles contained in Parts II and III can be used in the identification, selection and organization of learning experiences.

BIOLOGIC AND PHYSICAL SCIENCES

The nursing care statements contained in Part II can be helpful in the selection of patients for the purpose of teaching physiological nursing care. For instance, upon examining conditions that may interfere with an adequate oxygen supply, it will be noted that patients with many different conditions are likely to have problems in this area; these patients can provide good learning experiences for students. The instructor might select a patient who is unconscious or one who has a lung tumor, pneumonia, asthma, ascites or a patent ductus arteriosus. Which patient the instructor selects should be decided not only on the basis of the type of respiratory problem involved but also on the basis of other problems that the patient has and how well the student is prepared in the nursing care of patients with these other problems.

Obviously, the more problems a patient has, the more complex the nursing care becomes. The more serious the problems are, in terms of the immediate requirements of life (e.g., maintenance of an adequate oxygen supply, maintenance of the volume and pressure of circulating blood within certain limits), the more demanding the nursing care and, usually, the more complex. The more a patient depends upon others for meeting basic needs, such as elimination and locomotion, the greater the demands for nursing care.

SOCIAL SCIENCES

For several reasons, the social sciences as applied to general nursing practice are less amenable to consistent selection and organization of learning experiences than the natural sciences. With the exception of neuropsychiatric or psychiatric illness, the patient's primary presenting problem is physiological in nature, so that at all times, in health agencies used for teaching, one can find problems relative to the material outlined in Part II. Although every patient has some psychosocial disturbance by virtue of being a totally reacting organism in an abnormal situation (hospitalization), the nature and the severity of the disturbance varies with each individual patient, regardless of his presenting problem. This does not encourage the use of a predetermined organizational pattern for the selection of learning experiences according to major psychosocial needs. Furthermore, identification of the patient's problems in this area, being secondary to his presenting complaint, is not a part of the formal diagnosis; and such identification occurs, if at all, during the ensuing process of physiological nursing care. Unless the problem is outstanding, the identification of such problems usually is left to the discretion of the nurse and seldom receives medical attention or orders for care.

In some ways, the selection of learning experiences in the social science areas is helped rather than hindered by these factors. If we can assume that all patients have some degree of disturbance of psychosocial equilibrium as a result of physical illness and hospitalization, then we also can assume that every patient can provide the student with an opportunity to learn and apply social science principles. If this is so, the instructor's problem is not so much one of selection and organization as one of identification and effective utilization of constant opportunity and careful guidance of the student in successive learning experiences. The successive experiences provide natural opportunity for increasing the depth of understanding and the skill in meeting problem situations concerning the patient's psychosocial adjustment.

The authors believe that, where patients are concerned, it is impossible to avoid *potential* learning experiences at all levels of complexity involving social science principles, regardless of the rationale for the selection and organization of learning experiences. It is in the failure of the instructor to recognize and utilize experiences that we encounter an uneconomical use of student learning time and capabilities. For example, let us consider the patient's need for satisfying relationships with others. Whatever the patient's reason for seeking medical care, his need for satisfying relationships is not left at home. He will, if he is hospitalized, experience some feeling of separation, of being alone. Unless health team members make attempts to prevent it or unless it can be achieved through good physical care, he will feel uncared for. Because he is in an environment that includes many other people, usually strangers, he will have an increased need for the acceptance and approval of those people upon whom he must depend for his continued health and well-being. Since every patient has had different growth and development experiences, each demonstrates individual differences in the way he attempts to meet these needs; and since every patient is a member of some sociocultural group, his behavior indicates the influence of his particular group in meeting these needs. Further, the patient is in a new social situation where he has to learn the roles and functions of those around him and how he fits into the social structure of hospital life.

Unless the instructor deliberately avoids patients who demonstrate intensified, chronic or exaggerated needs in these areas, the law of averages would suggest it is impossible for the student not to encounter patients who demonstrate a range of possibilities, from highly satisfactory to acutely unsatisfactory relationships with others. The only real need for the deliberate selection of experiences for learning increasingly complex psychological nursing care occurs when extreme degrees of psychosocial need are encountered. If a student is only beginning to learn the principles involved in, for example, helping the patient to achieve and maintain satisfying relationships with others, it is easy enough to avoid her assignment to patients whose disturbances in this area are so great that they cause behavior that deviates widely from normal. Such an experience can be planned for later in the program, when the student may be assigned to a psychiatric unit, in which the patients' presenting problems are in this area. Similar examples could be given for all of the identified social science material in Part III. The crucial factor in guiding the student's learning of skill in applying social science principles is in the instructor's recognition of the constant opportunity and in her deliberate plans to capitalize on it. It seems quite reasonable to say that learning under such circumstances would be most effective, because it would help the student to recognize the interdependence of all aspects of human function, regardless of the specific acute problems.

If the instructor feels that it is necessary to have an organized outline or plan, she could utilize the identified principles to formulate a check list, together with a more formalized plan for teaching according to the kinds of problems that students are most likely to encounter at various stages in their growth and development as nurses. For example, the beginning student may encounter problems in human relationships when first meeting a patient face-to-face and having to communicate with that patient for purposes of observation and promoting comfort for both of them. Emphasis on learning in this first experience, together with formal classes or ward conferences, might well be directed toward acquiring a beginning skill in communication. As the student learns to be comfortable in simple verbal communication with a patient, further guidance and conference time could be planned to increase her understanding of the total communication process and to use communication for therapeutic purposes. This implies the need for additional understanding of the dynamics of verbal and nonverbal communication, including the use of symbols in communication, and of the dynamics of perception, as well as some understanding of specific problems that can be solved through effective communication.

In addition, by reviewing the plan for the teaching of physiological care, the instructor can foresee other problems that are likely to occur with regularity. For example, while students are having clinical experiences related to the maintenance of an adequate supply of oxygen, it is almost certain that they will encounter acute fear on the part of the patient because of the threat to his life. At this time, the instructor can plan to help the students learn some of the dynamics of behavior related to fear and some of the skills, based on principles, that the nurse needs in order to minimize fear. This method of organization has the advantage of being based on the students' motivation to solve the problems with which they are immediately faced.

The above discussion has covered a few ideas pertaining primarily to the identification, selection and organization of learning experiences in clinical nursing practice. The following discussion is limited to suggestions for helping nursing students to learn or apply scientific knowledge. It is the sincere belief of the authors that a professional nurse should base her nursing care on scientific facts, principles and hypotheses. The ability to apply such knowledge in giving nursing care enables the nurse to interpret and to follow medical orders intelligently, to perform and adapt nursing activities effectively and to be creative in the planning and the execution of the nursing care of the individual patient. This ability helps to prevent rigidity in thinking and acting; it frees the nurse from continual dependence upon others for solving nursing problems; it frees the nurse from the monotony of repetitious nursing activities which might be performed according to routine rather than reason. In short, this ability provides the nurse with one means of becoming a truly professional person.

It is customary to teach science to nursing students before they have their clinical practice; that is, before they have direct contact with patients. A supposed advantage of this pattern is that the student comes to the clinical nursing instructor possessing the important facts from the fields of anatomy, physiology, physics, chemistry, micro-biology, sociology and psychology, which can then be applied in learning and perform-ing nursing care. This seems to be an ideal method, but in actual practice it sometimes does not work. The instructors in the various science fields may not be familiar with what aspects of the science are important in nursing; or they may be familiar with them but must teach a science course that cannot be directed toward the specific learning needs of nursing students. The clinical instructors may be weak in their own science preparation, causing difficulty in the integration of science into the teaching of nursing. A nursing instructor may not believe that the ability to apply scientific knowledge in solving nursing problems is an objective of nursing education, or she may not know what science content to integrate or what methods to use for successful integration. The instructor may be unaware of how much science content or what specific science content the student had prior to her clinical experience. The students, themselves, may have learned relatively little science while taking the preclinical courses in an academic setting. They may have forgotten much of the memorized science content before they reach the clinical experience, or they may need to learn additional science content. Not infrequently, they need considerable guidance and practice in solving problems through systematic thinking, which requires the application of scientific facts and principles.

REVIEW OR LEARNING OF BIOLOGIC
AND PHYSICAL SCIENCE CONTENT

Let us look at a few of the possible ways in which the various types of instructional media can be very helpful to students in reviewing and learning science content that is important in nursing. Programs may be purchased or may be developed by the clinical instructors themselves. Study guides can be prepared for students to use in the review of science content. Class time can be planned for the express purpose of helping students to broaden and deepen their knowledge of science. Formal classes or informal conferences that are planned to explore specific patient problems provide an excellent means of helping students to recall and apply science facts and principles.

Study guides can be made specific enough to direct the students' independent study toward important new science content. Classes can be planned exclusively for the introduction of new content, and it may be desirable to have resource persons, such as science instructors, teach this type of class. If the amount of new content is not exten-sive, it can be integrated in nursing classes and conferences. When classes and confer-ences are planned and conducted so that the basic "whys" are an integral part of any discussion, new science content can be introduced very effectively.

All of these methods require that instructors be very clear about what science content is most important for the students. The material identified in Part II can be useful to instructors in developing learning tools, in selecting reading assignments and in planning and preparing for specific classes and conferences.

REVIEW OR LEARNING OF SOCIAL SCIENCE CONTENT

One of the most effective ways for reviewing or learning social science content is through the use of references and questions pertaining to specific patient problems, as the student encounters them in clinical practice. Theoretically, the most effective learning could be achieved if the individual student could be guided toward reference reading that would be in accord with the specific patient problem that she is concerned with at any given time. Practically, there is seldom a high enough ratio of instructors to students to make this entirely possible.

The authors have found that group discussion of prepared problems, accompanied by reading assignments, has been useful for purposes of both review and new learning. These prepared problems, or cases, can be constructed on the basis of actual problems that one or more of the students in the group are having to deal with at the time. For example, we can refer to the area of communication as it was discussed in relation to the selection and organization of learning experiences. If one or several of the students are experiencing some difficulty in communicating effectively with their patients, a case could be constructed that would include the common and the specific elements of the actual experiential problem. References could be given for the students to review or read preparatory to the group discussion. If this method is used, there should be some designated time, such as weekly or biweekly, for continuity in planning so that each case can build upon previous cases. The social science material as identified in Part III could serve as a resource for planning and constructing case materials and for selecting references.

Occasionally resource people, lectures or movies are helpful in acquainting the student with new facts and principles or in helping the student to look at previous learning in a new light. For example, an anthropologist might be called upon to discuss some of the problems of acculturation, especially as it pertains to health practices.

In addition to group discussion of actual patient problems, the student may be asked to select a nurse-patient situation in which she is involved, to give a written description of the situation, with particular emphasis on certain aspects of it, and to analyze the situation in terms of social science principles, supporting her analysis with reference materials. Some of the aspects she might be asked to emphasize are the forms of communication that took place, her own subjective feelings about the patient, behavior of the patient that indicated psychological disequilibrium or the influence of the various team members on the patient's behavior.

Perhaps one of the most useful methods for helping students to learn social science principles important to nursing is the same method by which the principles and hypotheses in Part III were acquired. If students are helped to identify psychosocial problems of specific patients and to analyze these problems in terms of underlying science principles, they would need to do less memorization of reference material which might or might not be useful at some later date.

Whatever methods are used for the introduction of new material or the review of previously encountered science content, the important element is pointing out or assisting the student to discover the relationship of the content to problems of nursing practice. Again, the material in Part III could be useful as a guide for helping students to look for such relationships.

APPLICATION OF SCIENTIFIC KNOWLEDGE

During the original study the authors found that the most effective method for teaching the application of scientific facts, principles and hypotheses in nursing was through the use of problem-solving techniques. As might be expected, the more practice the students had in using science to solve nursing problems, the more adept at the process they became. When the development of problem-solving abilities is an objective, it is important that instructors create an atmosphere, both in the classroom and in the clinical situation, that is conducive to the solution of problems by students. Encouraging students to look at situations analytically is essential. When an instructor volunteers a direct and positive answer to problems, the student's ability to solve problems is not allowed to develop.

It is believed that the science material can be helpful in planning learning experiences aimed at helping students to develop skills in problem-solving and in the use of science in solving problems. The nursing sections can be helpful in identifying nursing care related to psychosocial and physiological problems that patients may have, and the science sections can be used to identify specific science content that is relevant.

Not only can the material in Parts II and III be useful in the preparation of formal nursing classes, but it can also be helpful in the development of nursing care plans during the students' clinical experiences. Only as nursing students become increasingly aware of the many aspects of total patient care and understand the major objectives of this care, are they able to develop comprehensive nursing care plans for individual patients. Only as students develop the many skills and understandings that are involved in providing totality of care do they come to function in a full nursing capacity. The authors believe that the material in Parts II and III can serve as a guide for students to use while they are developing the many skills and understandings important in nursing.

Evaluation of the Attainment of Objectives

If objectives are well defined, the development of evaluation tools to measure the attainment of these objectives is markedly facilitated. The type of evaluative method selected will, of course, depend largely upon the kind of behavior that is to be measured. The discussion of general methods of evaluation is not within the scope of this book; however, suggestions are made relative to the possible uses of the science and nursing sections in the development of evaluation tools.

There are a number of criteria to take into consideration when evaluating the nursing care given to patients. Possible criteria include completeness of care, therapeutic effectiveness of care, safety of care for the patient and the staff, and the physical and psychological comfort of the patient. The sections of nursing care included in Parts II and III can be useful in deciding what to look for in relation to criteria such as these while the student's performance is being evaluated.

For paper and pencil tests, questions can be constructed that measure various aspects of the understanding of and the ability to apply scientific knowledge. The material contained in Parts II and III can be of use as a resource for the development of test items concerned with these factors.

Essay questions might ask that the student compare and contrast the nursing care of two or three patients with fairly similar physiological or psychosocial problems and that her answers be supported with scientific facts, principles or hypotheses. The student also might be asked to describe the nursing care of a patient who has a certain kind of physiological or psychosocial problem and to justify this care on the basis of scientific knowledge. A third type of essay question might ask the student to write possible nursing applications of a particular scientific fact or principle. Still another type would be to describe a certain patient situation and list possible nursing interventions. The student would be asked to select the "best" nursing action and to give reasons for that choice of action.

Objective questions can be constructed to determine both the student's understanding and her ability to apply scientific knowledge. One type of test experimented with at the University of Washington was called the Application of Sciences Test. Two sets of tests composed of multiple-choice items were constructed, each with a corresponding part for the natural and the social sciences. In one set of tests, the student was asked to select proper courses of action for given situations. In the second set, the student was asked to select science principles that would be the best guides to action in given situations. The items were constructed in such a way that the best answer in an item in the first test was based on the same fact or principle that would be the best guide for action in an item in the second test. Insofar as possible, the situations in the associated items were sufficiently different to avoid the possibility of choosing the correct answer because of the similarity of items. The second set of tests were given at some time after the first set. Theoretically, such tests can be used to measure not only a student's knowledge but also her ability to apply that knowledge.

Construction of any of these types of test items can be greatly facilitated by use of the material in Parts II and III. The material can help in identifying important areas within which questions can be developed, as well as important points to be included. It also provides a good source of ideas for alternative responses in the case of multiple-choice test items.

This chapter was written not to instruct clinical nursing teachers in the use of the science and nursing sections but to offer some suggestions of ways in which it might be helpful. Suggestions have been made relative to the use of the material for defining objectives, planning, selecting and organizing learning experiences and evaluating the attainment of objectives. The authors hope that these suggestions will prove helpful in the teaching of nursing students and that instructors will find other practical uses for the material.

Index